Health

—— AND ——

Numbers

A

Health

AND

Numbers

A Problems-Based Introduction to Biostatistics

Second Edition

Chap T. Le, Ph.D.

Distinguished Professor of Biostatistics
Director of Biostatistics
Comprehensive Cancer Center
University of Minnesota

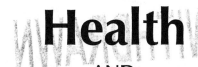**WILEY-LISS**

A JOHN WILEY & SONS, INC., PUBLICATION
New York • Chichester • Weinheim • Brisbane • Singapore • Toronto

Library of Congress Cataloging-in-Publication Data:

Le, Chap T.
    Health and numbers : a problems-based introduction to biostatistics /
    Chap T. Le
        p.   cm.
    Includes bibliographical references and index.
    ISBN 0-471-41661-4 (cloth : alk. paper)
        1.

Printed in the United States of America

10 9 8 7 6 5 4 3

*To my wife, Minhha,
and my daughters,
Mina and Jenna,
with love.*

Contents

Preface

A course in introductory biostatistics is often required for professional students in public health, dentistry, nursing, and even medicine, as well as for graduate students in nursing and other biomedical sciences. It is only a course or two, but the requirement is often considered as a roadblock causing anxiety in many quarters. The feelings are expressed in many ways and in many different settings but all leading to the same conclusion that simply surviving the experience is the only practical goal. And students need help, in the form of a user-friendly text, in order to do just that—namely, surviving. In the early 1990s, we decided that it was time to write our own text. *Health and Numbers: Basic Biostatistical Methods* was published in 1995, reflecting our experience after teaching introductory biostatistics courses for many years to students from various human health disciplines. This second edition, *Health and Numbers: A Problems-Based Introduction to Biostatistics*, should appeal to the same audience for which the first edition was written: professional and beginning graduate students in human health disciplines who need help to successfully pass and to benefit from the basic biostatistics course requirement. Our main objective is to avoid the perception that statistics is just a course with a bunch of formulas that students need to get over with, but to present it as a way of thinking, thinking about ways to gather and analyze data so as to benefit from taking the required course. And there is no better way to do that than making our book problem-based: Many problems with real data in various fields are provided at the end of all eight chapters as aids to learning how to use statistical procedures, still the nuts and bolts of elementary applied statistics. The first five chapters have been strengthened; the two chapters on hypothesis testing, Chapters 6 and 7, have been reorganized with newly added topics, and a separate chapter on regression and correlation, Chapter 8, has been added. Another new feature of this second edition consists of sections on *Notes on Computations* at the end of each chapter. These notes cover uses of Microsoft's Excel, but samples of SAS computer programs are also included at the end of many examples.

The "way of thinking" called statistics has become important to all professionals who not only are scientific or business-like, but also are caring people who want to help and make the world a better place. But what is it? What is biostatistics and what can it do? There are popular definitions and perceptions of statistics. We see "vital statistics" in the newspaper, announcements of life events such as births, marriages, and deaths. Motorists are warned to drive carefully, to avoid "becoming a statistic." The public use of the word is widely varied, most often indicating lists of numbers, or data. We have also heard people use the word *data* to describe a verbal report, a believable anecdote. For this book and its readers, we don't emphasize the definition of "statistics as things," but offer instead an active concept of "doing statistics." The doing of statistics is a way of thinking about numbers, with emphasis on relating their interpretation and meaning to the manner in which they are collected. Our working definition of statistics, as an activity, is that it is a way of thinking about data, its collection, its analysis, and its presentation. Formulas are only a part of that thinking, simply tools of the trade; they are needed but are not the only things you need to know.

To illustrate statistics as a way of thinking, let's start with a familiar scenario of our criminal court procedures. A crime has been discovered and a suspect has been identified. After a police investigation to collect evidence against the suspect, a prosecutor presents summarized evidence to a jury. The jurors learn about and debate the rule about convicting beyond a reasonable doubt and the rule about unanimous decision. After the debate, the jurors vote and a verdict is reached: guilty or not guilty. Why do we need to have this time-consuming, cost-consuming process called trial by jury? Well, the truth is often unknown, at least uncertain. Maybe only the suspect knows, and he does not talk. It is uncertain because of variability (every case is different) and because of incomplete information (missing key evidence?). Trial by jury is the way our society deals with uncertainties; its goal is to minimize mistakes.

How does society deal with uncertainties? We go through a process called trial by jury, consisting of these steps: (1) We form an assumption or hypothesis (that every person is innocent until proven guilty), (2) we gather data (evidence against the suspect), and (3) we decide whether the hypothesis should be rejected (guilty) or should not be rejected (not guilty). With such a well-established procedure, sometimes we do well and sometimes we don't. Basically, a successful trial should consist of these elements: (1) a probable cause (with a crime and a suspect), (2) a thorough investigation by police, (3) an efficient presentation by the prosecutor, and (4) a fair and impartial jury.

In the above-described context of a trial by jury, let us consider a few specific examples: (i) The *crime* is lung cancer and the *suspect* is cigarette smoking, or (ii) the *crime* is leukemia and the *suspect* is pesticides, or (iii) the *crime* is breast cancer and the *suspect* is a defective gene. The process is now called *research*, and the tool to carry out that research is biostatistics. In a simple way, biostatistics serves as the biomedical version of the trial-by-jury process. It is *the science of dealing with uncertainties using incomplete information.* Yes, even science is uncertain; scientists arrive at different conclusions in many different areas at different times; many studies are inconclusive (hung jury?). The reasons for uncertainties remain the same. Nature is complex and full of unexplained biological variability. But, most important of all, we always have to deal with incomplete information. It is often not practical to study the entire population; we have to rely on information gained from *sample(s)*.

How does science deal with uncertainties? We learn from how society deals with uncertainties; we go through a process called biostatistics, consisting of the following steps: (1) We form an assumption or a hypothesis (from the research question), (2) we gather data (from clinical trials, surveys, medical records abstractions), and (3) we make decision(s) (by doing statistical analysis/inference, a guilty verdict is referred to as *statistical significance*). Basically, a successful research should consist of the following elements: (1) a good research question (with well-defined objectives and endpoints), (2) a thorough investigation (by experiments or surveys), (3) an efficient presentation of data (organizing data, summarizing, and presenting data; an area called descriptive statistics), and (4) proper statistical inference. This book is a problems-based introduction to the last three elements; together they form a field called *biostatistics*. The coverage is rather brief on data collection, but very extensive on descriptive statistics (Chapters 1 and 2) and on methods of statistical inference (Chapters 4 to 8). Chapter 3, on probability and probability models, serves as the link between descriptive and inferential parts. Notes on computions are incorporated through the book.

The author would like to express his sincere appreciation to colleagues for feedback, to teaching assistants who helped with examples and exercises, and to many generations of students for various improvements from the first to the second edition. I have learned very much from my former students, and I hope that some of what they have taught me is reflected well in the first edition and even more so in the present edition of this book. Finally, my family tolerated patiently the pressures resulting from my long-term commitment to write books; to my wife and daughters, I will always be most grateful.

CHAP T. LE
Edina, Minnesota

1

Proportions, Rates, and Ratios

Most introductory textbooks in statistics and biostatistics start with methods for summarizing and presenting continuous data. We have decided, however, to adopt a different starting point because our focused areas are in biomedical sciences, and health decisions are frequently based on proportions, ratios, or rates. In this first chapter we will see how these concepts appeal to common sense, and we will learn their meaning and uses.

1.1. PROPORTIONS

Many outcomes can be classified as belonging to one of two possible categories: Presence and Absence, Nonwhite and White, Male and Female, Improved and Not-improved. Of course, one of these two categories is usually identified as of primary interest; for example, Presence in the Presence and Absence classification, Nonwhite in the White and Nonwhite classification. We can, in general, relabel the two outcome categories as Positive $(+)$ and Negative $(-)$. An outcome is positive if the primary category is observed, but is negative if the other category is observed.

It is obvious that in the summary to characterize observations made on a group of individuals, the number x of positive outcomes is not sufficient; the group size n, or total number of observations, should also be recorded. The number x tells us very little and only becomes meaningful after adjusting for the size n of the group; in other words, the two figures x and n are often combined into a *statistic*, called *proportion*:

$$p = \frac{x}{n}$$

The term "statistic" means a summarized figure from observed data. Clearly, $0 \leq p \leq 1$. This proportion p is sometimes expressed as a percentage and is calculated as follows:

$$\% = \frac{x}{n}(100)\%$$

Example 1.1

A study, published by the Urban Coalition of Minneapolis and the University of Minnesota Adolescent Health Program, surveyed 12,915 students in grades 7 through 12 in Minneapolis and St. Paul public schools. The report said minority students, about one-third of the group, were much less likely to have had a recent routine physical checkup. Among Asian students, 25.4% said they had not seen a doctor or a dentist in the last 2 years, followed by 17.7% of American Indians, 16.1% of Blacks, and 10% of Hispanics. Among Whites, it was 6.5%.

Proportion is a number used to describe a group of individuals according to a dichotomous characteristic under investigation. The following are a few illustrations of its use in the health sciences.

1.1.1. Comparative Studies

Comparative studies are intended to show possible differences between two or more groups. For example, the same survey of Example 1.1 provided the following figures concerning boys in the surveyed group who use tobacco at least weekly. Among Asians, it was 9.7%, followed by 11.6% of Blacks, 20.6% of Hispanics, 25.4% of Whites, and 38.3% of American Indians.

In addition to surveys that are cross-sectional, as seen in the above example, data for comparative studies may come from different sources; the two fundamental designs are *retrospective* and *prospective*. Retrospective studies gather past data from selected cases and controls to determine differences, if any, in the exposure to a suspected risk factor. They are commonly referred to as *case–control studies*. In a case–control study, cases of a specific disease are ascertained as they arise from population-based registers or lists of hospital admissions, and controls are sampled as either (a) disease-free individuals from the population at risk or (b) hospitalized patients having a diagnosis other than the one under study. The advantages of a retrospective study are that it is economical and it provides answers to research questions relatively quickly because the cases are already available. Major limitations are due to the inaccuracy of the exposure histories and uncertainty about the appropriateness of the control sample; these problems sometimes hinder retrospective studies and make them less preferred than prospective studies. The following is an example of a retrospective study in the field of occupational health.

Example 1.2

A case–control study was undertaken to identify reasons for the exceptionally high rate of lung cancer among male residents of coastal Georgia. Cases were identified from these sources:

1. Diagnoses since 1970 at the single large hospital in Brunswick
2. Diagnoses during 1975–1976 at three major hospitals in Savannah
3. Death certificates for the period 1970–1974 in the area

Controls were selected from admissions to the four hospitals and from death certificates in the same period for diagnoses other than lung cancer, bladder cancer, or chronic lung cancer. Data are tabulated separately for smokers and nonsmokers as follows:

Smoking	Shipbuilding	Cases	Controls
No	Yes	11	35
	No	50	203
Yes	Yes	84	45
	No	313	270

The exposure under investigation, "Shipbuilding," refers to employment in shipyards during World War II. By separate tabulation, with the first half of the table for nonsmokers and the second half for smokers, we treat *smoking* as a potential confounder. A confounder is a factor, an exposure by itself, not under investigation but related to the disease (in this case, lung cancer) and the exposure (shipbuilding); previous studies have linked smoking to lung cancer, and construction workers are more likely to be smokers. The term *exposure* is used here to emphasize that employment in shipyards is a suspected *risk* factor; however, the term is also even used in studies where the factor under investigation has beneficial effects.

In an examination of the smokers in the above data set, the numbers of people employed in shipyards, 84 and 45, tell us little because the sizes of the two groups, cases and controls, are different. Adjusting these absolute numbers for the group sizes, we have the following:

1. For the controls,

$$\text{Proportion of exposure} = \frac{45}{315}$$
$$= .143 \text{ or } 14.3\%$$

2. For the cases,

$$\text{Proportion of exposure} = \frac{84}{397}$$
$$= .212 \text{ or } 21.2\%$$

The results reveal different exposure histories: The proportion among cases was higher than that among controls. It is *not* in any way a conclusive proof, but it is a good *clue* indicating a possible relationship between the disease (lung cancer) and the exposure (shipbuilding).

Similar examination of the data for nonsmokers shows that, by taking into consideration the numbers of cases and of controls, we have the following figures for employment:

1. For the controls,

$$\text{Proportion of exposure} = \frac{35}{238}$$
$$= .147 \text{ or } 14.7\%$$

2. For the cases,

$$\text{Proportion of exposure} = \frac{11}{61}$$
$$= .180 \text{ or } 18.0\%$$

The results also reveal different exposure histories: The proportion among cases was higher than that among controls.

The above analyses also show that the difference between proportions of exposure among smokers, that is,

$$21.2 - 14.3 = 6.9\%$$

is different from the difference between proportions of exposure among nonsmokers, which is

$$18.0 - 14.7 = 3.3\%$$

The differences, 6.9% and 3.3%, are *measures* of the strength of the relationship between the disease and the exposure, one for each of the two strata—the two groups of smokers and nonsmokers, respectively. The above calculation shows that the possible effects of employment in shipyards (as a suspected risk factor) are different for smokers and non-smokers. This difference of differences, if confirmed, is called a "three-term interaction" or an "effect modification," where smoking alters the effect of employment in shipyards as a risk for lung cancer. In that case, *smoking* is not only a confounder, it is an *effect modifier* that modifies the effects of shipbuilding (on the possibility of causing lung cancer).

Another situation is provided in the following example concerning glaucomatous blindness.

_____

Example 1.3

Persons registered blind from glaucoma:

	Population	Cases	Cases per 100,000
White	32,930,233	2,832	8.6
Nonwhite	3,933,333	3,227	82.0

_____

For these *disease registry data*, direct calculation of a proportion results in a very tiny fraction—that is, the number of cases of the disease per person at risk. For convenience, this is multiplied by 100,000 and hence the result expresses the number of cases per 100,000 individuals. This data set also provides an example of the use of proportions as disease prevalence, which is defined as

$$\text{Prevalence} = \frac{\text{Number of diseased individuals at the time of investigation}}{\text{Total number of individuals examined}}$$

More details on *disease prevalence* and related concepts are in Section 1.2.2.

For blindness from glaucoma, calculations in Example 1.3 reveal a striking difference between the races: The blindness prevalence among nonwhites was over 8 times that among whites. The number "100,000" was selected arbitrarily; any power of 10 would be suitable so as to obtain a result between 1 and 100, sometimes between 1 and 1000; it is easier to state the result "82 cases per 100,000" than saying that the prevalence was .00082.

1.1.2. Screening Tests

Other uses of proportions can be found in the evaluation of screening tests or diagnostic procedures. Following these procedures, clinical observation or laboratory techniques, individuals are classified as healthy or as falling into one of a number of disease categories. Such tests are important in medicine and epidemiologic studies and may form the basis of early interventions. Almost all such tests are imperfect, in the sense that healthy individuals will occasionally be classified wrongly as being ill, while some individuals who are really ill may fail to be detected. That is, misclassification is unavoidable. Suppose that each individual in a large population can be classified as truly positive or negative for a particular disease; this true diagnosis may be based on more refined methods than are used in the test; or it may be based on evidence that emerges after passage of time—for instance, at autopsy. For each class of individuals, diseased and healthy, the test is applied and results are depicted as follows:

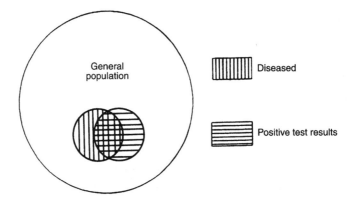

The two proportions fundamental to evaluating diagnostic procedures are *sensitivity* and *specificity.* The sensitivity is the proportion of diseased individuals detected as positive by the test

$$\text{Sensitivity} = \frac{\text{Number of diseased individuals who screen positive}}{\text{Total number of diseased individuals}}$$

(the corresponding errors are false negatives), whereas the specificity is the proportion of healthy individuals detected as negative by the test

$$\text{Specificity} = \frac{\text{Number of healthy individuals who screen negative}}{\text{Total number of healthy individuals}}$$

(the corresponding errors are false positives).

Clearly, it is desirable that a test or screening procedure be highly sensitive and highly specific. However, the two types of errors go in opposite directions; for example, an effort to increase sensitivity may lead to more false positives.

Example 1.4

A cytological test was undertaken to screen women for cervical cancer. Consider a group of 24,103 women consisting of 379 women whose cervices are abnormal (to an extent sufficient to justify concern with respect to possible cancer) and 23,724 women whose cervices are acceptably healthy. A test was applied, and results are tabulated in the table below (this study was performed with a rather old test, it is used here only for illustration):

True	Test −	Test +	Totals
−	23,362	362	23,724
+	225	154	379

The calculations

$$\text{Sensitivity} = \frac{154}{379}$$
$$= .406 \text{ or } 40.6\%$$
$$\text{Specificity} = \frac{23,362}{23,724}$$
$$= .985 \text{ or } 98.5\%$$

show that the above test is highly specific (98.5%) but not very sensitive (40.6%); there were more than half (59.4%) false negatives. The implications of the use of this test are as follows:

1. If a woman without cervical cancer is tested, the result would almost surely be negative, *but*
2. If a woman with cervical cancer is tested the chance is that the disease would go undetected because 59.4% of these cases would lead to false negatives.

Finally, it is important to note that throughout this section, proportions have been defined so that both the numerator and the denominator are counts or frequencies, and the numerator corresponds to a subgroup of the larger group involved in the denominator resulting in a number between 0 and 1 (or between 0 and 100%). It is straightforward to generalize this concept for use with characteristics having more than two outcome categories; for each category we can define a proportion, and these category-specific proportions add up to 1 (or 100%).

Example 1.5

An examination of the 668 children reported living in crack/cocaine households shows 70% Blacks, followed by 18% Whites, 8% American Indians, and 4% Other or Unknown.

1.1.3. Displaying Proportions

Perhaps the most effective and most convenient way of presenting data, especially discrete data, is through the use of graphs. Graphs convey the information, the general patterns in a set of data, at a single glance. Therefore, graphs are often easier to read than tables; the most informative graphs are simple and self-explanatory. Of course, in order to achieve that objective, graphs should be carefully constructed. Like tables, they should be clearly labeled and units of measurement and/or magnitude of quantities should be included. Remember that graphs must tell their own story; they should be complete in themselves and require little or no additional explanation.

Bar Charts

Bar charts are a very popular type of graph used to display several proportions for quick comparison. In a bar chart, the various groups are represented along the horizontal axis; they may be arranged alphabetically, or by the size of their proportions, or on some other rational basis. A vertical bar is drawn above each group such that the height of the bar is the proportion associated with that group. The bars should be of equal width and should be separated from one another so as not to imply continuity.

Example 1.6

We can present the data set on kids without a recent physical checkup (Example 1.1) by a bar chart as follows:

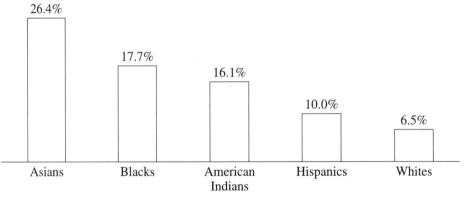

Kids without a recent physical checkup

Pie Charts

Pie charts are another popular type of graph. A pie chart consists of a circle; the circle is divided into wedges that correspond to the magnitude of the proportions for various categories. A pie chart shows the differences between the sizes of various categories or subgroups as a decomposition of the total. It is suitable, for example, for use in presenting a budget where we can easily see the difference between expenditures on health care and defense in the United States. In other words, a bar chart is a suitable graphic device when we have several groups, each associated with a different proportion, whereas a pie chart is more suitable when we have one group which is divided into several categories. The proportions of various categories in a pie chart should add up to 100%. Like bar charts, the categories in a pie chart are usually arranged by the size of the proportions. They may also be arranged alphabetically, or on some other rational basis.

Example 1.7

We can present the data set on the crack kids of Example 1.5 by a bar chart as follows:

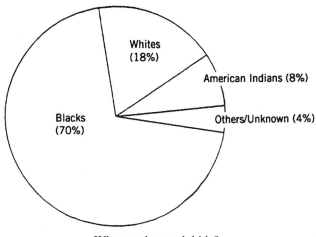

Who are the crack kids?

Another example of the pie chart's use is for presenting the proportions of deaths due to different causes.

Example 1.8

The following table provides the number of deaths due to different causes among Minnesota residents for the year 1975.

Cause of Death	Number of Deaths
Heart disease	12,378
Cancer	6,448
Cerebrovascular disease	3,958
Accidents	1,814
Others	8,088
Total	32,686

After calculating the proportion of deaths due to each cause, for example,

$$\text{Deaths due to cancer} = \frac{6,448}{32,686} = .197 \text{ or } 19.7\%$$

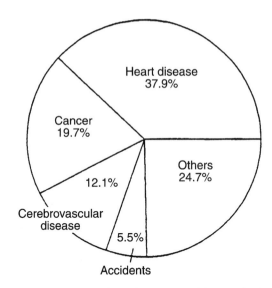

Causes of death for Minnesota residents, 1975

we can present the results as in the above pie chart:

Line Graphs

A line graph is similar to a bar chart, but the horizontal axis represents time. Different "groups" are consecutive years so that a line graph is suitable to illustrate how certain proportions change over time. In a line graph, the proportion associated with each year is represented by a point at the appropriate height; the points are then connected by straight lines.

Example 1.9

Between the years 1984 and 1987, the crude death rates for females in the United States are as follows:

Year	Crude death rate per 100,000 Population
1984	792.7
1985	806.6
1986	809.3
1987	813.1

The change in crude death rate for United States females can be represented by the following line graph:

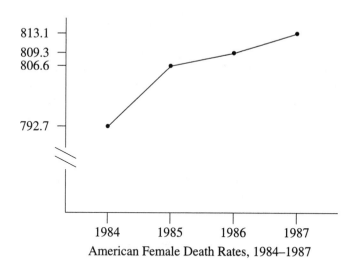

American Female Death Rates, 1984–1987

In addition to their use with proportions, line graphs can also be used to describe changes in the number of occurrences and with continuous measurements.

Example 1.10

The following line graph displays the trend in the reported rates of malaria that occurred in the United States between 1940 and 1989 (proportion × 100,000 as above).

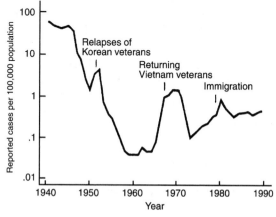

[htb]   Malaria rates in the United States, 1940–1989

1.2. RATES

The term *rate* is kind of confusing; sometimes it is used interchangeably with the term *proportion* as defined in the previous section, but sometimes it refers to a quantity of very different nature. The first subsection (1.2.1) on the *change rate* covers this special use and the next two subsections (1.2.2 and 1.2.3) focus on *rates* used interchangeably with *proportions* as measures of morbidity and mortality. Even when they refer to the same things—measures of morbidity and mortality—there is still some degree of difference between these two terms; as contrast to the static nature of proportions, rates are aimed at measuring the occurrences of events during or after a certain time period.

1.2.1. Changes

Familiar examples of rates include their use to describe changes after a certain period of time. The *change rate* is defined by

$$\text{Change rate } (\%) = \frac{\text{New value} - \text{Old value}}{\text{Old value}} \times 100\%$$

In general, change rates could exceed 100% and could be negative. *They are not proportions* (a proportion is a number between 0 and 1, or 0% and 100%). *Change rates* are mostly used for description and not involved in common *statistical analyses*.

Example 1.11

The following is a typical paragraph of a *news report*:

A total of 35,238 new AIDS cases was reported in 1989 by the Centers for Disease Control (CDC), compared to 32,196 reported during 1988. The 9% increase is the smallest since the spread of AIDS began in the early 1980s. For example, new AIDS cases were up 34% in 1988 and 60% in 1987.

In 1989, 547 cases of AIDS transmissions from mothers to newborns were reported, up 17% from 1988; while females made up just 3,971 of the 35,238 new cases reported in 1989, that was an increase of 11% over 1988.

In the above example:

1. The change rate for new AIDS cases was calculated as

$$\frac{35,238 - 32,196}{32,196} \times 100\% = 9.4\%$$

(this was *rounded down* to the reported figure of 9% in the news report).

2. For the new AIDS cases transmitted from mothers to newborns, we have

$$17\% = \frac{547 - (1988 \text{ cases})}{(1988 \text{ cases})} \times 100\%$$

leading to

$$1988 \text{ cases} = \frac{547}{1.17}$$
$$= 468$$

(a figure obtainable, as shown above, but usually not reported because of redundancy). Similarly, the number of new AIDS cases for the year 1987 is calculated as follows:

$$34\% = \frac{32,196 - (1987 \text{ total})}{(1987 \text{ total})} \times 100\%$$

or

$$1987 \text{ total} = \frac{32,196}{1.34}$$
$$= 24,027$$

3. Among the 1989 new AIDS cases, the proportion of females is

$$\frac{3,971}{35,238} = .113 \text{ or } 11.3\%$$

and the proportion of males is

$$\frac{35,238 - 3,971}{35,238} = .887 \text{ or } 88.7\%.$$

The proportions of females and males add up to 1.0 or 100%.

1.2.2. Measures of Morbidity and Mortality

The field of vital statistics makes use some special applications of rates, three kinds of which are commonly mentioned: crude, specific, and adjusted (or standardized). Unlike change rates, these measures are proportions. Crude rates are computed for an entire large group or population; they disregard factors such as age, sex, and race. Specific rates consider these differences among subgroups or categories of diseases. Adjusted or standardized rates are used to make valid summary comparisons between two or more groups possessing different age distributions.

The annual *crude death rate* is defined as the number of deaths in a calendar year, divided by the population on July 1 of that year (which is usually an estimate); the quotient is often multiplied by 1000, or another suitable power of 10, resulting in a number between 1 and 100, or 1 and 1000. For example, the 1980 population of California was 23,000,000 (as estimated by July 1) and there were 190,237 deaths during 1980, leading to

$$\text{Crude death rate} = \frac{190,247}{23,000,000} \times 1000$$

$$= 8.3 \text{ deaths per 1000 persons per year}$$

The age-specific and cause-specific death rates are similarly defined.

As for morbidity, the disease prevalence, as defined in the previous section, is a proportion used to describe the population at a certain point in time, whereas incidence is a rate used in connection with new cases:

$$\text{Incidence rate} = \frac{\text{Number of individuals who developed the disease over a defined period of time (a year, say)}}{\text{Number of individuals initially without the disease who were followed for the defined period of time}}$$

In other words, *prevalence* presents a snapshot of the population's morbidity experience at certain time point, whereas the *incidence* is aimed to investigate possible time trends.

For example, the 35,238 new AIDS cases in Example 1.7 and the national population without AIDS at the start of 1989 could be combined according to the above formula to yield an incidence of AIDS for the year.

Another interesting use of rates is in connection with cohort studies. Cohort studies are epidemiological designs in which one enrolls a group of persons and follows them over certain periods of time; examples include occupational mortality studies among others. The cohort study design focuses on a particular exposure rather than a particular disease as in case–control studies. Advantages of a longitudinal approach include the opportunity for more accurate measurement of exposure history and a careful examination of the time relationships between exposure and any disease under investigation. Each member of the cohort belongs to one of three types of termination:

1. Subjects still alive on the analysis date
2. Subjects who died on a known date within the study period
3. Subjects who are lost to follow-up after a certain date (these cases are a potential source of bias; effort should be expended on reducing the number of subjects in this category)

The contribution of each member is the length of follow-up time from enrollment to his/her termination. The quotient defined as the observed number of deaths for the cohort, divided by the total follow-up times (in person-years, say) is the *rate* to characterize the mortality experience of the cohort:

$$\text{Follow-up death rate} = \frac{\text{Number of deaths}}{\text{Total person-years}}$$

Rates may be calculated for total deaths and for separate causes of interest and they are usually multiplied by an appropriate power of 10, say 1000, to result in a single-digit or double-digit figure—for example, deaths per 1000 months of follow-up. Follow-up death rates may be used to measure effectiveness of medical treatment programs.

Example 1.12

In an effort to provide a complete analysis of the survival of patients with end-stage renal disease (ESRD), data were collected for a sample that included 929 patients who initiated hemodialysis for the first time at the Regional Disease Program in Minneapolis, Minnesota between 1 January 1976 and 30 June 1982; all patients were followed until 31 December 1982. Of these 929 patients, 257 are diabetics; among the 672 nondiabetics, 386 are classified as low risk (without co-morbidities such as arteriosclerotic heart disease, peripheral vascular disease, chronic obstructive pulmonary, and cancer). Results from these two subgroups were as follows (only some summarized figures are given here for illustration; details such as numbers of deaths and total treatment months for subgroups are not included):

Group	Age	Deaths/1000 Treatment Months
Low risk	1–45	2.75
	46–60	6.93
	61+	13.08
Diabetics	1–45	10.29
	46–60	12.52
	61+	22.16

For example, for the low risk patients over 60 years of age, there were 38 deaths during 2906 treatment months leading to:

$$\frac{38}{2906} \times 1000 = 13.08 \text{ deaths per 1000 treatment months}$$

1.2.3. Standardization of Rates

Crude rates, as measures of morbidity or mortality, can be used for population description and may be suitable for investigations of their variations over time; however, the comparisons of crude rates are often invalid because the populations may be different with respect to an important characteristic such as age, sex, or race (these are potential *confounders*). To overcome this difficulty, an adjusted (or standardized) rate is used in the comparison; the adjustment removes the difference in composition with respect to a confounder.

Example 1.13

The following table provides mortality data for Alaska and Florida for the year 1977.

Age Group	Alaska			Florida		
	No. of Deaths	Persons	Deaths per 100,000	No. of Deaths	Persons	Deaths per 100,000
0–4	162	40,000	405.0	2,049	546,000	375.3
5–19	107	128,000	83.6	1,195	1,982,000	60.3
20–44	449	172,000	261.0	5,097	2,676,000	190.5
45–64	451	58,000	777.6	19,904	1,807,000	1,101.5
65+	444	9,000	4,933.3	63,505	1,444,000	4,397.9
Totals	1,615	407,000	396.8	91,760	8,455,000	1,085.3

The above example shows that the 1977 crude death rate per 100,000 population for Alaska was 396.8 and for Florida was 1,085.3, almost a threefold difference. However, a closer examination shows the following:

1. Alaska had higher age-specific death rates for four of the five age groups, the only exception being 45–64 years.
2. Alaska had a higher percentage of its population in the younger age groups.

The findings make it essential to adjust the death rates of the two states in order to make a valid comparison. A simple way to achieve this, called the *direct method*, is to apply, to a common standard population, age-specific rates observed from the two populations under investigation. For this purpose, the population of the United States as of the last decennial census is frequently used. The procedure consists of the following steps:

1. The standard population is listed by the same age groups.
2. Expected number of deaths in the standard population is computed for each age group of each of the two populations being compared. For example, for age group 0–4, the United States population for 1970 was 84,416 (per 1 million); therefore, we have:

(i) Alaska rate = 405.0 per 100,000
    The expected number of deaths is

$$\frac{(84,416)(405.0)}{100,000} = 341.9$$

$$\cong 342$$

(ii) Florida rate = 375.3 per 100,000
     The expected number of deaths is

$$\frac{(84,416)(375.3)}{100,000} = 316.8$$

$$\cong 317$$

which is lower than the expected number of deaths for Alaska obtained for the same age group.

3. Obtain total number of expected deaths.
4. Age-adjusted death rate is

$$\text{Adjusted rate} = \frac{\text{Total number of expected deaths}}{\text{Total standard population}} \times 100,000$$

Detailed calculations are

		Alaska		Florida	
Age Group	1970 United States Standard Million	Age-Specific Rate	Expected Deaths	Age-Specific Rate	Expected Deaths
0–4	84,416	405.0	342	375.3	317
5–19	294,353	83.6	246	60.3	177
20–44	316,744	261.0	827	190.5	603
45–64	205,745	777.6	1,600	1,101.5	2,266
65+	98,742	4,933.3	4,871	4,397.9	4,343
Totals	1,000,000		7,886		7,706

The age-adjusted death rate per 100,000 population for Alaska is 788.6 and for Florida is 770.6. These age-adjusted rates are much closer than the crude rates, and the adjusted rate for Florida is *lower*. It is important to keep in mind that any population could be chosen as "standard" and, because of this, an adjusted rate is artificial; it does not reflect data from an actual population. The numerical values of the adjusted rates depend in large part on the choice of the standard population. They have real meaning only as relative comparisons.

The advantage of using the United States population as the standard is that we can adjust death rates of many states and compare them with each other. Any population could be selected and used as "standard." In the above example, it does not mean that there were only 1 million people in the United States in the year 1970; it only presents the *age distribution* of 1 million United States residents for that year. If all we want to do is to compare Florida versus Alaska, we could choose either one of the states as standard and adjust the death rate of the other; this practice would save half of the labor. For example, if we choose Alaska as the standard population, then the adjusted death rate for the state of Florida is calculated as follows:

	Alaska Population (Used as Standard)	Florida	
Age Group		Rate/100,000	Expected Number of Deaths
0–4	40,000	375.3	150
5–19	128,000	60.3	77
20–44	172,000	190.5	328
45–64	58,000	1,101.5	639
65+	9,000	4,397.9	396
Totals	407,000		1,590

The new adjusted rate

$$\frac{(1590)(100,000)}{407,000} = 390.7 \text{ per } 100,000$$

is not the same as that obtained using the 1970 United States population as standard (it was 770.6), but it also shows that after age adjustment the death rate in Florida (390.7 per 100,000) is somewhat lower than that of Alaska (396.8 per 100,000; there is no need for adjustment here because we use Alaska's population as the standard population).

1.3. RATIOS

In many cases, such as disease prevalence and disease incidence, proportions and rates are defined very similarly and the two terms, *proportions* and *rates* may even be used interchangeably. Ratio is a completely different term; it is a computation of the form

$$\text{Ratio} = \frac{a}{b}$$

where a and b are *similar quantities* measured from *different groups* or under *different circumstances*. An example is the male-to-female ratio of smoking rates; such a ratio is positive but may exceed 1.0.

1.3.1. Relative Risk

One of the most often used ratios in epidemiological studies is the *relative risk*, a concept for the comparison of two groups or populations with respect to a certain unwanted event (disease or death). The traditional method of expressing it in prospective studies is simply the ratio of the incidence rates:

$$\text{Relative risk} = \frac{\text{Disease incidence in group 1}}{\text{Disease incidence in group 2}}$$

However, ratio of disease prevalences as well as follow-up death rates can also be formed. Usually, group 2 is under standard conditions—such as non-exposure to a certain risk factor—against which group 1 (exposed) is measured. A relative risk that is greater than 1.0 indicates harmful effects, whereas a relative risk that is less than 1.0 indicates beneficial effects. For example, if group 1 consists of smokers while group 2 consists of nonsmokers, then we have a *relative risk due to smoking*. Using the data on end-stage renal disease (ESRN) of Example 1.12, we can obtain the following relative risks due to diabetes:

Age group	Relative Risk
1–45	3.74
46–60	1.81
61+	1.69

All three numbers are greater than 1 (indicating higher mortality for diabetics) and form a decreasing trend with increasing age.

1.3.2. Odds and Odds Ratio

The *relative risk*, also called risk ratio, is an important index in epidemiological studies because in such studies it is often useful to measure the *increased* risk (if any) of incurring a particular disease if a certain factor is present. In cohort studies such an index is readily obtained by observing the experience of groups of subjects with and without the factor as shown above. In a case–control study the data do not present an immediate answer to this type of question, and we now consider how to obtain a useful shortcut solution.

Suppose that each subject in a large study, at a particular time, is classified as positive or negative according to some risk factor and as having or not having a certain disease under investigation. For any such categorization the population may be enumerated in a 2×2 table, as follows:

	Disease		
Factor	$+$	$-$	Total
$+$	A	B	$A + B$
$-$	C	D	$C + D$
Total	$A + C$	$B + D$	$N = A + B + C + D$

The entries A, B, C, and D in the table are sizes of the four combinations of disease presence/absence, and factor presence/absence and the number N at the lower right corner of the table is the total population size. The relative risk is

$$RR = \frac{A}{A + B} \div \frac{C}{C + D}$$
$$= \frac{A(C + D)}{C(A + B)}$$

In many situations, the number of subjects classified as disease positive is small compared to the number classified as disease negative; that is,

$$C + D \cong D$$
$$A + B \cong B$$

($\cong$ means "almost equal to"), and therefore the relative risk can be approximated as follows:

$$RR \cong \frac{AD}{BC}$$
$$= \frac{A/B}{C/D} = \frac{A/C}{B/D}$$

where the slash denotes division. The resulting ratio, AD/BC, is an approximate relative risk, but it is often referred to as "odds ratio" because:

1. A/B and C/D are the odds in favor of having disease from groups with or without the factor.
2. A/C and B/D are the odds in favor of exposure to the factors from groups with or without the disease. These two odds can be easily estimated using case–control data, by using sample frequencies. For example, the odds A/C can be estimated by a/c, where a is the number of exposed cases and c is the number of exposed controls in the sample of cases in a case–control design.

For the many diseases that are rare, the terms "relative risk" and "odds ratio" are used interchangeably because of the above-mentioned approximation. The relative risk is an important epidemiological index used to measure seriousness, or the magnitude of the harmful effect of suspected risk factors. For example, if we have

$$RR = 3.0$$

we can say that the exposed individuals have a risk of contracting the disease which is approximately three times the risk of unexposed individuals. A perfect 1.0 indicates no effect, and beneficial factors result in relative risk values which are smaller than 1.0. From data obtained by a case–control or retrospective study, it is impossible to calculate the relative risk that we want, but if it is reasonable to assume that the disease is rare (prevalence is less than .05, say), then we can calculate the odds ratio as a "stepping stone" and use it as an approximate relative risk (we use the notation $\cong$ for this purpose). In these cases, we interpret the calculated odds ratio just as we would do with the relative risk.

Example 1.14

The role of smoking in the etiology of pancreatitis has been recognized for many years. In order to provide estimates of the quantitative significance of these factors, a hospital-based study was carried out in eastern Massachusetts and Rhode Island between 1975 and 1979. Ninety-eight patients who had a hospital discharge diagnosis of pancreatitis were included in this unmatched case–control study. The control group consisted of 451 patients admitted for diseases other than those of the pancreas and biliary tract. Risk factor information was obtained from a standardized interview with each subject, conducted by a trained interviewer.

The following are some data for the males:

Use of Cigarettes	Cases	Controls
Never	2	56
Ex-smokers	13	80
Current Smokers	38	81
Total	53	217

For the above data, the approximate relative risks or odds ratios are calculated as follows:

1. For ex-smokers,

$$RR_e \cong \frac{13/2}{80/56}$$
$$= \frac{(13)(56)}{(80)(2)}$$
$$= 4.55$$

(The subscript e in RR_e indicates that we are calculating the relative risk (RR) for exsmokers.)

2. For current smokers,

$$RR_c \cong \frac{38/2}{81/56}$$
$$= \frac{(38)(56)}{(81)(2)}$$
$$= 13.14$$

[The subscript c in RR_c indicates that we are calculating the relative risk (RR) for current smokers.] In these calculations, the nonsmokers (who never smoke) are used as references. These values indicate that the risk of having pancreatitis for current smokers is approximately 13.14 times the same risk for people who never smoke. The effect for ex-smokers is smaller (4.55 times), but it is still very high (as compared to 1.0—the no-effect baseline for relative risks and odds ratios). In other words, if the smokers quit smoking, they would reduce their own risk (from 13.14 times to 4.55 times), but *not* to the normal level for people who never smoke.

1.3.3. Generalized Odds for Ordered 2 × *k* Tables

It is interesting to note that an odds ratio can be interpreted as an odds for a different event. For example, consider again the same 2 × 2 table, as seen in the previous section:

Factor	Disease +	−	Total
+	A	B	$A + B$
−	C	D	$C + D$
Total	$A + C$	$B + D$	$N = A + B + C + D$

where entries A, B, C, and D in the table are sizes of the four combinations of disease presence/absence and factor presence/absence and N is the total population size.

The number of case–control pairs with different exposure histories is $(AD + BC)$; among them are AD pairs with an exposed case and BC pairs with an exposed control. Therefore AD/BC, the odds ratio of the previous section, can be seen as the odds of finding a pair with an exposed case among discordant pair (a *discordant pair* is a case–control pair with *different* exposure histories).

The above interpretation of the concept odds ratio as an ddds can be generalized as follows. The aim here is to present an efficient method for use with ordered $2 \times k$ contingency tables, tables with two rows and with k columns having a certain natural ordering. The summarized figure is the generalized odds formulated from the concept of odds ratio. Let us first consider an example concerning the use of seat belts in automobiles. Each accident in this example is classified according to whether a seat belt was used and the severity of injuries received: none, minor, major, or death. The data were as follows:

	Extent of Injury Received			
Seat Belt	None	Minor	Major	Death
Yes	75	160	100	15
No	65	175	135	25

To compare the extent of injury from those who used seat belts and those who did not, we can calculate the percent of seat belt users in each injury group from level "none" to level "death," and the results are:

$$\text{None:} \quad 75/(75 + 65) = 58\%$$

$$\text{Minor:} \quad 160/(100 + 175) = 48\%$$

$$\text{Major:} \quad 100/(100 + 135) = 43\%$$

$$\text{Death:} \quad 15/(15 + 25) = 38\%$$

What we are seeing here is a "trend" or an *association* indicating that the lower the percentage of seat belt users, the more severe the injury.

We now present the concept of generalized odds, a special statistic specifically formulated to measure the strength of such a "trend," and will use the same example and another one to illustrate its use. In general, consider an ordered $2 \times k$ table with frequencies:

	Column Level				
Row	1	2	$\cdots$	k	Total
1	a_1	a_2	$\cdots$	a_k	A
2	b_1	b_2	$\cdots$	b_k	B
Total	n_1	n_2	$\cdots$	n_k	N

The number of "concordances" is calculated by

$$C = a_1(b_2 + \cdots + b_k) + a_2(b_3 + \cdots + b_k) + \cdots + a_{k-1}b_k$$

(The term "concordance" pair as used in the above example corresponds to a less severe injury for the seat belt user.) The number of "discordances" is

$$D = b_1(a_2 + \cdots + a_k) + b_2(a_3 + \cdots + a_k) + \cdots + b_{k-1}a_k$$

In order to *measure* the degree of association, we use the index C/D and call it the *generalized odds*; if there are only two levels of injury, this new index is reduced to the familiar odds ratio. When data are properly arranged, by an a priori hypothesis, the products in the number of concordance pairs C (for example, a_1b_2) go from upper left to lower right direction, and the products in the number of discordance pairs D (for example b_1a_2) go from lower left to upper right direction. In that a priori hypothesis, column 1 is associated with row 1; In the above example, the use of seat belt (yes, first row) is hypothesized to be associated with less severed injury (none, first column). Under this hypothesis, the resulting generalized odds is greater than 1.

Example 1.15

For the above study on the use of seat belts in automobiles

Seat Belt	Extent of Injury Received			
	None	Minor	Major	Death
Yes	75	160	100	15
No	65	175	135	25

we have

$$C = 75(175 + 135 + 25) + 160(135 + 25) + (100)(25)$$
$$= 53,225$$
$$D = 65(160 + 100 + 15) + 175(100 + 15) + (135)(15)$$
$$= 40,025$$

leading to a generalized odds of

$$\theta = \frac{C}{D}$$
$$= \frac{53,225}{40,025}$$
$$= 1.33$$

That is, *given two persons with different levels of injury*, the (generalized) odds that the more severely injured did not wear a seat belt is 1.33. In other words, the people with more severe injuries would more likely be the ones who did not use a seat belt than the people with less severe injuries.

The following example shows the use of the generalized odds in case–control studies with an ordinal risk factor.

Example 1.16

A case–control study of the epidemiology of preterm delivery, defined as one with less than 37 weeks of gestation, was undertaken at Yale–New Haven Hospital in Connecticut during 1977. The study population consisted of 175 mothers of singleton preterm infants and 303 mothers of singleton full-term infants. The following table gives the distribution of mother's age.

Age	Cases	Controls
14–17	15	16
18–19	22	25
20–24	47	62
25–29	56	122
≥ 30	35	78

We have

$$C = (15)(25 + 62 + 122 + 78) + (22)(62 + 122 + 78) + (47)(122 + 78) + (56)(78)$$
$$= 23,837$$
$$D = (16)(22 + 47 + 56 + 35) + (25)(47 + 56 + 35) + (62)(56 + 35) + (122)(35)$$
$$= 15,922$$

leading to a generalized odds of

$$\theta = \frac{C}{D}$$
$$= \frac{23,837}{15,922}$$
$$= 1.50$$

This means that the odds that the younger mother has preterm delivery is 1.5. In other words, the younger mothers would more likely have preterm delivery.

The next example shows the use of the generalized odds for contingency tables with more than two rows of data.

Example 1.17

The following table shows the results of a survey, each subject of a sample of 282 adults was asked to indicate which of three policies they favored with respect to smoking in public places:

Highest Education Level	Policy Favored			
	No Restrictions on Smoking	Smoking Allowed in Designated Areas Only	No Smoking at All	Total
Grade school	15	40	10	65
High school	15	100	30	145
College graduate	5	44	23	72
Total	35	184	63	282

We have

$$C = (15)(100 + 30 + 44 + 23) + (40)(30 + 23) + (100)(23) = 8380$$
$$D = (5)(100 + 30 + 40 + 10) + (44)(30 + 10) + (100)(10) = 4410$$

leading to a generalized odds of

$$\theta = \frac{C}{D}$$
$$= \frac{8,380}{4,410}$$
$$= 1.90$$

This means that the odds that the more educated person favors more restriction for smoking in public places is 1.90. In other words, people with more education would prefer more restriction on smoking in public places.

1.3.4. The Mantel–Haenszel Method

In most investigations, we are concerned with one primary outcome, such as a disease, and focusing on one primary (risk) factor, such as an exposure with a possible harmful effect. There are situations, however, where an investigator may want to adjust for aconfounder that could influence the outcome of a statistical analysis. A confounder, or a confounding variable, is a variable that may be associated with either the disease or exposure or both. For example, in Example 1.2, a case–control study was undertaken to investigate the relationship between lung cancer and employment in shipyards during World War II among male residents of coastal Georgia. In this case, smoking is a possible counfounder; it has been found to be associated with lung cancer, and it may be associated with employment because construction workers are likely to be smokers. Specifically, we want to know the following:

1. Among smokers, whether or not shipbuilding and lung cancer are related
2. Among nonsmokers, whether or not shipbuilding and lung cancer are related

In fact, the original data were tabulated separately for three smoking levels (non-, moderate, and heavy); in Example 1.2, the last two tables were combined and presented together for simplicity. Assuming that the confounder, smoking, is not an effect modifier (i.e., smoking does not alter the relationship between lung cancer and shipbuilding), however, we do not want to reach separate conclusions, one at each level of smoking. In those cases, we want to pool data for a combined decision. When both the disease and the exposure are binary, a popular method to achieve this task is the Mantel–Haenszel method. This method provides one single estimate for the common odds ratio and can be summarized as follows:

1. We form 2×2 tables, one at each level of the confounder.
2. At a level of the confounder, we have

	Disease Classification		
Exposure	+	−	Total
+	a	b	r_1
−	c	d	r_2
Total	c_1	c_2	n

Because we assume that the counfounder is not an effect modifier, the odds ratio is constant across its levels. The odds ratio at each level is estimated by ad/bc; the Mantel–Haenszel procedure pools data across levels of the confounder to obtain a combined estimate (some kind of weighted average of level-specific odds ratios:

$$OR_{MH} = \frac{\sum \frac{ad}{n}}{\sum \frac{bc}{n}}$$

Example 1.18

A case–control study was conducted to identify reasons for the exceptionally high rate of lung cancer among male residents of coastal Georgia as first presented in Example 1.2. The primary risk factor under investigation was employment in shipyards during World War II, and data are tabulated separately for three levels of smoking as follows:

Smoking	Shipbuilding	Cases	Controls
No	Yes	11	35
	No	50	203
Moderate	Yes	70	42
	No	217	220
Heavy	Yes	14	3
	No	96	50

There are three 2 × 2 tables, one for each level of smoking. We begin with the 2 × 2 table for nonsmokers:

Shipbuilding	Cases	Controls	Total
Yes	11(a)	35(b)	46(r_1)
No	50(c)	203(d)	253(r_2)
Total	61(c_1)	238(c_2)	299(n)

We have, for the nonsmokers,

$$\frac{ad}{n} = \frac{(11)(203)}{299}$$
$$= 7.47,$$
$$\frac{bc}{n} = \frac{(35)(50)}{299}$$
$$= 5.85$$

The process is repeated for each of the other two smoking levels. For moderate smokers

$$\frac{ad}{n} = \frac{(70)(220)}{549}$$
$$= 28.05,$$
$$\frac{bc}{n} = \frac{(42)(217)}{549}$$
$$= 16.60$$

and for heavy smokers

$$\frac{ad}{n} = \frac{(14)(50)}{163}$$
$$= 4.29,$$
$$\frac{bc}{n} = \frac{(3)(96)}{163}$$
$$= 1.77$$

These results are combined to obtain a combined estimate for the common odds ratio:

$$OR_{MH} = \frac{7.47 + 28.05 + 4.28}{5.85 + 16.60 + 1.77}$$
$$= 1.64$$

This combined estimate of the odds ratio, 1.64, represents an approximate increase of 64% in lung cancer risk for those employed in the shipbuilding industry.

The following is another similar example aiming at the possible effects of oral contraceptive use on myocardial infarction. The presentation has been shortened, keeping only key figures.

Example 1.19

A case–control study was conducted to investigate the relationship between myocardial infarction (MI) and oral contraceptive use (OC). The data, stratified by cigarette smoking, were as follows:

Smoking	OC Use	Cases	Controls
No	Yes	4	52
	No	34	754
Yes	Yes	25	83
	No	171	853

An application of the Mantel–Haenszel procedure yields

	Smoking	
	No	Yes
$\dfrac{ad}{n}$	3.57	18.84
$\dfrac{bc}{n}$	2.09	12.54

The combined odds ratio estimate is

$$OR_{MH} = \frac{3.57 + 18.84}{2.09 + 12.54}$$
$$= 1.53$$

representing an approximate increase of 53% in myocardial infarction risk for oral contraceptive users.

1.3.5. Standardized Mortality Ratio

In a cohort study, the follow-up death rates are calculated and used to describe the mortality experience of the cohort under investigation. However, the observed mortality of the cohort is often compared with that expected from the death rates of the national population (used as *standard* or *baseline*). The basis of this method is the comparison of the observed number of deaths, d, from the cohort with the mortality that would have been expected if the group had experienced similar death rates to those of the national population of which the cohort is a part. Let e denote the expected number of deaths, then the comparison is based on the following ratio called the *standardized mortality ratio:*

$$\text{SMR} = \frac{d}{e}$$

The expected number of deaths is calculated using published national life tables and the calculation can be approximated as follows:

$$e \cong \lambda T$$

where T is the total follow-up time (person-years) from the cohort and λ the annual death rate (per person) from the referenced population. Of course, the annual death rate of the referenced population changes with age. Therefore, what we actually do in research is more complicated, although based on the same idea. First, we subdivide the cohort into many age groups, then calculate the product λT for each age group using the correct age-specific rate for that group, and add up the results.

Example 1.20

Some 7000 British workers exposed to vinyl chloride monomer were followed for several years to determine whether their mortality experience differed from those of the general population. The following data are for deaths from cancers, and they are tabulated separately for four groups based on years since entering the industry. This data display shows some interesting features:

1. For the group with 1–4 years since entering the industry, we have a death rate that is substantially less than that of the general population (SMR = .445 or 44.5%). This phenomenon, known as the "healthy worker effect," is most likely a consequence of a selection factor whereby workers are necessarily in better health (than people in the general population) at the time of their entry into the work force.
2. We see an attenuation of the healthy worker effect (i.e., a decreasing trend) with the passage of time, so that the cancer death rates show a slight excess after 15 years (vinyl chloride exposures are known to induce a rare form of liver cancer and to increase rates of brain cancer).

Deaths from Cancers	Years Since Entering the Industry				Total
	1–4	5–9	10–14	15+	
Observed	9	15	23	68	115
Expected	20.3	21.3	24.5	60.8	126.8
SMR (%)	44.5	70.6	94.0	111.8	90.7

Taking the ratio of two standardized mortality ratios is another way of expressing relative risk. For example, the relative risk of the 15+ years group is 1.58 times the risk of the risk of the 5–9 years group, since the ratio of the two corresponding mortality ratios is

$$\frac{111.8}{70.6} = 1.58$$

Similarly, the risk of the >15 years group is 2.51 times the risk of the 1 to 4 year group because the ratio of the two corresponding mortality ratios is

$$\frac{111.8}{44.5} = 2.51$$

1.4. NOTES ON COMPUTATIONS

Much of this book is concerned with arithmetic/algebraic procedures for data analysis. In many biomedical investigations, particularly those involving large quantities of data, the analysis—for example, regression analysis of Chapter 8—gives rise to difficulties in computational implementation. In these investigations it will be necessary to use statistical software specially designed to do these jobs. Most of the calculations described in this book can be readily carried out using statistical packages, and any student or practitioner of data analysis will find the use of such packages essential.

Some methods of survival analysis (section 2.3), some nonparametric methods (Sections 2.4 and 7.4), and some methods of multiple regression analysis (Section 8.2) may be best handled by a specialized package, such as SAS; in these sections, samples of programs are included in our examples where they were needed. However, students and investigators contemplating to use of one of these commercial programs should read the specifications of each program—maybe with help from the course instructor—before choosing options needed or suitable for any particular arithmetic/algebraic procedure. But these sections are exceptions, all other calculations described in this book can be readily carried out using Microsoft's Excel, a popular software available in every personal computers. Notes on the use of Excel are included in separate sections at the end of each chapter.

A *worksheet* or spreadsheet is a blank sheet where you do your work. An Excel *file* holds a stack of worksheets in a *workbook*. You can *name* a sheet, put data on it and *save*, and, later, *open* and use it. You can *move* or *size* your windows by *dragging* the borders. You can also scroll up and down, or left and right through an Excel worksheet using the "scroll bars" on the right side and at the bottom.

An Excel worksheet consists of *grid lines* forming *columns* and *rows*; columns are *lettered* and rows are *numbered*. The intersection of each column and row is a box called a *cell*. Every cell has an *address*, also called *cell reference*; to refer to a cell, enter the column letter followed by the row number. For example, *the intersection of column C and row 3 is cell C3*. Cells hold numbers, text, or formulas. To refer to a range of cells, enter the cell in the upper left corner of the range followed by a colon (:) and then enter the lower right corner of the range. For example, A1:B20 refers to the first 20 rows in both column A and B.

You can click a cell to make it *active* (for use); an active cell is where you enter or edit your data, and it's identified by a *heavy border*. You can also *define or select a range* by left clicking on the upper-left-most cell and dragging the mouse to the lower-right-most cell. To move around inside a selected range, press Tab or Enter to move forward one cell at a time.

Excel is a software to handle numbers; so, get a project and start typing. Conventionally, files for data analysis use rows for subjects and columns for factors. For example, you conduct a survey using a 10-item questionnaire and receive returns from 75 people; your data require a file with 75 rows and 10 columns—not counting labels for columns (factors' names) and rows (subjects' ID). If you made an error, it can fixed; e.g., hit the Del key, that wipes out the cell contents. You can change your mind again, deleting the delete by clicking the *Undo button* (reversed curved arrow). Remember, you can widen your columns by double-clicking their right borders.

The formula bar (near the top, next to an = sign) is a common way to provide the content of an active cell. Excel executes a formula from left to right and performs multiplication (∗) and division (/) before addition (+) and subtraction (−). Parentheses can/should be used to change the order of calculations. To use formulas (e.g., for data transformation), do it in one of two ways: (i) Click the cell you want to fill, then type an = sign followed by the formula in the formula bar (e.g., click C5, then type = A5 + B5); or (ii) click the cell you want to fill, then click the *paste function icon*, f∗, which will give you—in a box—a list Excel functions available for your use.

The *Cut and Paste* procedure greatly simplifies the typing necessary to form a chart or table or write numerous formulas. The procedure involves highlighting the cells that contain the information you want to copy, clicking on the cut button (scissors icon) or copy button (two page icon), selecting the cell(s) to which the information is to be placed, and clicking on the paste button (clipboard and page icon). The *Select and Drag* is very efficient for *data transformation*. Suppose you have the weight and height of 15 men, weights are in C6:C20 and heights are in D6:D20, and you need their body mass index. You can use the formula bar, for example, clicking E6 and typing = C6/(D6^2). The content of E6 now has the body mass index for the first man in your sample, but you do not have to repeat this process 15 times. Notice when you click on E6, there is a little box in the lower right corner of the cell boundary. If you move the mouse over this box, the cursor changes to a smaller plus sign. If you click on this box, you can then drag the mouse over the remaining cells; and once you release the button, the cells will be filled.

Bar and Pie Charts

Forming a bar chart or pie to display proportions is a very simple task. Just click any blank cell to start, and you'll be able to move your chart to any location when done. With data ready, click the *ChartWizard* icon (the one with multiple colored bars on the *standard toolbar* near the top). A box appears with choices including bar chart, pie chart, and line chart; the list is on the left side. Choose your chart type and follow instructions. There are many choices, including 3D! You can put data and charts side by side for impressive presentation.

Rate Standardization

This is a good problem to practice with Excel: Use it as a *calculator*. Recall this example:

- Florida's rate = 1085.3
- Alaska's rate = 396.8

If Florida has Alaska's population

Age Group	Alaska Population (Used as Standard)	Florida Rate/100,000	Florida Expected Number of Deaths
0–4	40,000	375.3	150
5–19	128,000	60.3	77
20–44	172,000	190.5	328
45–64	58,000	1,101.5	639
65+	9,000	4,397.9	396
Totals	407,000		1,590

then you can do the following:

- Use *formula* to calculate the first expected number.
- Use *drag and fill* to obtain other expected numbers.
- Select last column, then click *Autosum icon* ($\sum$) to obtain the total number of expected deaths.

Forming 2 × 2 Tables

Recall that in a *data file* you have one row for each subject and one column for each variable. Suppose *two* of those variables are categorical, say *binary*, and you want to *form a 2 × 2 table* so you can study their relationship—for example, to calculate an *odds ratio*.

- Step 0: Create a dummy factor, call it (say) *fake*, and fill up that column with "*1*" (you can enter "1" for the first subject, then *select and drag*).
- Step 1: *Activate* a cell (by clicking it), then click *Data* (on the bar above the standard toolbar, near the end); when a box appears, choose *PivotTable Report*. Click "*next*" (to indicate that data are here, in Excel), then *highlight* the area containing your data (including variable names on first row—use the mouse; or you could identify the *range of cells*—say, C5:E28) as a response to question on *range*. Then click "*next*" to bring in the *PivotTable Wizard*, which shows two groups of things:

  1. A *frame* for a 2 × 2 *table* with places identified as *row, column, and data*;
  2. Names of the factors you chose, say, *exposure, disease, and fake*.

- Step 2: *Drag* exposure to merge with row (or column), *drag* disease to merge with column (or row), and *drag* fake to merge with data. Then click *Finish*; a 2 × 2 *table* appears in the active cell you identified, complete with *cell frequencies, row and column totals*, and *grand total*.

Note: If you have another *factor*, besides exposure and disease, available in the data set—even a column for *names* or *IDs*—then there is no need to create the *dummy factor*. Complete step 1; then, in step 2, *drag that third factor*, say *ID*, to merge with "*data*" in the frame shown by the *PivotTable Wizard*; it appears as *sum ID*. Click on that item, then choose *count* (to replace *sum*).

EXERCISES

1.1. Self-reported injuries among left-handed and right-handed people were compared in a survey of 1896 college students in British Columbia, Canada. Ninety-three of the 180 left-handed students reported at least one injury, and 619 of the 1716 right-handed students reported at least one injury in the same period. Arrange the data into a 2 × 2 table and calculate the proportion of people with at least one injury during the period of observation for each group.

1.2. A study was conducted in order to evaluate the hypothesis that tea consumption and premenstrual syndrome are associated. One hundred eighty-eight nursing students and 64 tea factory workers were given questionnaires. The prevalence of premenstrual syndrome was 39% among the nursing students and 77% among the tea factory workers. How many people in each group have premenstrual syndrome? Arrange the data into a 2 × 2 table.

1.3. The relationship between prior condom use and tubal pregnancy was assessed in a population-based case–control study at Group Health Cooperative of Puget Sound during 1981–1986. The results are:

Condom use	Cases	Controls
Never	176	488
Ever	51	186

Calculate the proportion of subjects in each group who never used condoms.

1.4. Epidemic keratoconjunctivitis (EKC) or "shipyard eye" is an acute infectious disease of the eye. A case of EKC is defined as an illness

- consisting of redness, tearing, and pain in one or both eyes for more than 3 days' duration,
- diagnosed as EKC by an ophthalmologist.

In late October 1977, one (Physician A) of the two ophthalmologists providing the majority of specialized eye care to the residents of a central Georgia county (population 45,000) saw a 27-year-old nurse who had returned from a vacation in Korea with severe EKC. She received symptomatic therapy and was warned that her eye infection could spread to others; nevertheless, numerous cases of an illness similar to hers soon occurred in the patients and staff of the nursing home (Nursing Home A) where she worked (these individuals came to Physician A for diagnosis and treatment). The following table provides exposure history of 22 persons with EKC between October 27, 1977 and January 13, 1978 (when the outbreak stopped after proper control techniques were initiated). Nursing Home B, included in this table, is the only other area chronic-care facility.

Exposure Cohort	Number Exposed	Number of Cases
Nursing Home A	64	16
Nursing Home B	238	6

Calculate and compare the proportions of cases from the two nursing homes; what would be your conclusion?

1.5. In August 1976 tuberculosis was diagnosed in a high school student (index case) in Corinth, Mississippi. Subsequently, laboratory studies revealed that the student's disease was caused by drug-resistant tubercule bacilli. An epidemiologic investigation was conducted at the high school.

The following table gives the rate of positive tuberculin reactions, determined for various groups of students according to degree of exposure to the index case.

Exposure Level	Number Tested	Number Positive
High	129	63
Low	325	36

(a) Calculate and compare the proportions of positive cases for the two exposure levels; what would be your conclusion?

(b) Calculate the odds ratio associated with high exposure. Does this result support your conclusion in (a)?

1.6. Consider the data taken from a study that attempts to determine whether the use of electronic fetal monitoring (EFM) during labor affects the frequency of caesarean section deliveries. Of the 5824 infants included in the study, 2850 were electronically monitored and 2974 were not. The outcomes are as follows:

Caesarean Delivery	EFM Exposure		Total
	Yes	No	
Yes	358	229	587
No	2492	2745	5237
Total	2850	2974	5824

(a) Calculate and compare the proportions of caesarean delivery for the two exposure groups. What would be your conclusion?

(b) Calculate the odds ratio associated with EFM exposure. Does this result support your conclusion in (a)?

1.7. A study was conducted to investigate the effectiveness of bicycle safety helmets in preventing head injury. The data consist of a random sample of 793 individuals who were involved in bicycle accidents during a 1-year period.

Head Injury	Wearing Helmet		Total
	Yes	No	
Yes	17	218	235
No	130	428	558
Total	147	646	793

(a) Calculate and compare the proportions of head injury for the group with helmets versus the group without helmets. What would be your conclusion?

(b) Calculate the odds ratio associated with not using helmet. Does this result support your conclusion in (a)?

1.8. A case–control study was conducted in Auckland, New Zealand to investigate the effects of alcohol consumption on both nonfatal myocardial infarction and coronary death in the 24 hours after drinking, among regular drinkers. Data were tabulated separately for men and women.

• Men

Drink in the Last 24 hours	Myocardial Infarction		Coronary death	
	Controls	Cases	Controls	Cases
No	197	142	135	103
Yes	201	136	159	69

• Women

Drink in the Last 24 hours	Myocardial Infarction		Coronary death	
	Controls	Cases	Controls	Cases
No	144	41	89	12
Yes	122	19	76	4

(a) Refer to myocardial infarction (table on the left); calculate the odds ratio associated with drinking, separately for men and women.

(b) Compare the two odds ratios in (a); when the difference is properly confirmed, we have an effect modification.

(c) Refer to coronary deaths (table on the right), calculate the odds ratio associated with drinking, separately for men and women.

(d) Compare the two odds ratios in (c); when the difference is properly confirmed, we have an effect modification.

1.9. Data taken from a study to investigate the effects of smoking on cervical cancer are stratified by the number of sexual partners. Results are as follows:

Number of Partners	Smoking	Cancer Yes	Cancer No
Zero or one	Yes	12	21
	No	25	118
Two or more	Yes	96	142
	No	92	150

(a) Calculate the odds ratio associated with smoking, separately for the two groups, those with zero or one partners and those with two or more partners.

(b) Compare the two odds ratios in (a); when the difference is properly confirmed, we have an effect modification.

(c) Asuming that the odds ratios for the two groups, those with zero or one partners and those with two or more partners, are equal (in other words, the number of partners is not an effect modifier), calculate the Mantel–Haenszel estimate of this common odds ratio.

1.10. The following table provides the proportions of currently married women having an unplanned pregnancy; data are tabulated for several different methods of contraception.

Method of Contraception	Proportion with Unplanned Pregnancy
None	0.431
Diaphragm	0.149
Condom	0.106
IUD	0.071
Pill	0.037

Display these proportions in a bar chart.

1.11. The following table summarizes the coronary heart disease (CHD) and lung cancer mortality rates per 1000 person-years by number of cigarettes smoked per day at baseline for men participating in MRFIT (Multiple Risk Factor Intervention Trial, a very large controlled clinical trial focusing on the relationship between smoking and cardiovascular diseases).

	Total	CHD Deaths N	CHD Deaths Rate/1000 yr	Lung Cancer Deaths N	Lung Cancer Deaths Rate/1000 yr
Never-smokers	1859	44	2.22	0	0
Ex-smokers	2813	73	2.44	13	0.43
Smokers					
1–19 cig./day	856	23	2.56	2	0.22
20–39 cig./day	3747	173	4.45	50	1.29
≥ 40 cig./day	3591	115	3.08	54	1.45

For each cause of death, display the rates in a bar chart.

1.12. The following table provides data taken from a study on the association between race and use of medical care by adults experiencing chest pain in the past year.

Response	Black	White
MD seen in past year	35	67
MD seen, not in past year	45	38
MD never seen	78	39
Total	158	144

Display the proportions of the three response categories for each group, blacks and whites, in a separate pie chart.

1.13. The following frequency distribution provides the number of cases of pediatric AIDS between 1983 and 1989.

Year	Number of cases
1983	122
1984	250
1985	455
1986	848
1987	1412
1988	2811
1989	3098

Display the trend of numbers of cases using a line graph.

1.14. A study was conducted to investigate the changes between 1973 and 1985 in women's use of three preventive health services. The data were obtained from the National Health Survey; women were divided into subgroups according to age and race. The percentages (%) of women receiving a breast exam within the past 2 years are given below.

Age and Race	Breast Exam Within Past 2 Years	
	1973	1985
Total	65.5	69.6
Black	61.7	74.8
White	65.9	69.0
20–39 years	77.5	77.9
Black	77.0	83.9
White	77.6	77.0
40–59 years	62.1	66.0
Black	54.8	67.9
White	62.9	65.7
60–79 years	44.3	56.2
Black	39.1	64.5
White	44.7	55.4

Separately for each group, Blacks and Whites, display the proportions of women receiving a breast exam within the past two years in a bar chart so as to show the relationship between the examination rate and age. Mark the midpoint of each age group on the horizontal axis and display the same data using a line graph.

1.15. Consider the following data:

	Tuberculosis		
X ray	No	Yes	Total
Negative	1739	8	1747
Positive	51	22	73
Total	1790	30	1820

Calculate the sensitivity and specificity of X ray as a screening test for tuberculosis.

1.16. Sera from a T-lyphotropic virus type (HTLV-I) risk group (prostitute women) were tested with two commercial "research" enzyme-linked immunoabsorbent assays (EIA) for HTLV-I antibodies. These results were compared with a gold standard, and outcomes are shown below.

	Dupont's EIA			Cellular Product's EIA	
True	Positive	Negative	True	Positive	Negative
Positive	15	1	Positive	16	0
Negative	2	164	Negative	7	179

Calculate and compare the sensitivity and specificity of these two EIAs.

1.17. The following table provides the number of deaths for several leading causes among Minnesota residents for the year 1991.

Cause of Death	Number of Deaths	Rate per 100,000 Population
Heart disease	10,382	294.5
Cancer	8,299	?
Cerebrovascular cisease	2,830	?
Accidents	1,381	?
Other Causes	11,476	?
Total	34,368	?

(a) Calculate the percentage of total deaths for deaths from each cause and display the results in a pie chart.

(b) From death rate (per 100,000 population) for heart disease, calculate the population for Minnesota for the year 1991.

(c) From the result of (b), fill in the missing death rates (per 100,000 population) at the question marks in the above table.

1.18. The survey described in Example 1.1, continued in the comparative studies section (Section 1.1.1), provided percentages of boys from various ethnic groups who use tobacco at least weekly. Display these proportions in a bar chart similar to the one in Example 1.6.

1.19. A case–control study was conducted relating to the epidemiology of breast cancer and the possible involvement of dietary fats, along with other vitamins and nutrients. It included 2024 breast cancer cases who were admitted to Roswell Park Memorial Institute, Erie County, New York, from 1958 to 1965. A control group of 1463 was chosen from the patients having no neoplasms and no pathology of gastrointestinal or reproductive systems. The primary factors being investigated were vitamins A and E (measured in international units per month). The following are data for 1500 women over 54 years of age.

Vitamin A (IU/mo)	Cases	Controls
≤ 150,500	893	392
> 150,500	132	83
Total	1025	475

Calculate the odds ratio associated with a decrease in ingestion of foods containing vitamin A.

1.20. Refer to the data set in Example 1.2,

Smoking	Shipbuilding	Cases	Controls
No	Yes	11	35
	No	50	203
Yes	Yes	84	45
	No	313	270

(a) Calculate the odds ratio associated with employment in shipyards for nonsmokers.

(b) Calculate the same odds ratio for smokers.

(c) Compare the results of (a) and (b); when the difference is properly confirmed, we have a "three-term interaction" or "effect modification," where smoking alters the effect of employment in shipyards as a risk for lung cancer.

(d) Asuming that the odds ratios for the two groups, nonsmokers and smokers, are equal (in other words, smoking is not an effect modifier), calculate the Mantel–Haenszel estimate of this common odds ratio.

1.21. Although cervical cancer is not a major cause of death among American women, it has been suggested that virtually all such deaths are preventable. In an effort to find out who is being screened for the disease, data from the 1973 National Health Interview (a sample of the United States population) were used to examine the relationship between Pap testing and some socioeconomic factors. The following table provides the percentages of women who reported never having had a Pap test (these are from metropolitan areas):

Age and Income		White (%)	Black
25–44	Poor	13.0	14.2
	Nonpoor	5.9	6.3
45–64	Poor	30.2	33.3
	Nonpoor	13.2	23.3
65 and over	Poor	47.4	51.5
	Nonpoor	36.9	47.4

(a) Calculate the odds ratios associated with race (Black versus White) among
    (i) 25–44 Nonpoor
    (ii) 45–64 Nonpoor
    (iii) 65+ Nonpoor
    Briefly discuss a possible effect modification, if any.

(b) Calculate the odds ratios associated with income (Poor versus Nonpoor) among
    (i) 25–44 Black
    (ii) 45–64 Black
    (iii) 65+ Black
    Briefly discuss a possible effect modification, if any.

(c) Calculate the odds ratios associated with race (Black versus White) among
    (i) 65+ Poor
    (ii) 65+ Nonpoor
    and briefly discuss a possible effect modification.

1.22. Because incidence rates of most cancers rise with age, this must always be considered a confounder. The following are stratified data for an unmatched case–control study; the disease was esophageal cancer among men, and the risk factor was alcohol consumption.

Age		Daily Alcohol Consumption	
		80+ g	0–79 g
25–44	Cases	5	5
	Controls	35	270
45–64	Cases	67	55
	Controls	56	277
65+	Cases	24	44
	Controls	18	129

(a) Calculate the odds ratio associated with *high* alcohol consumption, separately for the three age groups.

(b) Compare the three odds ratios in (a); when the difference is properly confirmed, we have an effect modification.

(c) Asuming that the odds ratios for the three age groups are equal (in other words, age is not an effect modifier), calculate the Mantel–Haenszel estimate of this common odds ratio.

1.23. Postmenopausal women who develop endometrial cancer are, on the whole, heavier than women who do not develop the disease. One possible explanation is that heavy women are more exposed to endogenous estrogens which are produced in postmenopausal women by conversion of steroid precursors to active estrogens in peripheral fat. In the face of varying levels of endogenous estrogen production, one might ask whether the carcinogenic potential of exogenous estrogens would be the same in all women. A case–control study has been conducted to examine the relation between weight, replacement estrogen therapy, and endometrial cancer; results are as follows.

Weight (kg)		Estrogen Replacement	
		Yes	No
< 57	Cases	20	12
	Controls	61	183
57–75	Cases	37	45
	Controls	113	378
> 75	Cases	9	42
	Controls	23	140

(a) Calculate the odds ratio associated with estrogen replacement, separately for the three weight groups.

(b) Compare the three odds ratios in (a); when the difference is properly confirmed, we have an effect modification.

(c) Asuming that the odds ratios for the three weight groups are equal (in other words, weight is not an effect modifier), calculate the Mantel–Haenszel estimate of this common odds ratio.

1.24. The role of menstrual and reproductive factors in the epidemiology of breast cancer has been reassessed using pooled data from three large case–control studies of breast cancer from several Italian regions. The following are summarized data for age at menopause and age at first live birth.

Age at first live birth	Cases	Controls
< 22	621	898
22–24	795	909
25–27	791	769
≥ 28	1043	775

Age at menopause	Cases	Controls
< 45	459	543
45–49	749	803
≥ 50	1378	1167

(a) For each of the two factors (age at first live birth and age at menopause), choose the lowest level as the baseline and calculate the odds ratio associated with each other level.

(b) For each of the two factors (age at first live birth and age at menopause), calculate the generalized odds and give your interpretation. How does this result compare with those in (a)?

1.25. Risk factors of gallstone disease were investigated in male self-defense officials who received, between October 1986 and December 1990, a retirement health examination at the Self-Defense Forces Fukuoka Hospital, Fukuoka, Japan. The following are parts of the data:

Factor	Number of men surveyed	
	Total	Number with Gallstones
(a) Smoking		
Never	621	11
Past	776	17
Current	1342	33
(b) Alcohol		
Never	447	11
Past	113	3
Current	2179	47
(c) Body mass index (kg/m^2)		
< 22.5	719	13
22.5–24.9	1301	30
≥ 25.0	719	18

(a) For each of the three factors (smoking, alcohol, and body mass index), rearrange the data into a 3×2 table; the other column is for those without gallstones.

(b) For each of the three 3×2 tables in (a), choose the lowest level as the baseline and calculate the odds ratio associated with each other level.

(c) For each of the three 3×2 tables in (a), calculate the generalized odds and give your interpretation. How does this result compare with those in (b)?

1.26. Data were collected from 2197 white ovarian cancer patients and 8893 white controls in 12 different United States case–control studies conducted by various investigators in the period 1956–1986. These were used to evaluate the relationship of invasive epithelial ovarian cancer to reproductive and menstrual characteristics, exogenous estrogen use, and prior pelvic surgeries. The following are parts of the data related to unprotected intercourse and to history of infertility.

Duration of Unprotected Intercourse (Years)	Cases	Controls
< 2	237	477
2–9	166	354
10–14	47	91
≥ 15	133	174

History of Infertility	Cases	Controls
No	526	966
Yes		
No drug use	76	124
Drug use	20	11

(a) For each of the two factors (duration of unprotected intercourse and history of infertility; treating the latter as ordinal: no history, history but no drug use, and history with drug use), choose the lowest level as the baseline and calculate the odds ratio associated with each other level.

(b) For each of the two factors (duration of unprotected intercourse and history of infertility; treating the latter as ordinal: no history, history but no drug use, and history with drug use), calculate the generalized odds and give your interpretation. How does this result compare with those in (a)?

1.27. Postneonatal mortality due to respiratory illnesses is known to be inversely related to maternal age, but the role of young motherhood as a risk factor for respiratory morbidity in infants has not been thoroughly explored. A study was conducted in Tucson, Arizona aimed at the incidence of lower respiratory tract illnesses during the first year of life. In this study, over 1200 infants were enrolled at birth between 1980 and 1984 and the following data are concerned with wheezing lower respiratory tract illnesses (wheezing LRI: No/Yes).

Maternal Age (years)	Boys		Girls	
	No	Yes	No	Yes
< 21	19	8	20	7
21–25	98	40	128	36
26–30	160	45	148	42
> 30	110	20	116	25

(a) For each of the two groups, boys and girls, choose the lowest age group as the baseline and calculate the odds ratio associated with each age group.

(b) For each of the two groups, boys and girls, calculate the generalized odds and give your interpretation. How does this result compare with those in (a)?

(c) Compare the two generalized odds in (b) and draw your conclusion.

1.28. An important characteristic of glaucoma, an eye disease, is the presence of classical visual field loss. Tonometry is a common form of glaucoma screening whereby, for example, an eye is classified as positive if it has an intraocular pressure of 21 mmHg or higher at a single reading. Given the following data,

Field Loss	Test Result		
	Positive	Negative	
Yes	13	7	20
No	413	4567	4980

calculate the sensitivity and specificity of this screening test.

1.29. Recall the news report of Example 1.11: "A total of 35,238 new AIDS cases was reported in 1989 by the Centers for Disease Control (CDC), compared to 32,196 reported during 1988. The 9% increase is the smallest since the spread of AIDS began in the early 1980s. For example, new AIDS cases were up 34% in 1988 and 60% in 1987.

In 1989, 547 cases of AIDS transmissions from mothers to newborns were reported, up 17% from 1988; while females made up just 3971 of the 35,238 new cases reported in 1989, that was an increase of 11% over 1988."

From the above information, calculate the following:

(a) The number of new AIDS cases for the years 1987 and 1986

(b) The number of cases of AIDS transmission from mothers to newborns for 1988

1.30. In an effort to provide a complete analysis of the survival of patients with end-stage renal disease (ESRD), data were collected for a sample that included 929 patients who initiated hemodialysis for the first time at the Regional Disease Program in Minneapolis, Minnesota between 1 January 1976 and 30 June 1982; all patients were followed until 31 December 1982. Of these 929 patients, 257 are diabetics; among the 672 nondiabetics, 386 are classified as low risk (without co-morbidities such as arteriosclerotic heart disease, peripheral vascular disease, chronic obstructive pulmonary, and cancer). For the low-risk ESRD patients, we had the following follow-up data (in addition to those in Example 1.12):

Age (years)	Deaths	Treatment Months
21–30	4	1012
31–40	7	1387
41–50	20	1706
51–60	24	2448
61–70	21	2060
Over 70	17	846

Compute the follow-up death rate for each age group and the relative risk for group "over 70" versus "51–60."

1.31. Given the following mortality data for the State of Georgia for the year 1977:

Age Group	Deaths	Population
0–4	2,483	424,600
5–19	1,818	1,818,000
20–44	3,656	1,126,500
45–64	12,424	870,800
65+	21,405	360,800

(a) From the above mortality table, calculate the crude death rate for the State of Georgia.

(b) From the above mortality table and the following data mortality data for Alaska and Florida for the year 1977 (same data as given in Example 1.13),

	Alaska			Florida		
Age Group	No. of Deaths	Persons	Deaths per 100,000	No. of Deaths	Persons	Deaths per 100,000
0–4	162	40,000	405.0	2,049	546,000	375.3
5–19	107	128,000	83.6	1,195	1,982,000	60.3
20–44	449	172,000	261.0	5,097	2,676,000	190.5
45–64	451	58,000	777.6	19,904	1,807,000	1101.5
65+	444	9,000	4933.3	63,505	1,444,000	4397.9
Totals	1615	407,000	396.8	91,760	8,455,000	1085.3

calculate the age-adjusted death rate for Georgia and compare them to those for Alaska and Florida, with the U.S. population given in Example 1.13, reproduced below, being used as standard.

Age group	Population
0–4	84,416
5–19	294,353
20–44	316,744
45–64	205,745
65+	98,742
Totals	1,000,000

(c) Calculate, again, the age-adjusted death rate for Georgia with the Alaska population serving as the standard population. How does this adjusted death rate compare to the crude death rate of Alaska?

1.32. Refer to the same set of mortality data as in the above Excercise 1.31. Calculate and compare the age-adjusted death rates for the states of Alaska and Florida with the Georgia population serving as the standard population. How do mortality in these two states compare to the state of Georgia?

1.33. Some 7000 British workers exposed to vinyl chloride monomer were followed for several years to determine whether their mortality experience differed from those of the general population. In addition to data for deaths from cancers as seen in Example 1.20, the study also provided the following data for deaths due to circulatory disease:

Deaths	Years since entering the industry				Total
	1–4	5–9	10–14	15+	
Observed	7	25	38	110	180
Expected	32.5	35.6	44.9	121.3	234.1

Calculate the SMRs for each subgroup and the relative risk for group "15+" versus group "1–4."

1.34. A long-term follow-up study of diabetes has been conducted among Pima Indian residents of the Gila River Indian Community of Arizona since 1965. Subjects of this study, at least 5 years old and of at least half Pima ancestry, were examined approximately every 2 years; examinations included measurements of height and weight and a number of other factors. The following table relates diabetes incidence rate (new cases/1000 person-years) to body mass index (a measure of obesity defined as weight/(height)^2).

Body Mass Index	Incidence Rate
< 20	0.8
20–25	10.9
25–30	17.3
30–35	32.6
35–40	48.5
≥ 40	72.2

Display these rates by means of a bar chart.

1.35. In the course of selecting controls for a study to evaluate effect of caffeine-containing coffee on the risk of myocardial infarction among women 30–49 years of age, a study noted appreciable differences in coffee consumption among hospital patients admitted for illnesses not known to be related to coffee use. Among potential controls, the coffee consumption of patients who had been admitted to the hospital by conditions having an acute onset (such as fractures) was compared to that of patients admitted for chronic disorders.

Admission by	Cups of Coffee Per Day			Total
	0	1–4	≥ 5	
Acute conditions	340	457	183	980
Chronic conditions	2440	2527	868	5835

(a) Each of the above 6815 subject is considered as belonging to one of the three groups defined by the number of cups of coffee consumed per day (the three columns). Calculate, for each of the three groups, the proportion of subjects admitted because of an acute onset. Display these proportions by means of a bar chart.

(b) For those admitted because of their chronic conditions, express their coffee consumption by means of a pie chart.

(c) Calculate the general odds and give your interpretation; exposure is defined as having an acute condition.

1.36. In a seroepidemiologic survey of health workers representing a spectrum of exposure to blood and patients with hepatitis B virus (HBV), it was found that infection increased as a function of contact. The following table provides data for hospital workers with uniform socioeconomic status at an urban teaching hospital in Boston, Massachusetts.

Personnel	Exposure	n	HBV Positive
Physicians	Frequent	81	17
	Infrequent	89	7
Nurses	Frequent	104	22
	Infrequent	126	11

(a) Calculate the proportion of HBV positive workers in each subgroup.

(b) Calculate the odds ratios associated with frequent contacts (as compared to infrequent contacts); do this separately for physicians and nurses.

(c) Compare the two ratios obtained in (b); a large difference would indicate a "three-term interaction" or "effect modification," where frequent effects are different for physicians and nurses.

(d) Asuming that the odds ratios for the two groups, physicians and nurses, are equal (in other words, type of personnel is not an effect modifier), calculate the Mantel–Haenszel estimate of this common odds ratio.

1.37. The results of the Third National Cancer survey have shown substantial variation in lung cancer incidence rates for white males within Allegheny County, Pennsylvania, which may be due to different smoking rates. The following table gives the percentages of current smokers by age for two study areas.

Age	Lawrenceville		South Hills	
	n	%	n	%
35–44	71	54.9	135	37.0
45–54	79	53.2	193	28.5
55–64	119	43.7	138	21.7
≥ 65	109	30.3	141	18.4
Total	378	46.8	607	27.1

(a) Display the age distribution for Lawrenceville by means of a pie chart.

(b) Display the age distribution for South Hills by means of a pie chart. How does this chart compare to the one in (a)?

(c) Display the smoking rates for Lawrenceville and South Hills, side by side, by means of a bar chart.

1.38. Prematurity, which ranks as the major cause of neonatal morbidity and mortality, has traditionally been defined on the basis of a birth weight under 2500 g. But this definition encompasses two distinct types of infants: infants who are small because they are born early, and infants who are born at or near term but are small because their growth was retarded. "Prematurity" has now been replaced by

(a) "low birth weight" to describe the second type

(b) "preterm" to characterize the first type (babies born before 37 weeks of gestation)

A case–control study of the epidemiology of preterm delivery was undertaken at Yale–New Haven Hospital in Connecticut during 1977. The study population consisted of 175 mothers of singleton preterm infants and 303 mothers of singleton full-term infants. The following tables give the distribution of age and socioeconomic status.

Age	Cases	Controls
14–17	15	16
18–19	22	25
20–24	47	62
25–29	56	122
≥ 30	35	78

Socio-economic level	Cases	Controls
Upper	11	40
Upper middle	14	45
Middle	33	64
Lower middle	59	91
Lower	53	58
Unknown	5	5

(a) Refer to the age data (first table) and choose the "≥ 30" group as baseline, and then calculate the odds ratio associated with each other age group. Is it true, in general, that the younger the mother, the higher the risk?

(b) Refer to the socioeconomic data (second table) and choose the "lower" group as the baseline, and then calculate the odds ratio associated with each other group. Is it true, in general, that the poorer the mother, the higher the risk?

(c) Refer to the socioeconomic data (second table), calculate the generalized odds, and give your interpretation. Does this support the conclusion in (b)?

1.39. Sudden infant death syndrome (SIDS), also known as "sudden unexplained death," "crib death," or "cot death," claims the lives of an alarming number of apparently normal infants every year. In a study at the University of Connecticut School of Medicine, significant associations were found between SIDS and certain demographic characteristics. Some of the summarized data are given below:

		Number of deaths	
		Observed	Expected
Sex	Male	55	45
	Female	35	45
Race	Black	23	11
	White	67	79

(Expected deaths are calculated using Connecticut infant mortality data 1974–1976.)

(a) Calculate standardized mortality ratio (SMR) for each subgroup.

(b) Compare males versus females and blacks versus whites.

1.40. Adult male residents of 13 counties of western Washington state in whom testicular cancer had been diagnosed during 1977–1983 were interviewed over the telephone regarding their history of genital tract conditions, including vasectomy. For comparison, the same interview was given to a sample of men selected from the population of these counties by dialing telephone numbers at random. The following data are tabulated by religious background.

Religion	Vasectomy	Cases	Controls
Protestant	Yes	24	56
	No	205	239
Catholic	Yes	10	6
	No	32	90
Others	Yes	18	39
	No	56	96

Calculate the odds ratio associated with vasectomy for each religious group. Is there any evidence of an effect modification? If not, calculate the Mantel–Haenszel estimate of the common odds ratio.

1.41. The role of menstrual and reproductive factors in the epidemiology of breast cancer has been reassessed using pooled data from three large case–control studies of breast cancer from several Italian regions. The following are summarized data for age at menopause and age at first live birth.

Age	Cases	Controls
At first live birth		
< 22	621	898
22–24	795	909
25–27	791	769
≥ 28	1043	775
At menopause		
< 45	459	543
45–49	749	803
≥ 50	1378	1167

Find a way (or ways) to further summarize the data so as to express the observation that the risk of breast cancer is lower for women with younger ages at first live birth and younger ages at menopause.

1.42. In 1979 the United States Veterans Administration conducted a health survey of 11,230 veterans. The advantages of this survey are that it includes a large random sample with a high interview response rate and that it was done before the recent public controversy surrounding the issue of the health effects of possible exposure to Agent Orange. The following are data relating Vietnam service to eight post-

	Service in Vietnam	
Symptom	Yes	No
Nightmares		
Yes	197	85
No	577	925
Sleep problems		
Yes	173	160
No	599	851
Troubled memories		
Yes	220	105
No	549	906
Depression		
Yes	306	315
No	465	699
Temper control problems		
Yes	176	144
No	595	868
Life goal association		
Yes	231	225
No	539	786
Omit feelings		
Yes	188	191
No	583	821
Confusion		
Yes	163	148
No	607	864

traumatic stress disorder symptoms among the 1787 veterans who entered the military service between 1965 and 1975. Calculate the odds ratio for each symptom.

1.43. It has been hypothesized that dietary fiber decreases the risk of colon cancer, while meats and fats are thought to increase this risk. A large study was undertaken to confirm these hypotheses. Fiber and fat consumptions are classified as "low" or "high," and data are tabulated separately for males and females as follows ("low" means below median):

Diet	Males		Females	
	Cases	Controls	Cases	Controls
Low fat, high fiber	27	38	23	39
Low fat, low fiber	64	78	82	81
High fat, high fiber	78	61	83	76
High fat, low fiber	36	28	35	27

For each group (males and females), using "low fat, high fiber" as the baseline, calculate the odds ratio associated with each other dietary combination. Any evidence of an effect modification (interaction between consumption of fat and consumption of fiber)?

1.44. The following table compiles data from different studies designed to investigate the accuracy of death certificates. The results of 5373 autopsies were compared to the causes of death listed on the certificates. The results are:

Date of Study	Accurate Certificate		Total
	Yes	No	
1955–1965	2040	694	2734
1970–1971	437	203	640
1975–1978	1128	599	1727
1980	121	151	272

Find a graphical way to display the downward trend of accuracy over time.

1.45. A study was conducted to ascertain factors that influence a physician's decision to transfuse a patient. A sample of 49 attending physicians was selected. Each physician was asked a question concerning the frequency with which an unnecessary transfusion was given because another physician suggested it. The same question was asked of a sample of 71 residents. The data were as follows:

Type of Physician	Frequency of Unnecessary Transfusion				
	Very Frequent (1/week)	Frequent (1/2 weeks)	Occasionally (1/month)	Rarely (1/2 months)	Never
Attending	1	1	3	31	13
Resident	2	13	28	23	5

(a) Choose "never" as the baseline and calculate the odds ratio associated with each other frequency and "residency."

(b) Calculate the general odds and give your interpretation. Does this result agree with those in (a)?

1.46. When a patient is diagnosed as having cancer of the prostate, an important question in deciding on treatment strategy for the patient is whether or not the cancer has spread to the neighboring lymp nodes. The question is so critical in prognosis and treatment that it is customary to operate on the patient (i.e., perform a laparotomy) for the sole purpose of examining the nodes and removing tissue samples to examine under the microscope for evidence of cancer. However, certain variables that can be measured without surgery are predictive of the nodal involvement; and the purpose of the study presented here was to examine the data for 53 prostate cancer patients receiving surgery, to determine which of five preoperative variables are predictive of nodal involvement. The following table presents the comple data set. For each of the 53 patients, there are two continuous independent variables, age at diagnosis and level of serum acid phosphatase ($\times 100$; called "acid"), and three binary variables, X ray reading, pathology reading (grade) of a biopsy of the tumor obtained by needle before surgery, and a rough measure of the size and location of the tumor (stage) obtained by palpation with the fingers via the rectum. For these three binary independent variables a value of one signifies a positive or more serious state and a zero denotes a negative or less serious finding. In addition, the sixth column presents the finding at surgery—the primary outcome of interest which is binary: A value of one denotes nodal involvement, and a value of zero denotes no nodal involvement found at surgery. In this exercise we investigate the effects of the three binary preoperative variables (X ray, grade, and stage); the effects of the two continuous factors (age and acid phosphatase) will be studied in an exercise in the next chapter.

(a) Arrange the data on *nodes* and *X ray* into a 2 × 2 table, calculate the odds ratio associated with X ray, and give your interpretation.

(b) Arrange the data on *nodes* and *grade* into a 2 × 2 table, calculate the odds ratio associated with grade, and give your interpretation.

(c) Arrange the data on *nodes* and *stage* into a 2 × 2 table, calculate the odds ratio associated with stage, and give your interpretation.

Prostate Cancer Data

X ray	Grade	Stage	Age	Acid	Nodes
0	1	1	64	40	0
0	0	1	63	40	0
1	0	0	65	46	0
0	1	0	67	47	0
0	0	0	66	48	0
0	1	1	65	48	0
0	0	0	60	49	0
0	0	0	51	49	0

Prostate Cancer Data

X ray	Grade	Stage	Age	Acid	Nodes
0	0	0	66	50	0
0	0	0	58	50	0
0	1	0	56	50	0
0	0	1	61	50	0
0	1	1	64	50	0
0	0	0	56	52	0
0	0	0	67	52	0
1	0	0	49	55	0
0	1	1	52	55	0
0	0	0	68	56	0
0	1	1	66	59	0
1	0	0	60	62	0
0	0	0	61	62	0
1	1	1	59	63	0
0	0	0	51	65	0
0	1	1	53	66	0
0	0	0	58	71	0
0	0	0	63	75	0
0	0	1	53	76	0
0	0	0	60	78	0
0	0	0	52	83	0
0	0	1	67	95	0
0	0	0	56	98	0
0	0	1	61	102	0
0	0	0	64	187	0
1	0	1	58	48	1
0	0	1	65	49	1
1	1	1	57	51	1
0	1	0	50	56	1
1	1	0	67	67	1
0	0	1	67	67	1
0	1	1	57	67	1
0	1	1	45	70	1
0	0	1	46	70	1
1	0	1	51	72	1
1	1	1	60	76	1
1	1	1	56	78	1
1	1	1	50	81	1
0	0	0	56	82	1
0	0	1	63	82	1
1	1	1	65	84	1
1	0	1	64	89	1
0	1	0	59	99	1
1	1	1	68	126	1
1	0	0	61	136	1

Note: This is a very long data file; its electronic copy is available from the author upon contact, both Web-based form and Excel. Summaries would be easily formed using simple computer software.

- If you use Microft's Excel, 2 × 2 tables can be formed using *PivotTable wizard* in the *Data menu*.
- An SAS program for (a), for example, would include these intructions:

```
PROC FREQ;\\
 TABLES NOTES*XRAY/ OR;
```

2

Organization, Summarization, and Presentation of Data

A class of measurements or a characteristic on which individual observations or measurements are made is called a *variable*; examples include weight, height, and blood pressure, among others. Suppose we have a set of numerical values for a variable:

1. If each element of this set may lie only at a few isolated points, we have a *discrete* data set. Examples are race, sex, counts of events, or some sort of artificial grading.
2. If each element of this set may theoretically lie anywhere on the numerical scale, we have a *continuous* data set. Examples are blood pressure, cholesterol level, or time to a certain event such as death.

The previous chapter deals with the summarization and description of discrete data; in this chapter the emphasis is on continuous measurements.

2.1. TABULAR AND GRAPHICAL METHODS

There are different ways of organizing and presenting data; simple tables and graphs, however, are still very effective methods. They are designed to help the reader obtain an intuitive feeling for the data at a glance.

2.1.1. One-Way Scatter Plots

This method is the most simple type of graph that can be used to summarize a set of continuous observations. A one-way scatter plot uses a single horizontal axis to display the relative position of each data point. As an example, Figure 2.1 depicts the crude death rates for all 50 states and the District of Columbia, from a low of 393.9 per 100,000 population to a high of 1242.1 per 100,000 population.

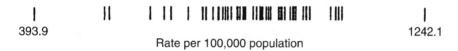

393.9   Rate per 100,000 population   1242.1

Figure 2.1. Crude death rates for the United States, 1988.

An advantage of a one-way scatter plot is that, because each observation is represented individually, no information is lost; a disadvantage is that it may be difficult to read (and to construct!) if values are close each other.

2.1.2. Frequency Distribution

There is no difficulty if the data set is small, because we can arrange those few numbers and write them, say, in increasing order; the result would be sufficiently clear; the above one-way scatter plot is an example. For fairly large data sets, a useful device for summarization is the formation of a *frequency table* or *frequency distribution*. This is a table showing the number of observations, called *frequency*, within certain ranges of values of the variable under investigation. For example, taking the variable to be the age at death, we have the following example; the second column of the table provides the frequencies.

Example 2.1

The following table gives the number of deaths by age for the state of Minnesota in 1987.

Age	Number of Deaths
Less than 1	564
1–4	86
5–14	127
15–24	490
25–34	667
35–44	806
45–54	1,425
55–64	3,511
65–74	6,932
75–84	10,101
85 and over	9,825
Total	34,524

If a data set is to be grouped to form a frequency distribution, difficulties should be recognized and an efficient strategy is needed for better communication. First, there is no clear-cut rule on the number of intervals or classes. With too many intervals, the data are not summarized enough for a clear visualization of how they are distributed. On the other hand, too few intervals are undesirable because the data are oversummarized and some of the details of the distribution may be lost. In general, between 5 and 15 intervals are acceptable; of course, this also depends on the number of observations.

The widths of the intervals must also be decided. Example 2.1 shows the special case of mortality data, where it is traditional to show infant deaths (deaths of persons who are born live but die before living 1 year). Without such specific reasons, intervals generally should be of the same width. This common width w may be determined by dividing the range R by k, the number of intervals:

$$w = \frac{R}{k}$$

where the range R is the difference between the smallest and the largest numbers in the data set. In addition, a width should be chosen so that it is convenient to use or easy to recognize, such as a multiple of 5 (or 1, for example, if the data set has a narrow range). Similar considerations apply to the choice of the beginning of the first interval; it is a convenient number that is low enough for the first interval to include the smallest observation. Finally, care should be taken in deciding in which interval to place an observation falling on one of the interval boundaries. For example, a consistent rule could be made so as to place such an observation in the interval of which the observation in question is the lower limit.

Example 2.2

The following are weights in pounds of 57 children at a day-care center:

68	63	42	27	30	36	28	32	79	27
22	23	24	25	44	65	43	25	74	51
36	42	28	31	28	25	45	12	57	51
12	32	49	38	42	27	31	50	38	21
16	24	69	47	23	22	43	27	49	28
23	19	46	30	43	49	12			

From the above data set we have the following:

1. The smallest number is 12 and the largest is 79 so that

$$R = 79 - 12$$

$$= 67$$

If 5 intervals are used, we would have

$$w = \frac{67}{5}$$
$$= 13.4$$

and if 15 intervals are used we would have

$$w = \frac{67}{15}$$
$$= 4.5$$

Between these two values, 4.5 and 13.4, there are two convenient (or conventional) numbers: 5 and 10. Because the sample size of 57 is not large, a width of 10 should be an apparent choice because it results in fewer intervals (the usual concept of "large" is "100 or more").

2. Because the smallest number is 12, we may begin our first interval at 10.
   These considerations, 1 and 2, lead to the following seven intervals:

10–19
20–29
30–39
40–49
50–59
60–69
70–79

3. Determining the frequencies or the number of values or measurements for each interval is merely a matter of examining the values one by one and of placing a tally mark beside the appropriate interval. When we do this we have the following table; the temporary column of tallies should be deleted from the final table.

Table 2.1. Frequency Distribution of Weights of 57 Children

Weight Interval (lb.)	Tally	Frequency	Relative Frequency (%)
10–19	ⵂ	5	8.8
20–29	ⵂ ⵂ ⵂ IIII	19	33.3
30–39	ⵂ ⵂ	10	17.5
40–49	ⵂ ⵂ III	13	22.8
50–59	IIII	4	7.0
60–69	IIII	4	7.0
70–79	II	2	3.5
Total		57	100.0

4. An optional, but recommended, step in the formulation of a frequency distribution is to present the proportion or *relative frequency* in addition to frequency, for each interval. These proportions, defined by

$$\text{Relative frequency} = \frac{\text{Frequency}}{\text{Total number of observations}}$$

were shown in the third column of Table 2.1 (as %) and would be very useful if we need to compare two data sets of different sizes.

***

Example 2.3

A study was conducted to investigate the possible effects of exercise on the menstrual cycle. From the data collected from that study, we obtained the menarchal age (in years) of 56 female swimmers who began their swimming training after they had reached menarche; these served as controls in order to compare with those who began their training prior to menarche.

14.0	16.1	13.4	14.6	13.7	13.2	13.7	14.3
12.9	14.1	15.1	14.8	12.8	14.2	14.1	13.6
14.2	15.8	12.7	15.6	14.1	13.0	12.9	15.1
15.0	13.6	14.2	13.8	12.7	15.3	14.1	13.5
15.3	12.6	13.8	14.4	12.9	14.6	15.0	13.8
13.0	14.1	13.8	14.2	13.6	14.1	14.5	13.1
12.8	14.3	14.2	13.5	14.1	13.6	12.4	15.1

From this data set we have the following:

1. The smallest number is 12.4 and the largest is 16.1 so that

$$R = 16.1 - 12.4$$

$$= 3.7$$

If five intervals are used, we would have

$$w = \frac{3.7}{5}$$

$$= .74$$

and if 15 intervals are used, we would have

$$w = \frac{3.7}{15}$$

$$= .25$$

Between these two values, .25 and .74, .5 seems to be a convenient number to use as the width; .25 is another choice but it would create many intervals (15) for such a small data set. (Another alternative is to express ages in months and not to deal with decimal numbers.)

2. Because the smallest number is 12.4, we may begin our intervals at 12.0, leading to the following intervals:

12.0–12.4
12.5–12.9
13.0–13.4
13.5–13.9
14.0–14.4
14.5–14.9
15.0–15.4
15.5–15.9
16.0–16.4

3. Count the number of swimmers whose ages belong to each of the above nine intervals, the frequencies, and obtain Table 2.2—completed with the last column for relative frequencies (expressed as %):

Table 2.2. Frequency Distribution of Menarchal Age of 56 Swimmers

Age (years)	Frequency	Relative Frequency (%)
12.0–12.4	1	1.8
12.5–12.9	8	14.3
13.0–13.4	5	8.9
13.5–13.9	12	21.4
14.0–14.4	16	28.6
14.5–14.9	4	7.1
15.0–15.4	7	12.5
15.5–15.9	2	3.6
16.0–16.4	1	1.8
Total	56	100.0

2.1.3. Histogram and the Frequency Polygon

A convenient way of displaying a frequency table is by means of a *histogram* and/or a *frequency polygon*. A histogram is a diagram in which

1. The horizontal scale represents the value of the variable marked at interval boundaries.
2. The vertical scale represents the frequency or relative frequency in each interval (see exceptions below).

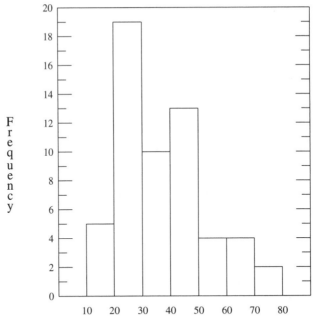

Figure 2.2. Distribution of weights of 57 children.

The histogram presents us with a graphic picture of the distribution of measurements. This picture consists of rectangular bars joining each other, one for each interval as shown in Figure 2.2 for the data set of Example 2.2. If disjoint intervals are used such as in Table 2.1, the horizontal axis is marked with true boundaries. A true boundary is the average of the upper limit of one interval and the lower limit of the next higher interval. For example, 19.5 serves as the true upper boundary of the first interval and true lower boundary for the second interval. In cases where we need to compare the shapes of the histograms representing different data sets, or if intervals are of unequal widths, the height of each rectangular bar should represent the density of the interval, where the interval density is defined by

$$\text{Density} = \frac{\text{Relative frequency } (\%)}{\text{Interval width}}$$

The unit for density is "percent per unit (of measurement)"—for example, percent per year. If we do this, the relative frequency is represented by the area of the rectangular bar and the total area under the histogram is 100%. It may be a good practice to always graph densities on the vertical axis with or without having equal class width; when class widths are equal, the shape of the histogram looks similar to the graph with relative frequencies on the vertical axis.

To draw a frequency polygon, we first place a dot at the midpoint of the upper base of each rectangular bar. The points are connected with straight lines. At the ends, the points are connected to the midpoints of the previous and succeeding intervals (these are make-up intervals with zero frequency, where widths are the widths of the first and last intervals, re-

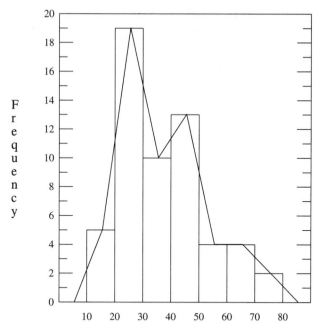

Figure 2.3. Distribution of weights of 57 children.

spectively). A frequency polygon as thus constructed is another way to portray graphically the distribution of a data set (see Figure 2.3). The frequency polygon can also be shown without the histogram on the same graph.

The frequency table and its graphical relatives, the histogram and the frequency polygon, have a number of applications, as explained below; the first leads to a research question and the second leads to a new analysis strategy.

1. When data are homogeneous, the table and graphs usually show a uni-modal pattern with one peak in the middle part. A bimodal pattern might indicate possible influence or effect of certain hidden factor or factors.

Example 2.4

The following table provides data on age and percentage saturation of bile for 31 male patients.

Age	% Saturation	Age	% Saturation	Age	% Saturation
23	40	55	137	48	78
31	86	31	88	27	80
58	111	20	88	32	47
25	86	23	65	62	74
63	106	43	79	36	58
43	66	27	87	29	88
67	123	63	56	27	73
48	90	59	110	65	118
29	112	53	106	42	67
26	52	66	110	60	57
64	88				

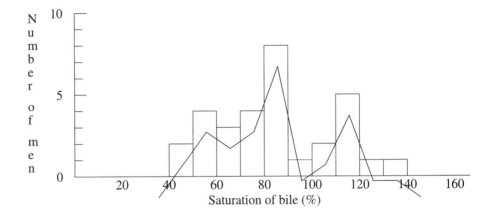

Figure 2.4. Frequency polygon for percentage saturation of bile in men.

Using 10% intervals, the above data set can be represented by a histogram or a frequency polygon as shown in Figure 2.4. This picture shows an apparent bimodal distribution; however, a closer examination shows that among the 9 patients with over 100% saturation, 8 (or 89%) are over 50 years of age. On the other hand, only 4 of 22 (or 18%) patients with less than 100 percent saturation are over 50 years of age. The two peaks in the diagram might correspond to the two age groups.

Another application concerns the symmetry of the distribution as depicted by the table or its graphs. A symmetric distribution is one in which the distribution has the same shape on both sides of the peak location. If there are more extremely large values, the distribution is then skewed to the right, or *positively* skewed. Examples include family income, antibody level after vaccination, and drug dose to produce a predetermined level of response, among others. It is common that for positively skewed distributions, subsequent statistical analyses should be performed on the log scale—for example, to calculate and/or to compare averages of log(dose).

Example 2.5

The distribution of family income for the United States in 1983 by race is shown below.

	Percent of families	
Income ($)	White	Nonwhite
0–14,999	13	34
15,000–19,999	24	31
20,000–24,999	26	19
25,000–34,999	28	13
35,000–59,999	9	3
60,000 and over	1	Negligible
Total	100	100

The distribution for nonwhite families is represented in the histogram in Figure 2.5, where the vertical axis represents the density (percent per thousand dollars). It is obvious that the distribution is not symmetric; it is very skewed to the right.

In this histogram, we graph the densities on the vertical axis. For example, for the second income interval (15,000–19,999), the relative frequency is 31% and the width of the

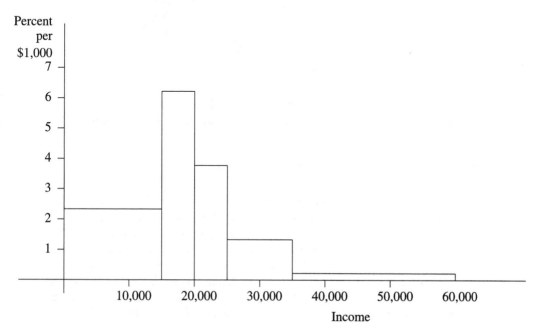

Figure 2.5. Income of U.S. nonwhite families, 1983.

interval is $5000 (31 percent per $5000), leading to the density

$$\frac{31}{5,000} \times 1000 = 6.2$$

or 6.2% per $1000 (we arbitrarily multiply by 1000—or any power of 10—just to obtain a larger number for easy graphing).

2.1.4. The Cumulative Frequency Graph and Percentiles

Cumulative relative frequency, or *cumulative percentage*, gives the percentage of individuals having a measurement less than or equal to the upper boundary of the class interval. Data from Table 2.1 are reproduced and supplemented with a column for cumulative relative frequency in Table 2.3.

Table 2.3. Distribution of Weights of 57 Children

Weight Interval (lbs)	Frequency	Relative Frequency (%)	Cumulative Relative Frequency (%)
10–19	5	8.8	8.8
20–29	19	33.3	42.1
30–39	10	17.5	59.6
40–49	13	22.8	82.4
50–59	4	7.0	89.4
60–69	4	7.0	96.4
70–79	2	3.5	$99.9 \cong 100.0$
Total	57	100.0	

This last column is easy to form; you do it by successively cumulating the relative frequencies of each of the various intervals. In the above example, the cumulative percentage for the first three intervals is

$$8.8 + 33.3 + 17.5 = 59.6$$

and we can say that 59.6% of the children in the data set have a weight of 39.5 pounds or less. Or, as another example, 96.4% of children weigh 69.5 pounds or less, and so on.

The cumulative relative frequency can be presented graphically as in Figure 2.6. This type of curve is called a *cumulative frequency graph*. To construct a cumulative frequency graph, we place a point with horizontal axis marked at the upper class boundary and vertical axis marked at the corresponding cumulative frequency. Each point represents the cumulative relative frequency for that interval, and the points are connected with straight lines. At the left end, it is connected to the lower boundary of the first interval. If disjoint intervals, such as

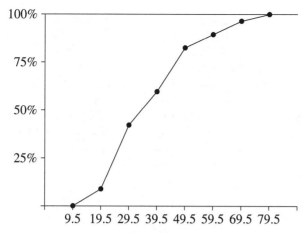

Figure 2.6. Cumulative distribution of weights of 57 children.

10–19

20–29

etc . . .

are used, points are placed at the true boundaries.

The cumulative percentages and their graphical representation, the cumulative frequency graph, have a number of applications.

1. When two cumulative frequency graphs, representing two different data sets, are placed on the same graph, they provide a rapid visual comparison without any need to compare individual intervals. Figure 2.7 gives such a comparison of family incomes using data of Example 2.4.

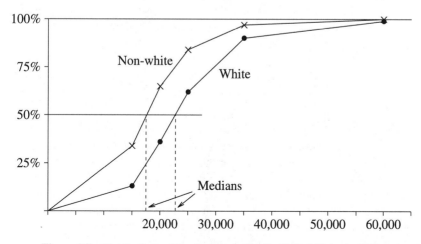

Figure 2.7. Distributions of family income for the United States in 1983.

2. The cumulative frequency graph provides a class of important statistics known as *percentiles* or *percentile scores*. The 90th percentile, for example, is the numerical value that exceeds 90% of the values in the data set and is exceeded by only 10% of them. Or, as another example, the 80th percentile is that numerical value that exceeds 80% of the values contained in the data set and is exceeded by 20% of them, and so on. The 50th percentile is commonly called the *median*. In our example of Figure 2.7, the median family income in 1983 for non-whites was about $17,500 as compared to a median of about $22,000 for white families. In order to get the median, we start at the 50% point on the vertical axis, and go horizontally until meeting the cumulative frequency graph; the projection of this intersection on the horizontal axis is the median. Other percentiles are obtained similarly.

The cumulative frequency graph also provides an important application in the formation of health norms (see Figure 2.8) for the monitoring of physical progress (weight and height) of infants and children. Here, the same percentiles, say 90th, of weight or height of groups of different ages are joined by a curve.

_____

Example 2.6

Figure 2.9 provides results from a study of Hmong refugees in the Minneapolis-St. Paul area where each dot represents the average height of five refugee girls of the same age. The graph shows that even though the refugee girls are small, mostly in the lowest 25%, they grow at the same rate as measured by the American standard. However, the pattern changes by the age of 15 years, when their average height drops to a level below the 5th percentile. In this example, we plot the *average* height of five girls instead of individual heights; because the Hmongs are small, individual heights are likely to be out of the chart. This concept of *average* or *mean* will be futher explained in the next section (2.2).

_____

2.1.5. Stem-and-Leaf Diagrams

A stem-and-leaf diagram is a graphical representation in which the data points are grouped in such a way that we can see the shape of the distribution while retaining the individual values of the data points. This is particularly convenient and useful for smaller data sets. Stem-and-leaf diagrams are similar to the frequency tables and histograms, but they also display each and every observation. Data on the weights of children from Example 2.2 are adopted here to illustrate the construction of this simple device. The weights (in pounds) of 57 children at a day-care center are as follows (p. 70):

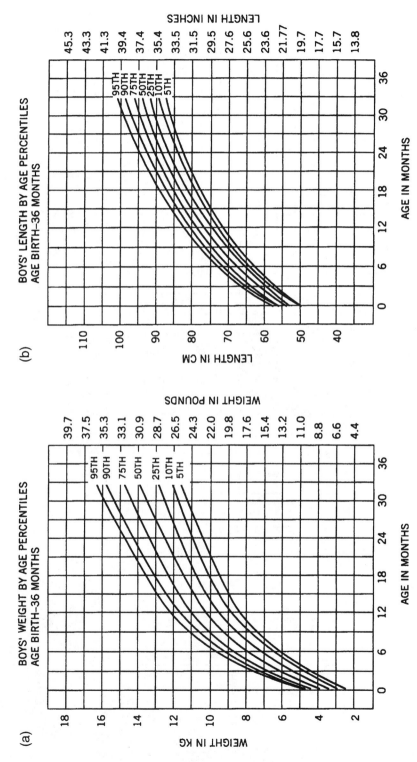

Figure 2.8. (a) Weight curve. (b) Height curve.

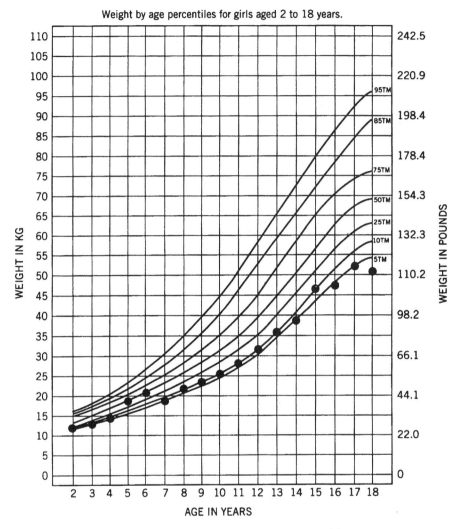

Figure 2.9. Mean stature by age for refugee girls.

68	63	42	27	30	36	28	32	79	27
22	23	24	25	44	65	43	25	74	51
36	42	28	31	28	25	45	12	57	51
12	32	49	38	42	27	31	50	38	21
16	24	69	47	23	22	43	27	49	28
23	19	46	30	43	49	12			

```
1              1 | 2 2 2 6 9
2              2 | 1 2 2 3 3 3 4 4 5 5 5 7 7 7 7 8 8 8 8
3              3 | 0 0 1 1 2 2 6 6 8 8
4    ⇒         4 | 2 2 2 3 3 3 4 5 6 7 9 9 9
5              5 | 0 0 1 7
6              6 | 3 5 8 9
7              7 | 4 9
Stems      Stems   Leaves
```

Figure 2.10. A typical stem-and-leaf diagram.

A stem-and-leaf diagram consists of a series of rows of numbers. The number used to label a row is called a *stem*, and the other numbers in the row are called *leaves*. There are no hard rules about how to construct a stem-and-leaf diagram. Generally, it consists of the following steps:

1. Choose some convenient/conventional numbers to serve as stems. The stems chosen are usually the first one or two digits of individual data points.
2. Reproduce the data graphically by recording the digit or digits following the stems as a leaf on the appropriate stem.

If the final graph is turned on its side, it looks similar to a histogram (Figure 2.10). The device is not practical for use with larger data sets because some stems are too long.

2.2. NUMERICAL METHODS

Although tables and graphs serve useful purposes, there are many situations that require other types of data summarization. What we need in many applications is the ability to summarize data by means of just a few numerical measures, particularly before inferences or generalizations are drawn from the data. Measures for describing the location (or typical value) of a set of measurements and their variation or dispersion are used for these purposes.

First, let us suppose we have n measurements in a data set; for example, here is a data set

$$\{8, 2, 3, 5\}$$

with $n = 4$. We usually denote these numbers as x_i's; thus we have for the above example: $x_1 = 8$, $x_2 = 2$, $x_3 = 3$, and $x_4 = 5$. If we add all the x_i's in the above data set, we obtain 18 as the sum. This addition process is recorded as

$$\sum x = 18$$

where the Greek letter Σ is the summation sign.

With the summation notation, we are now able to define a number of important summarized measures starting with the arithmetic average or *mean*.

2.2.1. Mean

Given a data set of size n,

$$\{x_1, x_2, \ldots, x_n\}$$

the mean of the x's will be denoted by $\bar{x}$ ("x-bar") and is computed by summing all the x's and dividing the sum by n. Symbolically,

$$\bar{x} = \frac{\sum x}{n}$$

It is important to know that $\sum$ stands for an operation (that of obtaining the sum of the quantities that follow), rather than a quantity itself. For example, considering the data set

$$\{8, 5, 4, 12, 15, 5, 7\}$$

we have

$$n = 7$$
$$\sum x = 56$$

leading to

$$\bar{x} = \frac{56}{7}$$
$$= 8$$

Occasionally, data—especially second-hand data—are presented in the grouped form of a frequency table. In these cases, the mean $\bar{x}$ can be approximated using the following formula ($\cong$ means "approximately equal to"):

$$\bar{x} \cong \frac{\sum (fm)}{n}$$

where f denotes the frequency (that is, the number of observations in an interval) m is the interval midpoint, and the summation is across the intervals. The midpoint for an interval is obtained by calculating the average of the interval lower true boundary and the upper true boundary. For example, if the first three intervals are

10–19

20–29

30–39

then the midpoint for the first interval is

$$\frac{9.5 + 19.5}{2} = 14.5$$

and for the second interval is

$$\frac{19.5 + 29.5}{2} = 24.5.$$

This process is illustrated in Table 2.4.

Table 2.4. Calculation of the Mean $\bar{x}$ Using Frequency Table 2.2

Weight Interval	Frequency, f	Interval Midpoint, m	fm
10–19	5	14.5	72.5
20–29	19	24.5	465.5
30–39	10	34.5	345.0
40–49	13	44.5	578.5
50–59	4	54.5	218.0
60–69	4	64.5	258.0
70–79	2	74.5	149.0
Totals	57		2086.5

$$\bar{x} \cong \frac{2086.5}{57}$$
$$= 36.6 \text{ lbs}$$

(If individual weights were used, we would have $\bar{x} = 36.7$ lb.)

Of course, the mean $\bar{x}$ obtained from this technique with a frequency table is different from the $\bar{x}$ using individual or raw data. However, the process saves some computational labor and the difference between the results, $\bar{x}$'s, is very small if the data set is large and the interval width is small.

As earlier indicated, a characteristic of some interest is the symmetry or lack of symmetry of a distribution and it was recommended that for very positively skewed distributions, analyses are commonly done on the log scale. After obtaining a mean on the log scale, we should take the antilog to return to the original scale of measurement; the result is called the *geometric mean* of the x's. The effect of this process is to minimize the influences of extreme observations (very large numbers in the data set). For example, considering the data set

$$\{8, 5, 4, 12, 15, 7, 28\}$$

with one unusually large measurement, we have the following table with natural logs presented in the second column:

	x	$\ln x$
	8	2.08
	5	1.61
	4	1.39
	12	2.48
	15	2.71
	7	1.95
	28	3.33
Totals	79	15.55

The mean is

$$\bar{x} = \frac{79}{7}$$
$$= 11.3$$

while on the log scale, we have

$$\frac{\sum \ln x}{n} = \frac{15.55}{7}$$
$$= 2.22$$

leading to a geometric mean of 9.22 which is less affected by the large measurements. Geometric mean is used extensively in microbiological and serological research in which distributions are often positively skewed.

Example 2.7

In some studies, the important number is the time to an event, such as death; it is called the *survival time*. The term survival time is conventional even though the primary event could be nonfatal such as a relapse or the appearance of the first disease symptom.

Similar to the cases of income and antibody level, the distributions of survival times are positively skewed; therefore, data are often summarized using median or geometric mean. The following is a typical example:

The remission times of 42 patients with acute leukemia were reported from a clinical trial undertaken to assess the ability of a drug called 6–mercaptopurine (6–MP) to maintain remission. Each patient was randomized to receive either 6–MP or placebo. The study was terminated after one year; patients have different follow-up time because they were enrolled sequentially at different times. Times to relapse in weeks for the 21 patients in the placebo group were:

$$1, 1, 2, 2, 3, 4, 4, 5, 5, 8, 8, 8, 8, 11, 11, 12, 12, 15, 17, 22, 23$$

The mean is

$$\bar{x} = \frac{\sum x}{n}$$
$$= 8.67 \text{ weeks}$$

while on the log scale, we have

$$\frac{\sum \ln x}{n} = 1.826$$

leading to a geometric mean of 6.21 which, in general, is less affected by the large measurements.

2.2.2. Other Measures of Location

Another useful measure of location is the *median*. If the observations in the data set are arranged in increasing or decreasing order, the median is the middle observation which divides the set into equal halves. If the number of observations n is odd, there will be a unique median, the $\frac{1}{2}(n+1)$th number from either end in the ordered sequence. If n is even, there is strictly no middle observation, but the median is defined by convention as the average of the two middle observations, the $\frac{1}{2}n$th and $\frac{1}{2}(n+1)$th from either end. In the previous section (Section 2.1), we showed a quicker way to get an approximate value for the median using the cumulative frequency graph (see Figure 2.6).

The two data sets $\{8, 5, 4, 12, 15, 7, 28\}$ and $\{8, 5, 4, 12, 15, 7, 49\}$, for example, have different means but the same median, 8. Therefore, the advantage of the median as a measure of location is that it is less affected by extreme observations. However, the median has some disadvantages in comparison with the mean:

1. It takes no account of the precise magnitude of most of the observations, and is therefore less efficient than the mean because it wastes information.
2. If two groups of observations are pooled, the median of the combined group cannot be expressed in terms of the medians of the two component groups. However, the mean can be so expressed. If component groups are of sizes n_1 and n_2 and have means $\bar{x}_1$ and $\bar{x}_2$, respectively, the mean of the combined group is

$$\bar{x} = \frac{n_1 \bar{x}_1 + n_2 \bar{x}_2}{n_1 + n_2}$$

3. In large data sets, the median requires more work to calculate than the mean and is not much use in the elaborate statistical techniques (it is still useful as a descriptive measure for skewed distributions).

A third measure of location, the *mode*, was briefly introduced in the section entitled "Histogram and Frequency Polygon" (Section 2.1.3). It is a value at which the frequency polygon reaches a peak. The mode is not widely used in analytical statistics, other than as a descriptive measure, mainly because of the ambiguity in its definition as the fluctuations of small frequencies are apt to produce spurious modes. Because of these reasons, the rest of this book is focused on only one measure of location, the mean.

2.2.3. Measures of Dispersion

When the mean $\bar{x}$ of a set of measurements has been obtained, it is usually a matter of considerable interest to measure the degree of variation or dispersion around this mean. Are the x's all rather close to $\bar{x}$ or are some of them dispersed widely in each direction? This question is important for purely descriptive reasons, but it is also important because the measurement of dispersion or variation plays a central part in the methods of statistical inference which will be described in subsequent chapters of this book.

An obvious candidate for the measurement of dispersion is the range R, defined as the difference between the largest value and the smallest value, which was introduced in the histogram section, Section 2.1.3. However, there are a few difficulties about the use of the range. The first is that the value of the range is determined by only two of the original observations. Secondly, the interpretation of the range depends, in a complicated way, on the number of observations, which is an undesirable feature.

An alternative approach is to make use of the *deviations* from the mean, $x - \bar{x}$; it is obvious that the greater the variation in the data set, the larger the magnitude of these deviations tends to be. From these deviations, the *variance* s^2 is computed by squaring each deviation, adding them, and dividing their sum by one less than n:

$$s^2 = \frac{\sum(x - \bar{x})^2}{n - 1}$$

The use of the divisor $(n - 1)$ instead of n is clearly not very important when n is large. It is more important for small values of n, and its justification will be briefly explained later in this section. It should be noted that

1. It would be no use to take the mean of deviations because

$$\sum(x - \bar{x}) = 0.$$

2. Taking the mean of the absolute values, e.g.,

$$\frac{\sum |x - \bar{x}|}{n}$$

is a possibility. However, this measure has the drawback of being difficult to handle mathematically, and we will not consider it further in this book.

The variance s^2 (s-squared) is measured in the square of the units in which the x's are measured. For example, if x is the time in seconds, the variance is measured in square seconds, (seconds)^2. It is convenient, therefore, to have a measure of variation expressed in the same units as the x's, and this can be easily done by taking the square root of the variance. This quantity is known as the *standard deviation*, and its formula is

$$s = \sqrt{\frac{\sum(x - \bar{x})^2}{n - 1}}$$

Consider again the data set

$$\{8, 5, 4, 12, 15, 5, 7\}$$

Calculation of the variance s^2 and standard deviation s is illustrated in Table 2.5.

In general, this calculation process is likely to cause some trouble. If the mean is not a "round" number, say $\bar{x} = 10/3$, it will need to be rounded off and errors arise in the subtraction of this figure from each x. This difficulty can be easily overcome with the use of the following short-cut formula for the variance:

$$s^2 = \frac{\sum x^2 - \frac{(\sum x)^2}{n}}{n - 1}$$

The previous example is reworked in Table 2.6, yielding identical results.

$$s^2 = \frac{(548) - (56)^2/7}{6}$$

$$= 16.67$$

Table 2.5. Calculation of Variance and Standard Deviation

x	$x - \bar{x}$	$(x - \bar{x})^2$
8	0	0
5	-3	9
4	-4	16
12	4	16
15	7	49
5	-3	9
7	-1	1
$\sum x = 56$		$\sum(x - \bar{x})^2 = 100$
$n = 7$		$s^2 = 100/6 = 16.67$
$\bar{x} = 8$		$s = \sqrt{16.67} = 4.08$

Table 2.6. Use of a Shortcut Formula for Variance

x	x^2
8	64
5	25
4	16
12	144
15	225
5	25
7	49
56	548

When data are presented in the grouped form of a frequency table, the variance is calculated using the following modified shortcut formula ($\cong$ means "approximately equal to"):

$$s^2 \cong \frac{\sum fm^2 - \frac{(\sum fm)^2}{n}}{n - 1}$$

where f denotes an interval frequency, m the interval midpoint calculated as in the previous section, and the summation is across the intervals. This approximation is illustrated in Table 2.7.

$$s^2 \cong \frac{89,724.25 - (2,086.5)^2/57}{56}$$

$$= 238.35$$

$$s \cong 15.4 \text{ lbs.}$$

(If individual weights were used, we would have $s = 15.9$ lb.)

It is often not clear to beginners why we use $(n - 1)$ instead of n as the denominator for s^2. This number $(n - 1)$ is called the "degrees of freedom" representing the "amount of

Table 2.7. Calculation of the Variance Using Frequency Table 2.2

Weight Interval	f	m	m^2	fm	fm^2
10–19	5	14.5	210.25	72.5	1,051.25
20–29	19	24.5	600.25	465.5	11,404.75
30–39	10	34.5	1,190.25	345.0	11,902.50
40–49	13	44.5	1,980.25	578.5	25,743.25
50–59	4	54.5	2,970.25	218.0	11,881.00
60–69	4	64.5	4,160.25	258.0	16,641.00
70–79	2	74.5	5,550.25	149.0	11,100.50
Totals	57			2,086.5	89,724.25

information" contained in the sample. The real explanation for $(n - 1)$ is hard to present at the level of this text; however, it may be seen this way. What we are trying to do with s is to provide a measure of variability, a measure of the "average gap" or "average distance" between numbers in the sample—and there are $(n - 1)$ "gaps" between n numbers. When $n = 2$ there is only one gap or distance beween the two numbers, and when $n = 1$ there is no variability to measure.

Finally, it is occasionally useful to describe the variation by expressing the standard deviation as a proportion or percentage of the mean. The resulting measure

$$CV = \frac{s}{\bar{x}} \times 100\%$$

is called the *coefficient of variation*. It is an *index*, a dimensionless quantity because the standard deviation is expressed in the same units as the mean and could be used to compare the difference in variation between two types of measurements. However, its use is rather limited and we will not present it at this level.

2.2.4. Box Plots

The box plot is a graphical representation of a data set that gives a visual impression of location, spread, and the degree and direction of skewness. It also allows for the identification of outliers. Box plots are similar to one-way scatter plots in that they require a single horizontal axis; however, instead of plotting each and every observation they display a summary of the data. A box plot consists of the following:

1. A central box extends from the 25th to the 75th percentiles. This box is divided into two compartments at the median value of the data set. The relative sizes of the two halves of the box provide an indication of the distribution symmetry. If they are approximately equal, the data set is roughly symmetric; otherwise, we are able to see the degree and direction of skewness (Figure 2.11).
2. The line segments projecting out from the box extend in both directions to the so-called *adjacent values*. The adjacent values are the points that are 1.5 times the length of the box beyond either quartile. All other data points outside this range are represented individually by little circles; these are considered to be outliers or extreme observations which are not typical of the rest of the data.

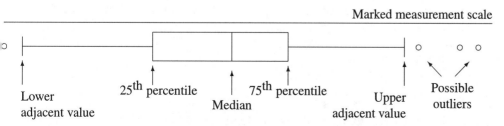

Figure 2.11. A typical box plot.

Figure 2.12. Crude death rates for the United States, 1988. A combination of one-way scatter and box plots.

Of course, it is possible to combine a one-way scatter plot and a box plot so as to convey an even greater amount of information (Figure 2.12). There are other ways of constructing box plots; for example, one may make it vertically or divided into different levels of outliers.

2.3. SURVIVAL CURVES

Methods discussed in this text have been directed to the analyses of *complete* data; this section is an exception, because it focuses on prospective studies.

In prospective studies, the important feature is not only the outcome event, such as death, but the time to that event, the *survival time* (Figure 2.13). In order to determine the survival time T, three basic elements are needed: (1) a time origin or starting point, (2) an ending event of interest, and (3) measurement scale for the passage of time—for example, the life span T from birth (starting point) to death (ending event) in years (measurement scale).

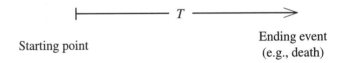

Figure 2.13. The survival time.

The time origin or starting point should be precisely defined, but it need not be birth; it could be the start of a new treatment (randomization date in a clinical trial) or the admission to a hospital or a nursing home. The ending event should also be precisely defined, but it need not be death; a nonfatal event such as the relapse of a disease (e.g., leukemia), the relapse from a smoking cessation, or the discharge to the community from a hospital or a nursing home satisfies the definition and is an acceptable choice. The use of calendar time in health studies is common and meaningful; however, other choices for a time scale are justified—for example, hospital cost (in dollars) from admission (starting point) to discharge (ending event).

2.3.1. Survival Data

A special source of difficulty in the analysis of survival data is the possibility that some individuals may not be observed for the full time to failure or event. The so-called "random

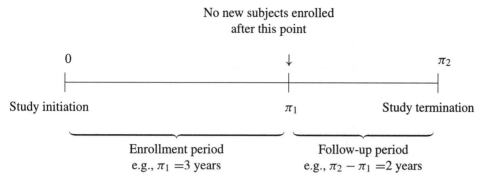

No new subjects enrolled
after this point

Figure 2.14. A clinical trial.

censoring" arises in medical applications with animal studies, epidemiological applications with human studies, or clinical trials. In these cases, observation is terminated before the occurrence of the event. In a clinical trial, for example, patients may enter the study at different times; then each is treated with one of several possible therapies after a randomization. Figure 2.14 shows a description of a typical clinical trial.

Of course, we want to observe their lifetimes from enrollment, but censoring may occur in one of the following forms:

- Loss to follow-up—the patient may decide to move elsewhere.
- Dropout—a therapy may have such bad effects that it is necessary to discontinue the treatment.
- Termination of the study (for data analysis at a predetermined time).
- Death due to a cause not under investigation (for example, suicide).

The censored observations are those subjects without the event under investigation. These subjects contain only partial information—for example, having survived 10 years or more (because the patient is still *alive*) or having no event at the end of the study which is 10 years after his/her enrollment. To make it possible for statistical analysis we make the crucial assumption that the prognosis for any individual who has survived to a certain time t should not be affected if the individual is censored at t. That is, an individual who is censored at t should be representative of all those subjects who survive to t. In other words, survival condition and reason of loss are independent; under this assumption, there is no need to distinguish the above four forms of censoring.

At the end of the study, our sample consists of n numbers, each is a time measurement, but some are times to an event some are censored observations. We can use "t" for time to an event and "$t+$" to denote a censored observation. The censored cases are important featues of survival data; with their presence all the methods of summarization we learned—such as $\bar{x}$ and s—become irrelevant. It is impossible to calculate $\bar{x}$ because the true survival time of a censored case is unknown.

Example 2.8

The remission times of 42 patients with acute leukemia were reported from a clinical trial undertaken to assess the ability of a drug called 6–mercaptopurine (6–MP) to maintain remission. Each patient was randomized to receive either 6–MP or placebo. The study was terminated after 1 year; patients have different follow-up time because they were enrolled sequentially at different times. Times in weeks were:

6–MP Group:
    6, 6, 6, 7, 10, 13, 16, 22, 23, 6+, 9+, 10+, 11+, 17+, 19+, 20+,
    25+, 32+, 32+, 34+, 35+

Placebo Group:
    1, 1, 2, 2, 3, 4, 4, 5, 5, 8, 8, 8, 8, 11, 11, 12, 12, 15, 17, 22, 23

---

in which, as explained, a $t+$ denotes a censored observation, that is, the case was censored after t weeks without a relapse. For example, "10+" is a case enrolled 10 weeks before study termination and still in remission at termination.

2.3.2. Survival Curve

The distribution of the survival time T from enrollment or starting point to the event of interest, considered as a random variable, is characterized by the *survival function*. The survival function, denoted $S(t)$, is defined as the probability that an individual survives longer than t units of time:

$$S(t) = \Pr(T > t)$$

$S(t)$ is also known as the *survival rate;* for example, if times are in years, then $S(2)$ is the 2-year survival rate, $S(5)$ is the 5-year survival rate, and so on. The 5-year survival rate is commonly used in cancer research as a measure of a treatment effectiveness. In clinical trials, the differences between survival rates are indications of a treatment effect. To express in a simple way, the t-year survival rate is defined by

$$\frac{\text{Number of individuals who survive longer than } t \text{ years}}{\text{Total number of individuals in the data set}}$$

The graph of $S(t)$ versus t is called the *survival curve*, as shown in Figure 2.15.

Without censoring, the calculation of survival rates is straightforward; for example, in the above placebo group,

$$\text{10-week survival rate} = \frac{8}{21} \times 100\% = 38.1\%$$

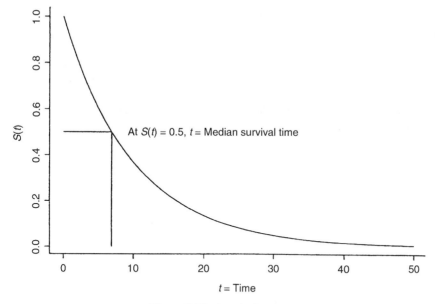

Figure 2.15. A typical curve.

because 8 of 21 cases survived 10 weeks or more. In the following sections we will discuss methods appropriate for censored data. The main objective is to take into account censored cases that contain only partial information.

Kaplan–Meier Method

We first introduce the *product-limit* (PL) method of estimating the survival rates; this is also called the *Kaplan–Meier* method. Let

$$t_1 < t_2 < \cdots < t_k$$

be the distinct observed death times (excluding censored observations) in a sample of size n from a homogeneous population with survival function $S(t)$ to be estimated ($k \leq n$). Let n_i be the number of subjects at risk at a time just prior to t_i ($1 \leq i \leq k$; these are cases whose duration time is at least t_i), and let d_i be the number of deaths at t_i. According to the Kaplan–Meier method, the survival function $S(t)$ is estimated by

$$\widehat{S}(t) = \prod_{t_i \leq t} \left(1 - \frac{d_i}{n_i}\right)$$

Its graph versus time is called the Kaplan–Meier curve. In the above formula, the notation $\prod$ denotes the product where we successively multiply terms from the beginning up to time t.

Example 2.9

Refer back to the clinical trial to evaluate the effect of 6-mercaptopurine (6-MP) to maintain remission from acute leukemia (Example 2.8). According to the product-limit method, survival rates for the 6-MP group are calculated by constructing a table such as Table 2.8 with five columns; to obtain $\widehat{S}(t)$, multiply all values in column 4 up to and including t. From Table 2.8, we have, for example:

Table 2.8. Survival Rates for 6-MP Group

(1)	(2)	(3)	(4)	(5)
t_i	n_i	d_i	$1 - \dfrac{d_i}{n_i}$	$\widehat{S}(t_i)$
6	21	3	.8571	.8571
7	17	1	.9412	$.8067 = (.8571)(.9412)$
10	15	1	.9333	$.7529 = (.8067)(.9333)$
13	12	1	.9167	$.6902 = (.7529)(.9167)$
16	11	1	.9091	$.6275 = (.6902)(.9091)$
22	7	1	.8571	$.5378 = (.6275)(.8571)$
23	6	1	.8333	$.4482 = (.5378)(.8333)$

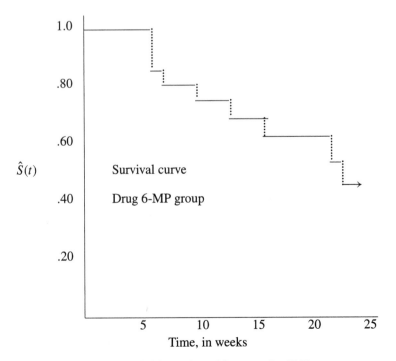

Figure 2.16. Kaplan–Meier curve for 6-MP group.

7-week survival rate is 80.67%
22-week survival rate is 53.78%

(the last column is only added to explain how to obtain the estimates).

Note: An SAS program would include these instructions:
```
PROC LIFETEST METHOD = KM;
TIME WEEKS*RELAPSE(0);
```
where WEEKS is the variable name for duration time, RELAPSE the variable name for survival status, "0" is the coding for censoring, and KM stands for Kaplan–Meier method.

Of course, we can always apply the same method to analyze any data set with or without censoring.

Example 2.10

Refer back to the clinical trial to evaluate the effect of 6-mercaptopurine (6-MP) to maintain remission from acute leukemia (Example 2.8). According to the product-limit method, the survival function of the placebo group is obtained as shown in Table 2.9. Kaplan–Meier curves for both groups, the 6-MP group and the placebo group, are shown together as Figure 2.17.

Table 2.9. Survival Rates for Placebo Group

(1)	(2)	(3)	(4)	(5)
t_i	η_i	d_i	$1 - \frac{d_i}{\eta_i}$	$\hat{S}(t_i)$
1	21	2	.9048	.9048
2	19	2	.8947	.8095
3	17	1	.9412	.7619
4	16	2	.8750	.6667
5	14	2	.8517	.5714
8	12	4	.6667	.3810
11	8	2	.7500	.2857
12	6	2	.6667	.1905
15	4	1	.7500	.1429
17	3	1	.6667	.0953
22	2	1	.5000	.0476
23	1	1	.0000	.0000

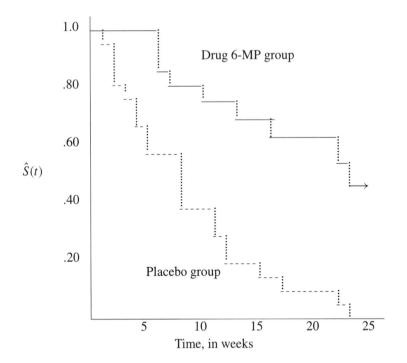

Figure 2.17. Kaplan–Meier curves.

Note: A SAS program would include these instructions:

```
PROC LIFETEST METHOD = KM;
TIME WEEKS*RELAPSE(0);
STRATA DRUG;
```

where KM stands for Kaplan–Meier method, WEEKS is the variable name for duration time, RELAPSE is the variable name for survival status, "0" is the coding for censoring, and DRUG is the variable name specifying groups to be compared.

Actuarial Method

The Kaplan–Meier method is applicable for any survival data set; however, for a large data set—say 100 or more patients—it may be much more convenient to group the times into intervals. The process is similar to the formation of a frequency table, and the method is referred to as the *actuarial method*. A concrete example is adapted (Table 2.9) to illustrate this method with eight columns following the outlines below:

(1) The choice of the time intervals will depend on the nature of the data and the size of the data set; guidelines given in the section entitled "Frequency Distribution" (Section 2.1.2) are equally applicable here.

(2) and (3) The patients are classified according to the time interval during which their condition was last reported. If the report was a death, the patient is counted in column (2); and if censored, the patient is counted in column (3). Time for each patient is calculated from his/her enrollment in the study.

(4) The number of patients living at the start of the intervals is obtained by cumulating columns (2) and (3) from the bottom. For example, the number alive at 10 years is $21 + 26 = 47$ and the number alive at 9 years is $47 + 2 + 5 + 54$, and so on.

(5) The number of patients at risk during interval t to $(t + 1)$ is given by

$$n' = n - c/2$$

The purpose of this formula is to provide a denominator for the next column. The adjustment from n to n' is needed because the c censored subjects are necessarily at risk for only part of the interval. The basic assumption here is that, on the average, these patients are at risk for half of the interval.

(6) The interval death rate is expressed as

$$q = d/n'$$

For example, during the first interval

$$q = \frac{90}{374.0}$$
$$= .2406$$

1. The interval survival rate is given by

$$p = 1 - q$$

Table 2.10. Survival of Patients with a Particular Form of Malignant Disease

(1)	(2)	(3)	(4)	(5)	(6)	(7)	(8)
			Living	No.	Interval	Interval	Survival
Time	Last Reported		at the	at	Death	Survival	Rate at
(Years)	Died	Censored	Start	Risk	Rate	Rate	t Years
t to $(t + 1)$	d	c	n	n'	q	p	%
0–1	90	0	374	374.0	.2406	.7594	100.0
1–2	76	0	284	284.0	.2676	.7324	75.9
2–3	51	0	208	208.0	.2452	.7548	55.6
3–4	25	12	157	151.0	.1656	.8344	42.0
4–5	20	5	120	117.5	.1702	.8298	35.0
5–6	7	9	95	90.5	.0773	.9227	29.1
6–7	4	9	79	74.5	.0537	.9463	26.8
7–8	1	3	66	64.5	.0155	.9845	25.4
8–9	3	5	62	59.5	.0504	.9496	25.0
9–10	2	5	54	51.5	.0388	.9612	23.7
10+	21	26	47	—	—	—	22.8

2. To obtain the survival rate at t years, multiply all values in the previous column, column (7), up to and including that for interval t to $(t + 1)$, as shown in Table 2.10.

Survival rate calculated by the actuarial method are displayed by a survival curve similar to that for rates obtained by the Kaplan–Meier method, but the dots in the diagram are connected by straight lines as shown in Figure 2.18.

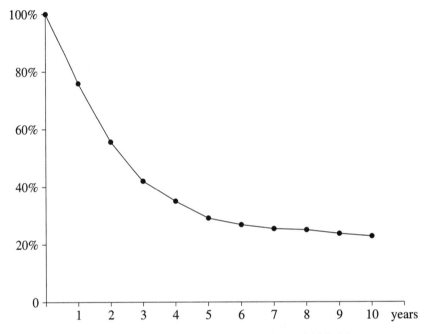

Figure 2.18. Survival curve for cancer patients of Table 2.8.

Note: The previous SAS program should be changed to:
PROC LIFETEST METHOD = AC;
where AC stands for Actuarial method of estmating the survival curve.

Finally, it is noted that this approximation—the actuarial method—is still useful even if the user has access to computer packages for constructing the Kaplan–Meier curve because it provides an estimate for the "hazard" or "risk" function which is not possible with the Kaplan–Meier method and which is useful and needed for certain more advanced analyses.

2.4. COEFFICIENTS OF CORRELATION

Methods discussed in this Chapter 2 has been directed to the analyses of data where a single continuous measurement was made on each element of a sample. However, in many important investigations we may have two measurements made—that is, where the sample consists of pairs of values and the research objective is concerned with the association between these variables. For example, what is the relationship between a mother's weight and her baby's weight? Section 1.3 was concerned with the association between dichotomous variables. For example, if we want to investigate the relationship between a disease and a certain risk factor, we could calculate an odds ratio to represent the strength of the relationship. This section deals with continuous measurements and the method is referred to as *correlation analysis*. Correlation is a concept, with common colloquial usage of association, such as "height and weight are correlated." The statistical procedure will give a technical meaning to it; we can actually calculate a number that tells the *strength* of the association.

When dealing with the relationship between two continuous variables, we first have to distinguish between a *deterministic* relationship and a *statistical* relationship. For a deterministic relationship, values of the two variables are related through an exact mathematical formula. For example, consider the relationship between hospital cost and number of days in hospital. If the costs are $100 for admission and $150 per day, then we can easily calculate the total cost given the number of days in hospital and if any set of data is plotted, say cost versus number of days, all data points fall perfectly on a straight line. A statistical relationship, unlike a deterministic one, is not a perfect one. In general, the points do not fall perfectly on any line or curve. Table 2.11 gives the values for the birth weight (x) and the increase in weight between 70th and 100th days of life, expressed as a percentage of the birth weight (y) for 12 infants:

Table 2.11. Birth Weight Data

x (oz)	y (%)
112	63
111	66
107	72
119	52
92	75
80	118
81	120
84	114
118	42
106	72
103	90
94	91

If we let each pair of numbers (x, y) be represented by a dot in a diagram with the x's on the horizontal axis, we have the figure shown below (Figure 2.19). The dots do not fall perfectly on a straight line, but rather scatter around one, very typical for statistical relationships. Because of this scattering of dots, the diagram is called a *scatter diagram*. The positions of the dots provide some information about the direction as well as the strength of the association under the investigation. If they tend to go from lower left to upper right, we have a positive association; if they tend to go from upper left to lower right, we have a negative association. The relationship becomes weaker and weaker as the distribution of

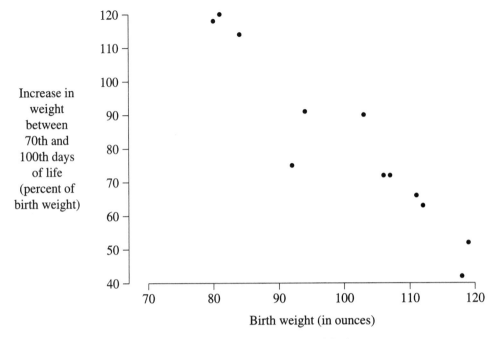

Figure 2.19. Scatter diagram for birth weight data.

the dots clusters less closely around the line, and it becomes virtually no correlation when the distribution approximates a circle or oval (the method is ineffective for measuring a relationship that is not linear).

2.4.1. Pearson's Correlation Coefficient

Consider again a scatter diagram, shown in Figure 2.20, where we added a vertical and a horizontal line through the point $(\bar{x}, \bar{y})$ and labeled the four quarters as I, II, III, and IV.

It can be seen that

- In quarters I and III,

$$(x - \bar{x})(y - \bar{y}) > 0$$

so that for positive association, we have

$$\sum(x - \bar{x})(y - \bar{y}) > 0.$$

Furthermore, this sum is large for stronger relationships because most of the dots, being closely clustered around the line, are in these two quarters.

- Similarly, in quarters II and IV,

$$(x - \bar{x})(y - \bar{y}) < 0$$

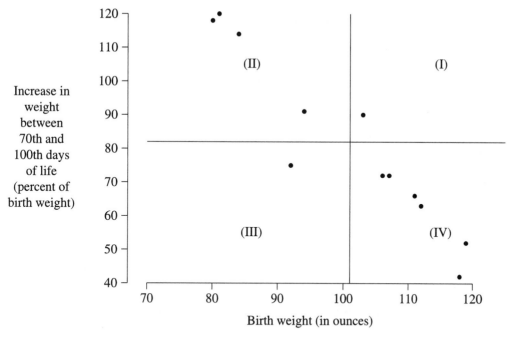

Figure 2.20. Scatter diagram divided into quadrants.

leading to

$$\sum(x - \bar{x})(y - \bar{y}) < 0$$

for negative association.

With a proper standardization, we obtain

$$r = \frac{\sum(x - \bar{x})(y - \bar{y})}{\sqrt{\left[\sum(x - \bar{x})^2\right]\left[\sum(y - \bar{y})^2\right]}}$$

so that

$$-1 \leq r \leq 1$$

This statistic r is called the *correlation coefficient* and is a popular measure for the strength of a statistical relationship; here is a shortcut formula:

$$r = \frac{\sum xy - \frac{(\sum x)(\sum y)}{n}}{\sqrt{\left[\sum x^2 - \frac{(\sum x)^2}{n}\right]\left[\sum y^2 - \frac{(\sum y)^2}{n}\right]}}$$

Meaningful interpretation of the correlation coefficient r is rather complicated at this level, we will revisit the topic in Chapter 8 in the context of regression analysis, a statistical method that is closely connected to correlation. Generally,

- Values near 1 indicate a strong positive association.
- Values near -1 indicate a strong negative association.
- Values around 0 indicate a weak association.

Interpretation of r should be made cautiously, however. It is true that a scatter plot of data which results in a correlation number of $+1$ or -1 has to lie in a perfectly straight line. But correlation of 0 doesn't mean that there is no association. It means there is no *linear* association. You can have a correlation near 0 and yet have a very strong association, such as the case when the data fall neatly on a sharply bending curve.

Example 2.11

Consider again the previous birth weight problem. We have

x	y	x^2	y^2	xy
112	63	12,544	3,969	7,056
111	66	12,321	4,356	7,326
107	72	11,449	5,184	7,704
119	52	14,161	2,704	6,188
92	75	8,464	5,625	6,900
80	118	6,400	13,924	9,440
81	120	6,561	14,400	9,720
84	114	7,056	12,996	9,576
118	42	13,924	1,764	4,956
106	72	11,236	5,184	7,632
103	90	10,609	8,100	9,270
94	91	8,836	8,281	8,554
Totals: 1,207	975	123,561	86,487	94,322

Using these five totals, we obtain

$$r = \frac{94,322 - \frac{(1,207)(975)}{12}}{\sqrt{\left[123,561 - \frac{(1,207)^2}{12}\right]\left[86,487 - \frac{(975)^2}{12}\right]}}$$

$$= -.946$$

indicating a very strong negative association.

The following example presents a problem with similar data structure where the target of investigation is a possible relationship between a woman's age and her systolic blood pressure.

Example 2.12

The following data represent systolic blood pressure readings on 15 women:

Age (x)	SBP (y)	Age (x)	SBP (y)
42	130	85	162
46	115	72	158
42	148	64	155
71	100	81	160
80	156	41	125
74	162	61	150
70	151	75	165
80	156		

We set up a work table as in the previous example:

	x	y	x^2	y^2	xy
	42	130	1,764	16,900	5,460
	46	115	2,116	13,225	5,290
	42	148	1,764	21,904	6,216
	71	100	5,041	10,000	7,100
	80	156	6,400	24,336	12,480
	74	162	5,476	26,224	11,988
	70	151	4,900	22,801	10,570
	80	156	6,400	24,336	12,480
	85	162	7,225	26,224	13,770
	72	158	5,184	24,964	11,376
	64	155	4,096	24,025	9,920
	81	160	6,561	25,600	12,960
	41	125	1,681	15,625	5,125
	61	150	3,721	22,500	9,150
	75	165	5,625	27,225	12,375
Totals	984	2,193	67,954	325,889	146,260

Using these totals, we obtain

$$r = \frac{146,260 - \frac{(984)(2,193)}{15}}{\sqrt{\left[67,954 - \frac{(984)^2}{15}\right]\left[325,889 - \frac{(2,193)^2}{15}\right]}}$$

$$= .566$$

indicating a moderately positive association.

2.4.2. Nonparametric Correlation Coefficients

Suppose the data set consists of n pairs of observations $\{(x_i, y_i)\}$ expressing a possible relationship between two continuous variables. We characterize the strength of such a relationship by calculating the coefficient of correlation

$$r = \frac{\sum(x - \bar{x})(y - \bar{y})}{\sqrt{\left[\sum(x - \bar{x})^2\right]\left[\sum(y - \bar{y})^2\right]}}$$

called the Pearson's correlation coefficient. Like other common statistics, such as the mean $\bar{x}$ and the standard deviation s, the correlation coefficient r is very sensitive to extreme observations. We may be interested in calculating a measure of association that is more robust with respect to outlying values. There are not one but two nonparametric procedures: the *Spearman's rho* and the *Kendall's tau* rank correlations.

The Spearman's rho

The Spearman's rank correlation is a direct nonparametric counterpart of the Pearson's correlation coefficient. To perform this procedure, we first arrange the x values from smallest to largest and assign a rank from 1 to n for each value; let R_i be the rank of value x_i. Similarly, we arrange the y values also from smallest to largest and assign a rank from 1 to n for each value; let S_i be the rank of value y_i. If there are tied observations, we assign an average rank averaging the ranks that the tied observations jointly take. For example, if the second and third measurements are equal, they both are assigned 2.5 as their common rank. The next step is to replace, in the formula of the Pearson's correlation coefficient r, x_i by its rank R_i and y_i by its rank S_i. The result is the Spearman's rho, a popular rank correlation:

$$\rho = \frac{\sum(R_i - \bar{R})(S_i - \bar{S})}{\sqrt{\left[\sum(R_i - \bar{R})^2\right]\left[\sum(S_i - \bar{S})^2\right]}}$$

$$= 1 - \frac{6\sum(R_i - S_i)^2}{n(n^2 - 1)}$$

The second expression is simpler and easier to use.

Example 2.13

Consider again the birth weight problem of Example 2.11. We have

Birth Weight		Increase in Weight			
x (oz)	Rank R	y (%)	Rank S	$R - S$	$(R - S)^2$
112	10	63	3	7	49
111	9	66	4	5	25
107	8	72	5.5	2.5	6.25
119	12	52	2	10	100
92	4	75	7	−3	9
80	1	118	11	−10	100
81	2	120	12	−10	100
84	3	114	10	−7	49
118	11	42	1	10	100
106	7	72	5.5	1.5	2.25
103	6	90	8	−2	4
94	5	91	9	−4	16
				Total	560.50

Substituting the value of $\sum (R_i - S_i)^2$ into the formula for rho (ρ), we obtain

$$\rho = 1 - \frac{(6)(560.5)}{(12)(143)}$$

$$= -.96$$

which is very close to the value of r (−.946) obtained in example 2.11. This closeness is true when there are few or no extreme observations.

The Kendall's Tau

Unlike the Spearman's rho, the other rank correlation—the Kendall's tau τ—is defined and calculated very differently, even though they often yield similar numerical results. The above birth weight problem of Example 2.11 is adapted to illustrate this method with the following steps:

1. First, the x and y values are presented in two rows; the x values in the first row are arranged from smallest to largest.

2. For each y value in the second row, we count the following:
   (a) The number of larger y values to its right (third row). The sum of these is denoted by C.
   (b) The number of smaller y-values to its right (fourth row). The sum of these is denoted by D.
   C and D are called the numbers of concordant pairs and discordant pairs.
3. The Kendall's rank correlation is defined by

$$\tau = \frac{C - D}{\frac{1}{2}n(n - 1)}$$

Example 2.14

For the above birth weight problem, we have

												Total
x:	80	81	84	92	94	103	106	107	111	112	118	119	
y:	118	120	114	75	91	90	72	72	66	63	42	52	
C:	1	0	0	2	0	0	0	0	0	0	0	0	3
D:	10	10	9	6	7	6	4	4	3	2	0	0	61

The value of Kendall's tau is

$$\tau = \frac{3 - 61}{\frac{1}{2}(12)(11)}$$
$$= -.88$$

Note: A SAS program would include these instructions:
```
PROC CORR PEARSON SPEARMAN KENDALL;
VAR BWEIGHT INCREASE;
```
If there are more than two variable names listed, the CORR procedure will compute correlation coefficients between all pairs of variables.

2.5. NOTES ON COMPUTATIONS

Section 1.4 covered basic techniques for Microsoft's Excel: How to open/form a spreadsheet, save, and retrieve it. Topics included data entry steps—such as *select and drag*, use of *formula bar*, and bar and pie charts. This short section focuses on continuous data covering topics such as the construction of histograms, basic descriptive statistics, and correlation analysis.

Histograms

With a frequency table ready, click the *ChartWizard* icon (the one with multiple colored bars on the *standard toolbar* near the top). A box appears with choices (as when you learned to form a bar chart or pie chart); select the column chart type. Then click on *next*.

- For the data range, highlight the frequency column. This can be done by clicking on the first observation and dragging the mouse to the last observation. Then click on *next*,
- To remove the gridlines, click on the gridline tab and uncheck the box. To remove the legend, you can do the same using the legend tab. Now click *finish*.
- The problem is that there are still gaps. To remove these, double click on a bar of the graph and a new set of options should appear. Click on the options tab and change the gap width from 150 to 0.

Descriptive Statistics:

- First, click the cell you want to fill, then click the *paste function icon*, f*, which will give you—in a box—a list Excel functions available for your use.
- The item you need in this list is *Statistical*; upon hitting this, a new list appears with *function names*, each for a statistical procedure.
- The following procedures/names we learn in this chapter (alphabetically): *AVERAGE, GEOMEAN, MEDIAN, STDEV,* and *VAR.*

  (i) AVERAGE: provides the sample mean,
  (ii) GEOMEAN: provides the geometric mean,
  (iii) MEDIAN: provides the sample median,
  (iv) STDEV: provides the standard deviation, and
  (v) VAR: provides the variance.

In each case, you can only obtain one statistic at a time. First, you have to enter the *range* containing your sample—for example, D6:D20 (you can see what you are entering on the *formula bar*); the computer will return with numerical value for the requested statistic in a *preselected* cell.

Pearson's Coefficient of Correlation

- First, click the cell you want to fill, then click the *paste function icon*, f*, which will give you—in a box—a list Excel functions available for your use.
- The item you need in this list is *Statistical*; upon hitting this, a new list appears with *function names*, each for a statistical procedure. Click *CORREL*, for correlation.
- In the newly appeared box, move the cursor to fill in the X and Y ranges in the two rows marked as *Array 1* and *Array 2*. The computer will return with numerical value for the requested statistic, the Pearson's correlation coefficient r, in a *preselected* cell.

EXERCISES

2.1. The following table gives the values of serum cholesterol levels for 1067 U.S. men, aged 25 to 34 years.

Cholesterol Level (mg/100 ml)	Number of Men
80–119	13
120–159	150
160–199	442
200–239	299
240–279	115
280–319	34
320–399	14
Total	1,067

(a) Plot the histogram, the frequency polygon, and the cumulative frequency graph.

(b) Find, approximately, the median using your cumulative frequency graph.

2.2. The following table provides the relative frequencies of blood lead concentrations for two groups of workers in Canada, one examined in 1979 and the other in 1987.

Blood Lead (μg/dl)	Relative Frequency (%) 1979	1987
0–19	11.5	37.8
20–29	12.1	14.7
30–39	13.9	13.1
40–49	15.4	15.3
50–59	16.5	10.5
60–69	12.8	6.8
70–79	8.4	1.4
80+	9.4	0.4

(a) Plot the histogram and frequency polygon for each year on separate graphs.

(b) Plot the two cumulative frequency graphs in one figure.

(c) Find and compare the medians.

2.3. A study on the effects of exercise on the menstrual cycle provides the following ages (years) of menarche (the beginning of menstruation) for 96 female swimmers who began training prior to menarche:

15.0	17.1	14.6	15.2	14.9	14.4	14.7	15.3
13.6	15.1	16.2	15.9	13.8	15.0	15.4	14.9
14.2	16.5	13.2	16.8	15.3	14.7	13.9	16.1
15.4	14.6	15.2	14.8	13.7	16.3	15.1	14.5
16.4	13.6	14.8	15.5	13.9	15.9	16.0	14.6
14.0	15.1	14.8	15.0	14.8	15.3	15.7	14.3
13.9	15.6	15.4	14.6	15.2	14.8	13.7	16.3
15.1	14.5	13.6	15.1	16.2	15.9	13.8	15.0
15.4	14.9	16.2	15.9	13.8	15.0	15.4	14.9
14.2	16.5	13.4	16.5	14.8	15.1	14.9	13.7
16.2	15.8	15.4	14.7	14.3	15.2	14.6	13.7
14.9	15.8	15.1	14.6	13.8	16.0	15.0	14.6

(a) Form a frequency distribution including relative frequencies and cumulative relative frequencies.

(b) Plot the frequency polygon and the cumulative frequency graph.

(c) Find the median and 95th percentile.

2.4. The following are the menarchal ages (in years) of 56 female swimmers who began training after they had reached menarche.

14.0	16.1	13.4	14.6	13.7	13.2	13.7	14.3
12.9	14.1	15.1	14.8	12.8	14.2	14.1	13.6
14.2	15.8	12.7	15.6	14.1	13.0	12.9	15.1
15.0	13.6	14.2	13.8	12.7	15.3	14.1	13.5
15.3	12.6	13.8	14.4	12.9	14.6	15.0	13.8
13.0	14.1	13.8	14.2	13.6	14.1	14.5	13.1
12.8	14.3	14.2	13.5	14.1	13.6	12.4	15.1

(a) Form a frequency distribution using the same age intervals as in Exercise 2.3. (These intervals may be different from those in Example 2.3.)

(b) Display in the same graph two cumulative frequency graphs, one for the group trained before menarche and one for the group trained after menarche. Compare these two graphs and draw your conclusion.

(c) Find the median and 95th percentile and compare to the results of the previous exercise.

2.5. The following table shows the daily fat intake (grams) of a group of 150 adult males.

22	62	77	84	91	102	117	129	137	141
42	56	78	73	96	105	117	125	135	143
37	69	82	93	93	100	114	124	135	142
30	77	81	94	97	102	119	125	138	142
46	89	88	99	95	100	116	121	131	152
63	85	81	94	93	106	114	127	133	155
51	80	88	98	97	106	119	122	134	151
52	70	76	95	107	105	117	128	144	150

68	79	82	96	109	108	117	120	147	153
67	75	76	92	105	104	117	129	148	164
62	85	77	96	103	105	116	132	146	168
53	72	72	91	102	101	128	136	143	164
65	73	83	92	103	118	127	132	140	167
68	75	89	95	107	111	128	139	148	168
68	79	82	96	109	108	117	130	147	153

(a) Form a frequency distribution including relative frequencies and cumulative relative frequencies.

(b) Plot the frequency polygon and investigate the symmetry of the distribution.

(c) Plot the cumulative frequency graph and find the 25th and 75th percentiles. Also calculate the *mid-range* = 75th percentile − 25th percentile (this is another good descriptive measure of variation; it is similar to the *range* but is less affected by extreme observations).

2.6. Refer to the data on daily fat intake of Exercise 2.5.

(a) Calculate the mean using raw data.

(b) Calculate, approximately, the mean using the frequency table as obtained in Exercise 2.5.

2.7. Using the income data of Example 2.5,

(a) Plot the histogram for the white families. Does it have the same shape as that for nonwhite families as seen in Figure 2.5?

(b) Plot and compare the two cumulative frequency graphs, whites versus nonwhites, confirming the results seen in Figure 2.7.

(c) Calculate, approximately, the means of the two groups and compare the results to the medians referred in the section just before Example 2.6.

2.8. Refer to the percentage saturation of bile for the 31 male patients in Example 2.4.

(a) Calculate the mean, the variance, and the standard deviation.

(b) The frequency polygon of Figure 2.3 is based on the following grouping (arbitrary choices):

Interval (%)	Frequency
40–49	2
50–59	4
60–69	3
70–79	4
80–89	8
90–99	1
100–109	2
110–119	5
120–129	1
130–139	1
140–149	0

Plot the cumulative frequency graph and obtain, approximately, the median from this graph. How does the answer compare to the exact median (the 16th largest saturation percentage)?

2.9. The same study referenced in Example 2.4 also provided data (percentage saturation of bile) for 29 women. These percentages were

65	58	52	91	84	107
86	98	35	128	116	84
76	146	55	75	73	120
89	80	127	82	87	123
142	66	77	69	76	

(a) Form a frequency distribution using the same intervals as in Example 2.4 and Exercise 2.8.
(b) Plot in the same graph and compare the two frequency polygons and cumulative frequency graphs: men and women.
(c) Calculate the mean, the variance, and the standard deviation using these new data for women and compare the results to those for men in Exercise 2.8.
(d) Calculate and compare the two coefficients of variation, men versus women.

2.10. The following frequency distribution was obtained for the preoperational percentage hemoglobin values of a group of subjects from a village where there has been a malaria eradication program (MEP):

Hemoglobin (%)	30–39	40–49	50–59	60–69	70–79	80–89	90–99
Frequency	2	7	14	10	8	2	2

The results in another group was obtained after MEP and are given below:

43	63	63	75	95	75	80	48	62	71	76	90
51	61	74	103	93	82	74	65	63	53	64	67
80	77	60	69	73	76	91	55	65	69	84	78
50	68	72	89	75	57	66	79	85	70	59	71
87	67	72	52	35	67	99	81	97	74	61	62

(a) Form a frequency distribution using the same intervals as in the first table.
(b) Plot in the same graph and compare the two cumulative frequency graphs: before and after the malaria eradication program.

2.11. In a study of water pollution, a sample of mussels was taken and lead concentration (milligrams per gram dry weight) was measured from each one. The following data were obtained:

$$\{113.0, 140.5, 163.3, 185.7, 202.5, 207.2\}$$

Calculate the mean $\bar{x}$, variance s^2, and standard deviation s.

2.12. Consider this data taken from a study that examines the response to ozone and sulfur dioxide among adolescents suffering from asthma. The following are measurements of forced expiratory volume (liters) for 10 subjects:

$$\{3.50, 2.60, 2.75, 2.82, 4.05, 2.25, 2.68, 3.00, 4.02, 2.85\}$$

Calculate the mean $\bar{x}$, variance s^2, and standard deviation s.

2.13. The percentage of ideal body weight was determined for 18 randomly selected insulin-dependent diabetics. The outcomes (%) are:

107	119	99	114	120	104	124	88	114
116	101	121	152	125	100	114	95	117

Calculate the mean $\bar{x}$, variance s^2, and standard deviation s.

2.14. A study on birthweight provided the following data (in ounces) on 12 newborns:

$$\{112, 111, 107, 119, 92, 80, 81, 84, 118, 106, 103, 94\}$$

Calculate the mean $\bar{x}$, variance s^2, and standard deviation s.

2.15. The following are the activity values (micromoles per minute per gram of tissue) of a certain enzyme measured in normal gastric tissue of 35 patients with gastric carcinoma:

.360	1.189	.614	.788	.273	2.464	.571
1.827	.537	.374	.449	.262	.448	.971
.372	.898	.411	.348	1.925	.550	.622
.610	.319	.406	.413	.767	.385	.674
.521	.603	.533	.662	1.177	.307	1.499

Calculate the mean $\bar{x}$, variance s^2, and standard deviation s.

2.16. The following data represent systolic blood pressure readings on 15 women:

Age (x)	SBP (y)	Age (x)	SBP (y)
42	130	85	162
46	115	72	158
42	148	64	155
71	100	81	160
80	156	41	125
74	162	61	150
70	151	75	165
80	156		

Calculate the mean $\bar{x}$, variance s^2, and standard deviation s for systolic blood pressure and for age.

2.17. The ages (in days) at time of death for samples of 11 girls and 16 boys who died of sudden infant death syndrome are shown below:

Females	Males	
53	46	115
56	52	133
60	58	134
60	59	175
78	77	175
87	78	
102	80	
117	81	
134	84	
160	103	
277	114	

Calculate the mean $\bar{x}$, variance s^2, and standard deviation s for each group.

2.18. A study was conducted to investigate whether oat bran cereal helps to lower serum cholesterol in men with high cholesterol levels. Fourteen men were randomly placed on a diet which included either oat bran or corn flakes; after 2 weeks, their low-density lipoprotein cholesterol levels were recorded. Each man was then switched to the alternative diet. After a second 2-week period, the LDL cholesterol level of each individual was again recorded. The data were as follows:

	LDL (mmol/liter)	
Subject	Corn Flakes	Oat Bran
1	4.61	3.84
2	6.42	5.57
3	5.40	5.85
4	4.54	4.80
5	3.98	3.68
6	3.82	2.96
7	5.01	4.41
8	4.34	3.72
9	3.80	3.49
10	4.56	3.84
11	5.35	5.26
12	3.89	3.73
13	2.25	1.84
14	4.24	4.14

Calculate the low-density lipoprotein cholesterol level (LDL) difference (corn flake − oat bran) for each of the 14 men, then the mean $\bar{x}$, variance s^2, and standard deviation s for this sample of differences.

2.19. An experiment was conducted at the University of California at Berkeley to study the psychological environment effect on the anatomy of the brain. A group of 19 rats was randomly divided into two groups. Twelve animals in the treatment group lived together in a large cage, furnished with playthings which were changed daily, while animals in the control group lived in isolation with no toys. After a month, the experimental animals were killed and dissected. The following table gives the cortex weights (the thinking part of the brain) in milligrams:

Treatment	Control
707	669
740	650
745	651
652	627
649	656
676	642
699	698
696	
712	
708	
749	
690	

Calculate the mean $\bar{x}$, variance s^2, and standard deviation s of the cortex weight separately for each group.

2.20. Ozone levels around Los Angeles have been measured as high as 220 parts per billion (ppb). Concentrations this high can cause the eyes to burn and are a hazard to both plant and animal life. But what about other cities? The following are data (in ppb) on the ozone level obtained in a forested area near Seattle, Washington:

160	165	170	172	161
176	163	196	162	160
162	185	167	180	168
163	161	167	173	162
169	164	179	163	178

(a) Calculate $\bar{x}$, s^2, and s; compare the mean to that of Los Angeles.

(b) Calculate the coefficient of variation.

2.21. The systolic blood pressures (in mmHg) of 12 women between the ages of 20 and 35 were measured before and after administration of a newly developed oral contraceptive. Focus on the column of differences in the following table, and calculate the mean $\bar{x}$, variance s^2, and standard deviation s:

Subject	Before	After	After–Before Difference, d_i
1	122	127	5
2	126	128	2
3	132	140	8
4	120	119	−1
5	142	145	3
6	130	130	0
7	142	148	6
8	137	135	−2
9	128	129	1
10	132	137	5
11	128	128	0
12	129	133	4

2.22. A group of 12 hemophiliacs, all under 41 years of age at the time of HIV seroconversion, were followed from primary AIDS diagnosis until death (ideally we should take, as a starting point, the time at which an individual contracts AIDS rather than the time at which the patient is diagnosed, but this information is unavailable). Survival times (in months) from diagnosis until death of these hemophiliacs were: 2, 3, 6, 6, 7, 10, 15, 15, 16, 27, 30, and 32. Calculate the mean, geometric mean, and median.

2.23. Refer to the survival data for hemophiliacs in Exercise 2.22, and calculate and graph the Kaplan–Meier curve.

2.24. Suppose that we are interested in studying patients with systemic cancer who subsequently develop a brain metastasis; our ultimate goal is to prolong their lives by controlling the disease. A sample of 23 such patients, all of whom were treated with radiotherapy, were followed from the first day of their treatment until recurrence of the original tumor. Recurrence is defined as the reappearance of a metastasis in exactly the same site, or, in the case of patients whose tumor never completely disappeared, enlargement of the original lesion. Times to recurrence (in weeks) for the 23 patients were: 2, 2, 2, 3, 4, 5, 5, 6, 7, 8, 9, 10, 14, 14, 18, 19, 20, 22, 22, 31, 33, 39, 195. Calculate the mean, geometric mean, and median.

2.25. A laboratory investigator interested in the relationship between diet and the development of tumors divided 90 rats into three groups and fed them with low-fat, saturated-, and unsaturated-fat diets, respectively. The rats were the same age and species and were in similar physical condition. An identical amount of tumor cells were injected into a foot pad of each rat. The tumor-free time is the time from injection of tumor cells to the time that a tumor develops; all 30 rats in the unsaturated-fat diet group developed tumors; tumor-free times (in days) were: 112, 68, 84, 109, 153, 143, 60, 70, 98, 164, 63, 63, 77, 91, 91, 66, 70, 77, 63, 66, 66, 94, 101, 105, 108, 112, 115, 126, 161, and 178. Calculate the mean, geometric mean, and median.

2.26. Refer to tumor-free times for rats in the unsaturated-fat diet group of Exercise 2.25, and calculate and graph the Kaplan–Meier curve.

2.27. The following data are taken from a study that compares adolescents who have bulimia to healthy adolescents with similar body compositions and levels of physical activity. The following table provides measures of daily caloric intake for random samples of 23 bulimic adolescents and 15 healthy ones:

Daily Caloric Intake (kcal/kg)				
Bulimic Adolescents			Healthy Adolescents	
15.9	17.0	18.9	30.6	40.8
16.0	17.6	19.6	25.7	37.4
16.5	28.7	21.5	25.3	37.1
18.9	28.0	24.1	24.5	30.6
18.4	25.6	23.6	20.7	33.2
18.1	25.2	22.9	22.4	33.7
30.9	25.1	21.6	23.1	36.6
29.2	24.5		23.8	

(a) Calculate and compare the means.

(b) Calculate and compare the variances.

2.28. Two drugs, amantadine (A) and rimantadine (R), are being studied for use in combating the influenza virus. A single 100-mg dose is administered orally to healthy adults. The response variable is the time (in minutes) required to reach maximum concentration. Results are as follows:

Drug					
A			R		
105	123	124	221	227	280
126	108	134	261	264	238
120	112	130	250	236	240
119	132	130	230	246	283
133	136	142	253	273	516
145	156	170	256	271	
200					

(a) Calculate and compare the means.

(b) Calculate and compare the variances and the standard deviations

(c) Calculate and compare the medians.

2.29. Data are shown below for two groups of patients who died of acute myelogenous leukemia. Patients were classified into the two groups according to the presence or absence of a morphologic characteristic of white cells. Patients termed "AG positive" were identified by the presence of Auer rods and/or significant granulature of the leukemic cells in the bone marrow at diagnosis. For the AG-negative patients these factors were absent. Leukemia is a cancer characterized by an overproliferation of white blood cells; the higher the white blood count (WBC), the more severe the disease.

(AG Positive) $N = 17$		(AG Negative) $N = 16$	
White Blood Count WBC	Survival Time (weeks)	White Blood Count WBC	Survival Time (weeks)
2,300	65	4,400	56
750	156	3,000	65
4,300	100	4,000	17
2,600	134	1,500	7
6,000	16	9,000	16
10,500	108	5,300	22
10,000	121	10,000	3
17,000	4	19,000	4
5,400	39	27,000	2
7,000	143	28,000	3
9,400	56	31,000	8
32,000	26	26,000	4
35,000	22	21,000	3
100,000	1	79,000	30
100,000	1	100,000	4
52,000	5	100,000	43
100,000	65		

(a) Calculate the mean $\bar{x}$, variance s^2, and standard deviation s for survival time, separately for each group (AG positive and AG negative).

(b) Calculate the mean, geometric mean, and median for white blood count, separately for each group (AG positive and AG negative).

2.30. Refer to the survival data for acute myelogenous leukemia patients of Exercise 2.29, and calculate and graph (in the same figure) the two Kaplan–Meier curves (one for AG-positive patients and one for AG-negative patients). How do they compare?

2.31. Given the small data set

$$9, 13, 13^+, 18, 23, 28^+, 31, 34, 45^+, 48, 161^+,$$

calculate and graph the Kaplan–Meier curve.

2.32. Consider the following small *life table*:

$[t, t+1)$	d	c	n
0–1	47	19	126
1–2	5	17	60
2–3	2	15	38
3–4	2	9	21
4–5	4	6	10

Complete the table with needed columns, calculate estimated survival rates at t's using the actuarial method, and graph this estimated survival curve similar to the one shown in Figure 2.18.

2.33. In Exercise 2.25, we described a diet study and tumor-free times were given for the 30 rats fed with unsaturated-fat diet. Tumor-free times (days) for the other two groups are as follows:

Low-fat: 140, 177, 50, 65, 86, 153, 181, 191, 77, 84, 87, 56, 66, 73, 119, 140^+ and 14 rats at 200^+

Saturated-fat: 124, 58, 56, 68, 79, 89, 107, 86, 142, 110, 96, 142, 86, 75, 117, 98, 105, 126, 43, 46, 81, 133, 165, 170^+ and 6 rats at 200^+

(140^+ and 170^+ were due to accidental deaths without evidence of tumor.) Calculate and graph the two Kaplan–Meier curves, one for rats fed with low-fat diet and one for rats fed with saturated-fat diet. Put these two curves and the one from Exercise 2.26 in the same figure, and draw your conclusion.

2.34. Consider this example:

Subject	Starting	Ending	Status (A/D)
1	01/80	01/90	A
2	06/80	07/88	D
3	11/80	10/84	D
4	08/81	02/88	D
5	04/82	01/90	A
6	06/83	11/85	D
7	10/85	01/90	A
8	02/86	06/88	D
9	04/86	12/88	D
10	11/86	07/89	D

(Analysis date: 01/90; A = Alive, D = Dead)

For each subject, determine the time (in months) to death (D) or to the ending date (for survivors whose status were marked as "A"); then calculate and graph the Kaplan–Meier curve (try this using an SAS computer program if you can).

2.35. Refer to the data on systolic blood pressure (in mmHg) of 12 women in Exercise 2.21. Calculate the Pearson's correlation coefficient, the Kendall's tau and the Spearman's rho rank correlation coefficients representing the strength of the relationship between systolic blood pressures measured before and after administration of the oral contraceptive.

2.36. The following are the heights (measured to the nearest 2 cm) and the weights (measured to the nearest kg) of 10 men and 10 women.

Men:

Height:	162	168	174	176	180	180	182	184	186	186
Weight:	65	65	84	63	75	76	82	65	80	81

Women:

Height:	152	156	158	160	162	162	164	164	166	166
Weight:	52	50	47	48	52	55	55	56	60	60

(a) Draw a scatter diagram, for men and women separately, to show the association, if any, between the height and the weight.

(b) Calculate the Pearson's correlation coefficient, the Kendall's tau and the Spearman's rho rank correlation coefficients of height and weight for men and women separately.

2.37. The following data give the net food supply (x, number of calories per person per day) and the infant mortality rate (y, number of infant deaths per 1000 live births) for certain selected countries before World War I:

Country	x	y	Country	x	y
Argentina	2730	98.8	Iceland	3160	42.4
Australia	3300	39.1	India	1970	161.6
Austria	2990	87.4	Ireland	3390	69.6
Belgium	3000	83.1	Italy	2510	102.7
Burma	1080	202.1	Japan	2180	60.6
Canada	3070	67.4	New Zealand	3260	32.2
Chile	2240	240.8	Netherlands	3010	37.4
Cuba	2610	116.8	Sweden	3210	43.3
Egypt	2450	162.9	England	3100	55.3
France	2880	66.1	USA	3150	53.2
Germany	2960	63.3	Uruguay	2380	94.1

(a) Draw a scatter diagram to show the association, if any, between between the avarage daily number of calories per person and the infant mortality rate.

(b) Calculate the Pearson's correlation coefficient, the Kendall's tau, and the Spearman's rho rank correlation coefficients.

2.38. In an assay of heparin, a standard preparation is compared with a test preparation by observing the log clotting times (y, in seconds) of blood containing different doses of heparin (x is log dose, replicate readings are made at each dose level):

Log Clotting Times				
Standard		Test		Log Dose
1.806	1.756	1.799	1.763	0.72
1.851	1.785	1.826	1.832	0.87
1.954	1.929	1.898	1.875	1.02
2.124	1.996	1.973	1.982	1.17
2.262	2.161	2.140	2.100	1.32

(a) Draw a scatter diagram to show the association, if any, between the log clotting times and log dose separately for the standard preparation and the test preparation. Do they appear to be linear ?

(b) Calculate the (Pearson's) correlation coefficient for log clotting times and log dose separately for the standard preparation and the test preparation. Do they appear to be different?

2.39. When a patient is diagnosed as having cancer of the prostate, an important question in deciding on treatment strategy for the patient is whether or not the cancer has spread to the neighboring lymph nodes. The question is so critical in prognosis and treatment that it is customary to operate on the patient (i.e., perform a laparotomy) for the sole purpose of examining the nodes and removing tissue samples to examine under the microscope for evidence of cancer. However, certain variables that can be measured without surgery are predictive of the nodal involvement; and the purpose of the study presented here was to examine the data for 53 prostate cancer patients receiving surgery, to determine which of five preoperative variables are predictive of nodal involvement. Table 2.12 presents the complete data set. For each of the 53 patients, there are two continuous independent variables (i.e., preoperative factors), age at diagnosis and level of serum acid phosphatase ($\times 100$; called "acid"), and three binary variables, X-ray reading, pathology reading (grade) of a biopsy of the tumor obtained by needle before surgery, and a rough measure of the size and location of the tumor (stage) obtained by palpation with the fingers via the rectum. For these three binary independent variables a value of 1 signifies a positive or more serious state and a 0 denotes a negative or less serious finding. In addition, the sixth column presents the finding at surgery—the primary outcome of interest which is binary: A value of 1 denotes nodal involvement, and a value of 0 denotes no nodal involvement found at surgery.

In the last exercise of Chapter 1 (1.46), we investigated the effects of the three binary preoperative variables (X ray, grade, and stage); in this exercise, we focus on the effects of the two continuous factors (age and acid phosphatase). The 53 patients are divided into two groups by the finding at surgery, a group with nodal involvement and a group without (denoted by 1 or 0 in the sixth column). For each group and for each of the two factors, age at diagnosis and level of serum acid phosphatase, calculate the mean $\bar{x}$, the variance s^2, and the standard deviation s.

2.40. Refer to the data on cancer of the prostate in Exercise 2.39, investigate the relationship between age at diagnosis and level of serum acid phosphatase by calculating the Pearson's correlation coefficient and draw your conclusion. Repeat this analysis but analyze data separately for the two groups, the group with nodal involvement and the

Table 2.12. Prostate Cancer Data

X ray	Grade	Stage	Age	Acid	Nodes	X ray	Grade	Stage	Age	Acid	Nodes
0	1	1	64	40	0	0	0	0	60	78	0
0	0	1	63	40	0	0	0	0	52	83	0
1	0	0	65	46	0	0	0	1	67	95	0
0	1	0	67	47	0	0	0	0	56	98	0
0	0	0	66	48	0	0	0	1	61	102	0
0	1	1	65	48	0	0	0	0	64	187	0
0	0	0	60	49	0	1	0	1	58	48	1
0	0	0	51	49	0	0	0	1	65	49	1
0	0	0	66	50	0	1	1	1	57	51	1
0	0	0	58	50	0	0	1	0	50	56	1
0	1	0	56	50	0	1	1	0	67	67	1
0	0	1	61	50	0	0	0	1	67	67	1
0	1	1	64	50	0	0	1	1	57	67	1
0	0	0	56	52	0	0	1	1	45	70	1
0	0	0	67	52	0	0	0	1	46	70	1
1	0	0	49	55	0	1	0	1	51	72	1
0	1	1	52	55	0	1	1	1	60	76	1
0	0	0	68	56	0	1	1	1	56	78	1
0	1	1	66	59	0	1	1	1	50	81	1
1	0	0	60	62	0	0	0	0	56	82	1
0	0	0	61	62	0	0	0	1	63	82	1
1	1	1	59	63	0	1	1	1	65	84	1
0	0	0	51	65	0	1	0	1	64	89	1
0	1	1	53	66	0	0	1	0	59	99	1
0	0	0	58	71	0	1	1	1	68	126	1
0	0	0	63	75	0	1	0	0	61	136	1
0	0	1	53	76	0						

group without. Does the nodal involvement seem to have any effect on the strength of this relationship?

2.41. The purpose of this study was to examine the data for 44 physicians working for an emergency room at a major hospital so as to determine which of a number of factors are related to the number of complaints received during the previous year. In addition to the number of complaints, data available consist of the number of visits—which serves as the *size* for the observation unit, the physician—and four other factors under investigation. Table 2.13 presents the comple data set. For each of the 44 physicians there are two continuous explanatory factors, the revenue (dollars per hour) and work load at the emergency service (hours), and two binary variables, gender (Female/Male) and residency training in emergency services (No/Yes).

Divide the number of complaints by the number of visits and use this ratio (number of complaints per visit) as the primary *outcome* or *endpoint* X.

(a) For each of the two binary factors, gender (Female/Male) and residency training in emergency services (No/Yes), which divide the 44 physicians into two

Table 2.13. Emergence Service Data

Number of Visits	Complaints	Residency	Gender	Revenue	Hours
2014	2	Y	F	263.03	1287.25
3091	3	N	M	334.94	1588.00
879	1	Y	M	206.42	705.25
1780	1	N	M	226.32	1005.50
3646	11	N	M	288.91	1667.25
2690	1	N	M	275.94	1517.75
1864	2	Y	M	295.71	967.00
2782	6	N	M	224.91	1609.25
3071	9	N	F	249.32	1747.75
1502	3	Y	M	269.00	906.25
2438	2	N	F	225.61	1787.75
2278	2	N	M	212.43	1480.50
2458	5	N	M	211.05	1733.50
2269	2	N	F	213.23	1847.25
2431	7	N	M	257.30	1433.00
3010	2	Y	M	326.49	1520.00
2234	5	Y	M	290.53	1404.75
2906	4	N	M	268.73	1608.50
2043	2	Y	M	231.61	1220.00
3022	7	N	M	241.04	1917.25
2123	5	N	F	238.65	1506.25
1029	1	Y	F	287.76	589.00
3003	3	Y	F	280.52	1552.75
2178	2	N	M	237.31	1518.00
2504	1	Y	F	218.70	1793.75
2211	1	N	F	250.01	1548.00
2338	6	Y	M	251.54	1446.00
3060	2	Y	M	270.52	1858.25
2302	1	N	M	247.31	1486.25
1486	1	Y	F	277.78	933.75
1863	1	Y	M	259.68	1168.25
1661	0	N	M	260.92	877.25
2008	2	N	M	240.22	1387.25
2138	2	N	M	217.49	1312.00
2556	5	N	M	250.31	1551.50
1451	3	Y	F	229.43	973.75
3328	3	Y	M	313.48	1638.25
2927	8	N	M	293.47	1668.25
2701	8	N	M	275.40	1652.75
2046	1	Y	M	289.56	1029.75
2548	2	Y	M	305.67	1127.00
2592	1	N	M	252.35	1547.25
2741	1	Y	F	276.86	1499.25
3763	10	Y	M	308.84	1747.50

subgroups—say men and women, calculate the mean $\bar{x}$ and standard deviation s for the above endpoint X.

(b) Investigate the relationship between the outcome, number of complaints per visit, and each of the two continuous explanatory factors, the revenue (dollars per hour) and work load at the emergency service (hours), by calculating the Pearson's correlation coefficient and draw your conclusion.

(c) Draw a scatter diagram to show the association, if any, between the number of complaints per visit and work load at the emergency service. Does it appear to be linear?

2.42. There have been times that the city of London experiened periods of dense fog. The following table shows such data for a 15-day very severe period which include the number of deaths in each day (y), the mean atmospheric smoke (x_1, in mg/m^3), and the mean atmospheric sulfur dioxide content (x_2, in parts/million):

Number of Deaths	Smoke	Sulphur Dioxide
112	0.30	0.09
140	0.49	0.16
143	0.61	0.22
120	0.49	0.14
196	2.64	0.75
294	3.45	0.86
513	4.46	1.34
518	4.46	1.34
430	1.22	0.47
274	1.22	0.47
255	0.32	0.22
236	0.29	0.23
256	0.50	0.26
222	0.32	0.16
213	0.32	0.16

(a) Calculate Pearson's correlation coefficient for y and x_1 alone.

(b) Calculate Pearson's correlation coefficient for y and x_2 alone.

CHAPTER

3

Probability and Probability Models

3.1. PROBABILITY

Most of Chapter 1 dealt with proportions. A proportion is defined to represent the relative size of the portion of a population with certain (binary) characteristics. For example, *disease prevalence* is the proportion of a population with a disease. Similarly, we can talk about the proportion of positive reactors to certain screening test, the proportion of males in colleges, and so on. A proportion is used as a descriptive measure for a target population with respect to a binary or dichomous characteristic. It is a number between 0 and 1 (or 100%); the larger the number, the larger the subpopulation with the characteristic, for example, 70% male means *more* males (than 50%).

Consider now a population with certain binary characteristic. A random selection is defined as one in which each individual has an equal chance of being selected. What is the *chance* that an individual with the characteristic will be selected? (For example, what is the chance to have, say, a diseased person?) The answer depends on the size of the subpopulation to which he/she belongs, i.e., the proportion. The larger the proportion, the higher the chance (for such an individual being selected). That *chance* is measured by the proportion, a number between 0 and 1, but called the *probability*. *Proportion* measures "size," a descriptive statistic; *probability* measures "chance." When we are concerned about the outcome (still *uncertain* at this stage) with a random selection, a proportion (static, no action) becomes a probability (action about to be taken). Think of this simple example about a box containing 100 marbles, 90 of which are red and the other 10 are blue. If the question is "Are there red marbles in the box?," then someone who saw the box's contents would answer "90 percent." But if the question is "If I take one marble at random, do you think I would have a red one?," the answer would be "90% chance." The first number, 90%, represents a proportion; the second number, 90%, indicates the probability. In addition, if we keep taking random selections (called repeated sampling), the *accumulated long-term relative frequency* with which the event occurs (i.e., characteristic be observed) is *equal*

114

the proportion of the subpopulation with that characteristic. Because of this observation, sometimes *proportion* and *probability* are used interchangeably.

The following sections of this chapter deal with the concept of *probability* and some simple applications in making health decisions.

3.1.1. The Certainty of Uncertainty

Even science is uncertain. Scientists are sometimes wrong. They arrive at different conclusions in many different areas: the effects of certain food ingredients or of low-level radioactivity, the role of fats in diets, and so on. Many studies are inconclusive. For example, for decades surgeons believed that a radical mastectomy was the only treatment for breast cancer. Only recently were carefully designed clinical trials conducted to show that less drastic treatments seem equally effective.

Why is it that science is not always certain? Nature is complex and full of *unexplained biological variability*. In addition, almost all methods of observation and experiment are imperfect. Observers are subject to human bias and error. Science is a continuing story; subjects vary; measurements fluctuate. Biomedical science, in particular, contains controversy and disagreement; with the best of intentions, biomedical data—medical histories, physical examinations, interpretations of clinical tests, descriptions of symptoms and diseases—are somewhat inexact. But, most important of all, we always have to deal with incomplete information: It is either impossible, or too costly, or too time-consuming to study the entire population; we often have to rely on information gained from a *sample*—that is, a subgroup of the population under investigation. So some uncertainty almost always prevails.

Science and scientists cope with uncertainty by using the concept of *probability*. By calculating probabilities, they are able to describe what has happened and predict what should happen in the future under similar conditions.

3.1.2. Probability

The target population of a specific research effort is the entire set of subjects at which the research is aimed. For example, in a screening for cancer in a community, the target population will consist of all persons in that community who are at risk for the disease. For one cancer site, the target population might be all women over the age of 35; for another site, all men over the age of 50.

The *probability* of an event, such as a screening test being positive, in a target population is defined as the relative frequency (i.e., proportion) with which the event occurs in that target population. For example, the probability of having a disease is the disease prevalence. For another example, suppose that out of $N = 100,000$ persons of a certain target population, a total of 5500 are positive reactors to a certain screening test; then the probability of being positive, denoted by Pr(positive), is

$$\text{Pr}(\text{Positive}) = \frac{5500}{100,000}$$
$$= .055 \text{ or } 5.5\%$$

A probability is thus a descriptive measure for a target population with respect to a certain event of interest. It is a number between 0 and 1 (or 0% and 100%); the larger the number, the larger the subpopulation with the event. For the case of a continuous measurement, we have the probability of being within a certain interval. For example, the probability of a serum cholesterol level between 180 and 210 (mg/100 ml) is the proportion of people in a certain target population having their cholesterol levels falling between 180 and 210 (mg/100 ml). This is measured, in the context of a histogram of Chapter 2, by the area of a rectangular bar for the class (180–210). Now of critical importance in the interpretation of probability is the concept of random sampling so as to associate the concept of probability with uncertainty and chance.

Let the size of the target population be N (usually a very large number), a sample is any subset—say n in number ($n < N$)—of the target population. Simple random sampling from the target population is sampling so that every possible sample of size n has an equal chance of selection. For simple random sampling:

1. Each individual draw is uncertain with respect to any event or characteristic under investigation (e.g., having a disease), but
2. In repeated sampling from the population, the accumulated long-run relative frequency with which the event occurs is the population relative frequency of the event.

The physical process of random sampling can be carried out as follows (or in a fashion logically equivalent to the following steps).

Step 1: A list of all N subjects in the population is obtained. Such a list is termed a *frame* of the population. The subjects are thus available to an arbitrary numbering (e.g., from 000 to $N = 999$). The frame is often based on a directory (telephone, city, etc.) or hospital records.

Step 2: A tag is prepared for each subject carrying a number $1, 2, \ldots, N$.

Step 3: The tags are placed in a receptacle (e.g., a box) and mixed thoroughly.

Step 4: A tag is drawn blindly. The number on the tag then identifies the subject from the population; this subject becomes a member of the sample.

Steps 2 to 4 can also be implemented using a table of random numbers (Appendix A). Arbitrarily pick a 3-digit column (or 4-digit column if the population size is larger), and a number arbitrarily selected in that column serves to identify the subject from the population. In practice, this process has been computerized.

We can now link the concepts of probability and random sampling as follows. In the above example of cancer screening in a community of $N = 100,000$ persons, the calculated probability of .055 is interpreted as "the probability of a randomly drawn person from the target population having a positive test result is .055 or 5.5%." The rationale is as follows. On an initial draw the chosen subject may or may not be a positive reactor. However, if this process—of randomly drawing one subject at a time from the population—is repeated over and over again a large number of times, the accumulated long-run relative frequency of positive receptors in the sample will approximate .055.

3.1.3. Statistical Relationship

The data from the cancer screening test of Example 1.4 are reproduced here as follows:

		Test Result, X		
		+	−	Total
Disease	+	154	225	379
Y	−	362	23,362	23,724
Total		516	23,587	24,103

In this design, each member of the population is characterized by two variables: the test result X and the true disease status Y. Following our above definition, the probability of a positive test result, denoted $\Pr(X = +)$, is

$$\Pr(X = +) = \frac{516}{24,103}$$
$$= .021$$

and the probability of a negative test result, denoted $\Pr(X = -)$, is

$$\Pr(X = -) = \frac{23,587}{24,103}$$
$$= .979$$

and similarly the probabilities of having $(Y = +)$ and not having $(Y = -)$ the disease are given by

$$\Pr(Y = +) = \frac{379}{24,103}$$
$$= .015$$
$$\Pr(Y = -) = \frac{23,724}{24,103}$$
$$= .985$$

Note that the sum of the probabilities for each variable is unity:

$$\Pr(X = +) + \Pr(X = -) = 1.0$$
$$\Pr(Y = +) + \Pr(Y = -) = 1.0$$

This is an example of the *Addition Rule* of probabilities for mutually exclusive events: One of the two events $(X = +)$ or $(X = -)$ is certain to be true for a randomly selected individual from the population.

Furthermore, we can calculate the *joint probabilities*. These are the probabilities for two events—such as having the disease *and* having a positive test result—occurring simultaneously. With two variables, X and Y, there are four conditions of outcomes and the associated joint probabilities are

$$\Pr(X = +, Y = +) = \frac{154}{24,103}$$

$$= .006$$

$$\Pr(X = +, Y = -) = \frac{362}{24,103}$$

$$= .015$$

$$\Pr(X = -, Y = +) = \frac{225}{24,103}$$

$$= .009$$

and

$$\Pr(X = -, Y = -) = \frac{23,362}{24,103}$$

$$= .970$$

The second of the four joint probabilities, .015, represents the probability of a randomly drawn person from the target population having a positive test result, but being healthy (that is, a *false positive*). These joint probabilities and the above marginal probabilities separately calculated for X and Y are summarized and displayed as follows:

	X		
Y	+	−	Total
+	.006	.009	.015
−	.015	.970	.985
Total	.021	.979	1.00

Observe that the four cell probabilities add to unity, i.e., one of the four events ($X = +, Y = +$) or ($X = +, Y = -$) or ($X = -, Y = +$) or ($X = -, Y = -$) is certain to be true for a randomly selected individual from the population. Also note that the joint probabilities in each row (or column) add up to the above *marginal* or *univariate probability* at the margin of that row (or column). For example,

$$\Pr(X = +, Y = +) + \Pr(X = -, Y = +) = \Pr(Y = +)$$

$$= .015.$$

We now consider a third type of probability. For example, the *sensitivity* is expressible as

$$\text{Sensitivity} = \frac{154}{379}$$
$$= .406$$

calculated for the event $(X = +)$ using the subpopulation having $(Y = +)$. That is, of the total number of 379 individuals with cancer, the proportion with a positive test result is .406 or 40.6%. This number, denoted by $\Pr(X = + \mid Y = +)$, is called a *conditional probability* $(Y = +$ being the condition) and is related to the other two types of probability, namely,

$$\Pr(X = + \mid Y = +) = \frac{\Pr(X = +, Y = +)}{\Pr(Y = +)}$$

or

$$\Pr(X = +, Y = +) = \Pr(X = + \mid Y = +)\Pr(Y = +)$$

Clearly, we want to distinguish this conditional probability, $\Pr(X = + \mid Y = +)$, from the *marginal probability* $\Pr(X = +)$. If they are equal,

$$\Pr(X = + \mid Y = +) = \Pr(X = +)$$

the two events $(X = +)$ and $(Y = +)$ are said to be *independent* (because the condition $Y = +$ does not change the probability of $X = +$) and we have the *Multiplication Rule* for probabilities of independent events:

$$\Pr(X = +, Y = +) = \Pr(X = +)\Pr(Y = +)$$

If the two events are not independent, they have a statistical relationship or we say that they are *statistically associated*. For the above screening example,

$$\Pr(X = +) = .021$$
$$\Pr(X = + \mid Y = +) = .406$$

clearly indicating a strong statistical relationship (because $\Pr(X = + \mid Y = +) \neq \Pr(X = +)$). Of course, it makes sense to have a strong statistical relationship here, otherwise the screening is useless. However, it should be emphasized that a statistical association does not necessarily mean there is a cause and effect. Unless a relationship is so strong and so constantly repeated that the case is overwhelming, a statistical relationship, especially those observed from a sample (because the totality of population information is rarely available), is only a clue, meaning more study or confirmation is needed.

It should be noted that there are several different ways to check for the presence of a statistical relationship.

1. *Calculation of Odds Ratio.* When X and Y are independent, or not statistically associated, the odds ratio equals 1. Here we refer to the odds ratio value for the population; this value is defined as

$$\text{Odds ratio} = \frac{\frac{\Pr(X=+|Y=+)}{\Pr(X=-|Y=+)}}{\frac{\Pr(X=+|Y=-)}{\Pr(X=-|Y=-)}}$$

and can be expressed, equivalently, in terms of the joint probabilities as

$$\text{Odds ratio} = \frac{\Pr(X=+,Y=+)\,\Pr(X=-,Y=-)}{\Pr(X=+,Y=-)\,\Pr(X=-,Y=+)}$$

and the above example yields

$$\text{OR} = \frac{(.006)(.970)}{(.015)(.009)}$$
$$= 43.11$$

clearly indicating a statistical relationship.

2. *Comparison of Conditional Probability and Unconditional (or Marginal) Probability.* For example, $\Pr(X=+\mid Y=+)$ versus $\Pr(X=+)$.

3. *Comparison of Conditional Probabilities.* For example, $\Pr(X=+\mid Y=+)$ versus $\Pr(X=+\mid Y=-)$. The above screening example yields

$$\Pr(X=+\mid Y=+) = .406$$

whereas

$$\Pr(X=+\mid Y=-) = \frac{362}{23,724}$$
$$= .015$$

again clearly indicating a statistical relationship. It should also be noted that we illustrate the concepts using data from a cancer screening test, but these concepts apply to any cross-classification of two binary factors or variables. The primary aim is to determine whether a statistical relationship is present; Exercise 3.1, for example, deals with relationships between health services and race.

The next two subsections present some applications of those simple probability rules introduced in the previous section: the problem of *when* to use screening tests and the problem of *how* to measure agreement.

3.1.4. Using Screening Tests

We have introduced the concept of *conditional probability.* However, it is important to distinguish the two conditional probabilities, $\Pr(X=+\mid Y=+)$ and $\Pr(Y=+\mid X=+)$.

In Example 1.4, reintroduced in Section 3.1.3, we have

$$\Pr(X = + \mid Y = +) = \frac{154}{379}$$
$$= .406$$

whereas

$$\Pr(Y = + \mid X = +) = \frac{154}{516}$$
$$= .298$$

Within the context of screening test evaluation:

1. $\Pr(X = + \mid Y = +)$ and $\Pr(X = - \mid Y = -)$ are the sensitivity and specificity, respectively.
2. $\Pr(Y = + \mid X = +)$ and $\Pr(Y = - \mid X = -)$ are called the *positive predictivity* and *negative predictivity*.

With positive predictivity (or *positive predictive value*), the question is, given that the test X suggests cancer, what is the probability that, in fact, cancer is present? Rationales for these predictive values are that a test passes through several stages. Initially, the original test idea occurs to some researcher. It then must go through a developmental stage. This may have many aspects (in biochemistry, microbiology, etc.), one of which is in biostatistics, namely, trying the test out on a pilot population. From this developmental stage, efficiency of the test is characterized by the sensitivity and specificity. An efficient test will then go through an applicational stage with an actual application of X to a target population; and here we are concerned with its predictive values. The following simple example shows that, unlike sensitivity and specificity, the positive and negative predictive values depend not only on the efficiency of the test but also on the disease prevalence of the target population.

	Population A			Population B	
	X			Y	
Y	+	−	Y	+	−
+	45,000	5,000	+	9,000	1,000
−	5,000	45,000	−	9,000	81,000

In both cases, the test is 90% sensitive and 90% specific. However,

1. Population A has a prevalence of 50%, leading to a positive predictive value of 90%.
2. Population B has a prevalence of 10%, leading to a positive predictive value of 50%.

The conclusion is clear: If a test—even a highly sensitive and highly specific one—is applied to a target population in which the disease prevalence is low (for example, population screening for a rare disease), the positive predictive value is low. (How does this relate to an important public policy: Should we conduct random testing for AIDS?)

In the actual application of a screening test to a target population (the applicational stage), data on the disease status of individuals are not available (otherwise, screening would not be needed). However, disease prevalences are often available from national agencies and health surveys. Predictive values are then calculated from

$$\frac{\text{Positive}}{\text{predictivity}} = \frac{(\text{Prevalence})(\text{Sensitivity})}{(\text{Prevalence})(\text{Sensitivity}) + (1 - \text{Prevalence})(1 - \text{Specificity})}$$

and

$$\frac{\text{Negative}}{\text{predictivity}} = \frac{(1 - \text{Prevalence})(\text{Specificity})}{(1 - \text{Prevalence})(\text{Specificity}) + (\text{Prevalence})(1 - \text{Sensitivity})}$$

These formulas, called *Bayes' theorem*, allow us to calculate the predictive values without having data from the application stage. All we need are the disease prevalence (obtainable from federal health agencies) and sensitivity and specificity; these were obtained after the developmental stage. It is not too hard to prove these formulas using the addition and multiplication rules of probability. For example, we have

$$\Pr(Y = + \mid X = +)$$
$$= \frac{\Pr(X = +, Y = +)}{\Pr(X = +)}$$
$$= \frac{\Pr(X = +, Y = +)}{\Pr(X = +, Y = +) + \Pr(X = +, Y = -)}$$
$$= \frac{\Pr(Y = +)\Pr(X = + \mid Y = +)}{\Pr(Y = +)\Pr(X = + \mid Y = +) + \Pr(Y = -)\Pr(X = + \mid Y = -)}$$
$$= \frac{\Pr(Y = +)\Pr(X = + \mid Y = +)}{\Pr(Y = +)\Pr(X = + \mid Y = +) + (1 - \Pr(Y = +))(1 - \Pr(X = - \mid Y = -))}$$

which is the first equation for posity predictivity. You can also see, instead of going through formal proofs, our illustration of their validity using the above Population B data:

(i) Direct calculation of positive predictivity yields

$$\frac{9,000}{18,000} = .5$$

(ii) Use of prevalence, sensitivity, and specificity yields

$$\frac{(\text{Prevalence})(\text{Sensitivity})}{(\text{Prevalence})(\text{Sensitivity}) + (1 - \text{Prevalence})(1 - \text{Specificity})}$$
$$= \frac{(.1)(.9)}{(.1)(.9) + (1 - .1)(1 - .9)} = .5$$

3.1.5. Measuring Agreement

Many research studies rely on an observer's judgment to determine whether a disease, a trait, or an attribute is present or absent. For example, results of ear examinations will sure have effects on a comparison of competing treatments for ear infection. Of course, the basic concern is the issue of reliability. Section 1.1.2 and the above subsection on screening tests dealt with an important aspect of reliability, the validity of the assessment. However, in order to judge a method's validity, an exact method for classification, or a *gold standard*, must be available for the calculation of sensitivity and specificity. When an exact method is *not* available, reliability can only be judged *indirectly* in terms of *reproducibility*; the most common way for doing that is measuring the agreement between examiners.

For simplicity, assume that each of two observers independently assigns each of n items or subjects to one of two categories. The sample may then be enumerated in a 2×2 table as follows:

	Observer 2	Observer 2	
Observer 1	Cat. 1	Cat. 2	Total
Cat. 1	n_{11}	n_{12}	n_{1+}
Cat. 2	n_{21}	n_{22}	n_{2+}
Total	n_{+1}	n_{+2}	n

or, in terms of the cell probabilities;

	Observer 2	Observer 2	
Observer 1	Cat. 1	Cat. 2	Total
Cat. 1	p_{11}	p_{12}	p_{1+}
Cat. 2	p_{21}	p_{22}	p_{2+}
Total	p_{+1}	p_{+2}	1.0

Using these frequencies, we can define:

1. An overall proportion of *concordance*:

$$C = \frac{n_{11} + n_{22}}{n}$$

2. And category-specific proportions of concordance:

$$C_1 = \frac{2n_{11}}{2n_{11} + n_{12} + n_{21}}$$

$$C_2 = \frac{2n_{22}}{2n_{22} + n_{12} + n_{21}}$$

The distinction between concordance and association is that for two responses to be perfectly associated we only require that we can predict the category on one response from the category of the other response, while for two responses to have a perfect concordance, they must fall into the identical category. However, the proportions of concordance, overall or category-specific, do not measure agreement. Among other reasons, they are affected by the marginal totals. One possibility is to compare the overall concordance,

$$\theta_1 = \sum_i p_{ii}$$

where p's are the proportions in the above second 2×2 table, with the *chance concordance*,

$$\theta_2 = \sum_i p_{i+} p_{+i}$$

that occurs if the row variable is independent of the column variable, because if two events are independent, the probability of their joint occurrence is the product of their individual or marginal probabilities (the Multiplication Rule). This leads to a measure of agreement,

$$\kappa = \frac{\theta_1 - \theta_2}{1 - \theta_2}$$

called the *Kappa statistic*, $0 \leq \kappa \leq 1$, which can be expressed as

$$\kappa = \frac{2[n_{11}n_{22} - n_{12}n_{21}]}{n_{1+}n_{+2} + n_{+1}n_{2+}}$$

and the following are guidlines for the evaluation of Kappa in clinical research:

$\kappa > .75$:	*excellent*	reproducibility
$.40 \leq \kappa \leq .75$:	*good*	reproducibility
$0 \leq \kappa < .40$:	*marginal/poor*	reproducibility

In general, reproducibility not good, indicating the need for multiple assessment.

Example 3.1

Two nurses perform ear examinations focusing on the color of the eardrum (tympanic membrane); each independently assigns each of 100 ears to one of two categories: (1) normal or gray, or (2) not normal (white, pink, orange, or red). The data were:

Nurse 1	Nurse 2		Total
	Normal	Not Normal	
Normal	35	10	45
Not normal	20	35	55
Total	55	45	100

The result

$$\kappa = \frac{2[(35)(35) - (20)(10)]}{(45)(45) + (55)(55)}$$

$$= 0.406$$

indicates that the agreement is barely acceptable.

It should also be pointed out that:

1. Kappa statistic, as a measure for agreement, can also be used when there are more than two categories for classification:

$$\kappa = \frac{\sum_i p_{ii} - \sum_i p_{i+} p_{+i}}{1 - \sum_i p_{i+} p_{+i}}$$

2. We can form category-specific kappa statistics; for example, with two categories, we have

$$\kappa 1 = \frac{p_{11} - p_{1+} p_{+1}}{1 - p_{1+} p_{+1}}$$

$$\kappa 2 = \frac{p_{22} - p_{2+} p_{+2}}{1 - p_{2+} p_{+2}}$$

3. The major problem with Kappa is that it approaches zero (even with high degree of agreement) if the prevalence is near 0 or near 1.

3.2. THE NORMAL DISTRIBUTION

3.2.1. Shape of the Normal Curve

The histogram of Figure 2.1 is reproduced here as Figure 3.1 (for numerical details, see Table 2.1). A close examination shows that, in general, the relative frequencies (or densi-

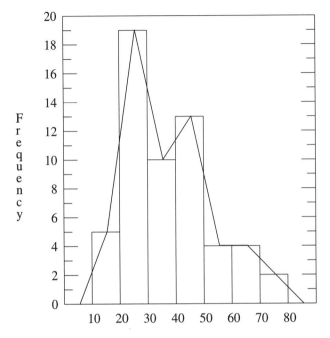

Figure 3.1. Distribution of weights of 57 children.

ties) are greatest in the vicinity of the intervals 20–29, 30–39, and 40–49, and they decrease as we go toward both extremes of the range of the measurements.

Figure 3.1 shows a distribution based on a total of 57 patients; the frequency distribution consists of intervals with a width of 10 lb. Now imagine that we increase the number of children to 50,000 and decrease the width of the intervals to .01 lb. The histogram would now look more like the one in Figure 3.2.

In Figure 3.2, the step to go from one rectangular bar to the next is very small. Finally, suppose we increase the number of children to ten million and decrease the width of the

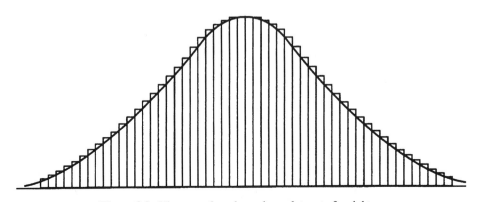

Figure 3.2. Histogram based on a large data set of weights.

interval to .00001 lb. You can now imagine a histogram with bars having practically no widths and the steps have all but disappeared. And if we continue to increase the size of the data set and decrease the interval width, we eventually arrive at a smooth curve that is superimposed on the histogram of Figure 3.2. It is called a *density curve.* You may have already heard about the normal distribution before you took a course in statistics; it is described as a bell-shaped distribution, sort of like a handlebar moustache, similar to that in Figure 3.2. The name may suggest that most distributions in nature are normal. Strictly speaking, that is false. Even more strictly speaking, they *cannot be exactly normal.* Some, such as heights of adults of a particular sex and race, are amazingly close to normal, *but never exactly.*

The normal distribution is extremely useful in statistics, but for a very different reason—not because it occurs in nature. Mathematicians proved that, for samples that are "big enough," values of their sample means $\bar{x}$ (including sample proportions as a special case) are approximately distributed as normal, even if the samples are taken from really strangely shaped distributions. This important result was called the *Central Limit Theorem.* It is as important to statistics as the understanding of germs is to the understanding of disease. Keep in mind that "normal" is just a name for this curve; if an attribute is not distributed normally, it does not imply that it is "abnormal." Many statistics texts provide statistical procedures for finding out whether a distribution is normal, but they are beyond the level of this text.

From now on, in order to distinguish samples from populations (a sample is a subgroup of a population), we adopt the following set of notations:

Quantity	Notation	
	Sample	Population
Mean	$\bar{x}$ (x-bar)	μ (mu)
Variance	s^2 (s-squared)	σ^2 (sigma-squared)
Standard deviation	s	σ
Proportion	p	π (pi)

Quantities in the third column (μ, σ^2, and π) are parameters representing numerical properties of populations; μ and σ^2 are for continuously measured information and π is for binary information. Quantities in the second column ($\bar{x}$, s^2, and p) are statistics representing summarized information from samples. Parameters are fixed (constants) but unknown, and each statistic can be used as an estimate for the parameter listed in the same row of the above table. For example, $\bar{x}$ is used as an estimate of μ; this topic will be discussed with more details in Chapter 4. A major problem in dealing with statistics, such as $\bar{x}$ and p, is that if we take a different sample—even using the same sample size—values of a statistic change from sample to sample. The *Central Limit Theorem* tells us that if sample sizes are fairly large, values of $\bar{x}$ (or p) in repeated sampling have a very nearly normal distribution. Therefore, in order to handle variability due to *chance,* so as to be able to declare—for example—that a certain observed difference is more than would occur by chance but is real, we first have to learn how to calculate probabilities associated with *normal curves.*

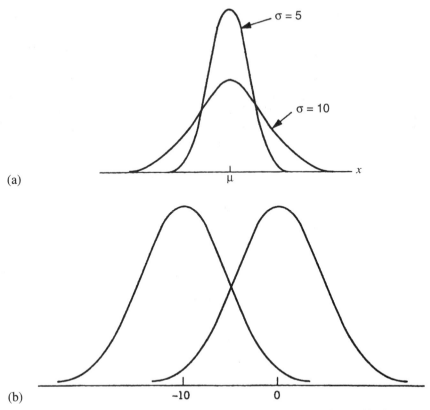

Figure 3.3. The family of normal curves. (a) Two normal distributions with the same mean but different variances. (b) Three normal distributions with the same variance but different means.

The term *normal curve*, in fact, refers not to one curve but to a family of many curves, each characterized by a mean μ and a variance σ^2. In the special case where $\mu = 0$ and $\sigma^2 = 1$, we have the *standard normal curve*. For a given μ and a given σ^2, the curve is bell-shaped with the tails dipping down to the baseline. In theory, the tails get closer and closer to the baseline but never touch it, proceeding to infinity in either direction. In practice, we ignore that and work within practical limits.

The peak of the curve occurs at the mean μ (which for this special distribution is also median and mode), and the height of the curve at the peak depends, inversely, on the variance σ^2. Figure 3.3 shows some of these curves.

3.2.2. Areas Under the Standard Normal Curve

A variable that has a normal distribution with mean $\mu = 0$ and variance $\sigma^2 = 1$ is called the *standard normal variate* and is commonly designated by the letter Z. As with any continuous variable, probability calculations here are always concerned with finding the probability that the variable assumes any value in an interval between two specific points a and b. The probability that a continuous variable assumes a value between two points a and

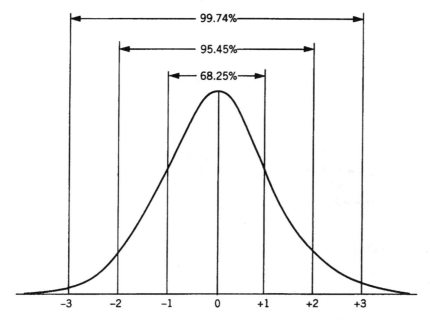

Figure 3.4. The standard normal curve and some important divisions.

b is the area under the graph of the density curve between a and b; the vertical axis of the graph represents the densities as defined in Chapter 2. The total area under any such curve is unity (or 100%) and Figure 3.4 shows the standard normal curve with some important divisions. For example, about 68% of the area is contained within ± 1, that is.

$$\Pr(-1 < z < 1) = .6826$$

and about 95% is contained within ± 2, that is,

$$\Pr(-2 < z < 2) = .9545$$

More areas under the standard normal curve have been computed and are available in tables, one of which is our Appendix B. The entries in the table of Appendix B give the area under the standard normal curve between the mean ($z = 0$) and a specified positive value of z. Graphically, it is represented by the shaded region of the following graph.

Using the table of Appendix B and the symmetric property of the standard normal curve, we will show how some other areas are computed (with access to some computer packaged program, these can be easily obtained (see Section 3.5); however, we believe that these practices do add to the learning even they may be no longer needed).

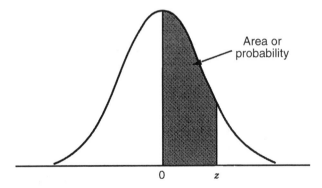

Figure 3.5. The area under standard normal curve as in Appendix B.

How to Read the Table

The entries in the table, Appendix B, give the area under the standard normal curve between zero and a positive value of z. Suppose we are interested in the area between $z = 0$ and $z = 1.35$ (numbers are first rounded off to two decimal places). To do this, first find the row marked with 1.3 in the left-hand column of the table, and then find the column marked with .05 in the top row of the table ($1.35 = 1.30 + .05$). Then looking in the body of the table, we find that the "1.30 row" and the ".05 column" intersect at the value .4115. This number, .4115, is the desired area between $z = 0$ and $z = 1.35$. A portion of Appendix B relating to these steps is shown below.

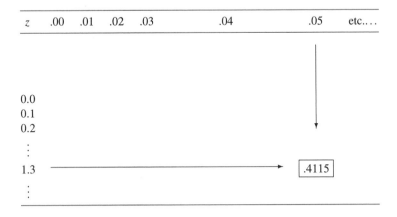

Another example: The area between $z = 0$ and $z = 1.23$ is .3907; this value is found at the intersection of the "1.2 row" and the ".03 column" of the table.

Inversely, given the area between zero and some positive value z, we can find that value of z. Suppose we are interested in a z value so that the area between zero and z is .20. To find this z value, we look into the body of the table to find the tabulated area value nearest to .20, which is .2019. This number is found at the intersection of the ".5 row" and the ".03 column." Therefore, the desired z value is .53 ($.53 = .50 + .03$).

Example 3.2

What is the probability of obtaining a z value between -1 and 1? We have

$$\Pr(-1 \leq z \leq 1) = \Pr(-1 \leq z \leq 0) + \Pr(0 \leq z \leq 1)$$
$$= 2 \times \Pr(0 \leq z \leq 1)$$
$$= (2)(.3413)$$
$$= .6826$$

which confirms the number listed in Figure 3.4. This area is shown graphically as follows:

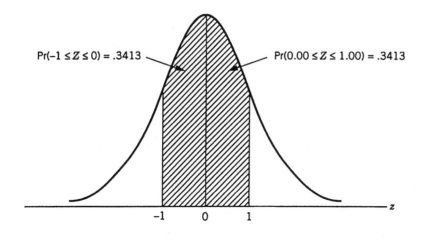

Example 3.3

What is the probability of obtaining a z value of at least 1.58? We have

$$\Pr(z \geq 1.58) = .5 - \Pr(0 \leq z \leq 1.58)$$
$$= .5 - .4429$$
$$= .0571$$

and this probability is shown below.

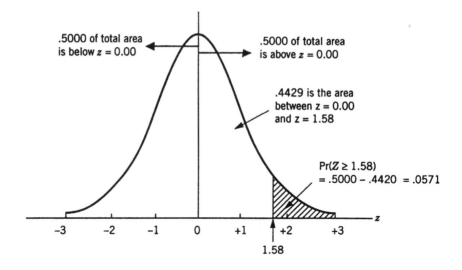

.5000 of total area is below z = 0.00

.5000 of total area is above z = 0.00

.4429 is the area between z = 0.00 and z = 1.58

Pr(Z ≥ 1.58) = .5000 − .4420 = .0571

−3   −2   −1   0   +1   +2   +3   z

1.58

Example 3.4

What is the probability of obtaining a z value of $-.5$ or larger? We have

$$\Pr(z \geq -.5) = \Pr(-.5 \leq z \leq 0) + \Pr(0 \leq z)$$
$$= \Pr(0 \leq z \leq .5) + \Pr(0 \leq z)$$
$$= .1915 + .5$$
$$= .6915$$

and this probability is shown below.

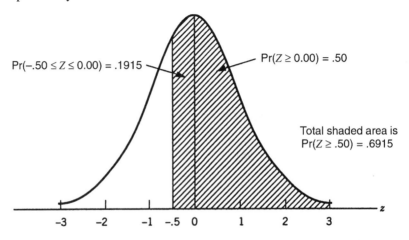

Pr(−.50 ≤ Z ≤ 0.00) = .1915

Pr(Z ≥ 0.00) = .50

Total shaded area is Pr(Z ≥ .50) = .6915

−3   −2   −1   −.5   0   1   2   3   z

Example 3.5

What is the probability of obtaining a z value between 1.0 and 1.58? We have

$$\Pr(1.0 \leq z \leq 1.58) = \Pr(0 \leq z \leq 1.58) - \Pr(0 \leq z \leq 1.0)$$
$$= .4429 - .3413$$
$$= .1016$$

and this probability is shown below.

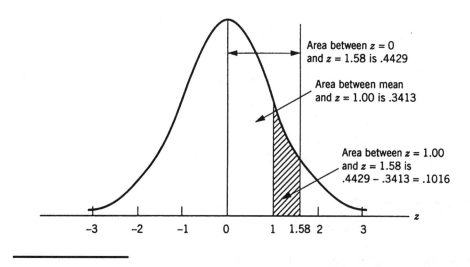

Example 3.6

Find a z value such that the probability of obtaining a larger z value is only .10. We have

$$\Pr(z \geq \, ?) = .10$$

and this is illustrated below. Scanning the table in Appendix B, we find .3997 (area between 0 and 1.28), so that

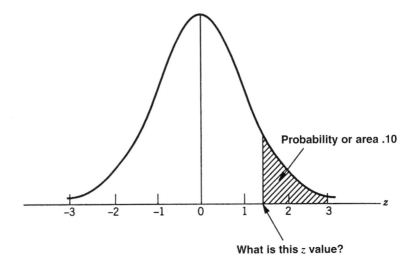

$$Pr(z \geq 1.28) = .5 - Pr(0 \leq z \leq 1.28)$$
$$= .5 - .3997$$
$$\cong .10$$

In terms of the question asked, there is approximately a .1 probability of obtaining a z value 1.28 or larger.

3.2.3. The Normal As a Probability Model

The reason we have been discussing the standard normal distribution so extensively with many examples is that probabilities for all normal distributions are computed using the standard normal distribution. That is, when we have a normal distribution with a given mean μ and a given standard deviation σ (or variance σ^2), we answer probability questions about the distribution by first converting to the standard normal viz.

$$z = \frac{x - \mu}{\sigma}$$

Here we interpret the z value (or z score) as the number of standard deviations from the mean.

Example 3.7

If the total cholesterol values for a certain target population are approximately normally distributed with a mean of 200 (mg/100 ml) and a standard deviation of 20 (mg/100 ml), then the probability that an individual picked at random from this population will have a cholesterol value greater than 240 (mg/100 ml) is

$$\Pr(x \geq 240) = \Pr\left(\frac{x - 200}{20} \geq \frac{240 - 200}{20}\right)$$

$$= \Pr(z \geq 2.0)$$

$$= .5 - \Pr(z \leq 2.0)$$

$$= .5 - .4772$$

$$= .0228 \text{ or } 2.28\%$$

Example 3.8

The following is a model for hypertension and hypotension (*Journal of the American Medical Association*, 1964). This is presented here as a simple illustration on the use of the normal distribution; the acceptance of the model itself is not universal.

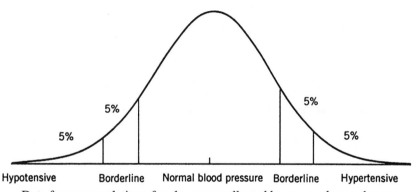

Data from a population of males were collected by age as shown above.

Means and standard deviation of systolic blood pressure
for males by age groups

Age in Years	Mean (mmHg)	Standard Deviation
16	118.4	12.17
17	121.0	12.88
18	119.8	11.95
19	121.8	14.99
20–24	123.9	13.74
25–29	125.1	12.58
30–34	126.1	13.61
35–39	127.1	14.20
40–44	129.0	15.07
45–54	132.3	18.11
55–64	139.8	19.99

From this table, using the same table of Appendix B, systolic blood pressure limits for each group can be calculated as follows:

Age	Hypotension if below	Lowest healthy	Highest healthy	Hypertension if above
16	98.34	102.80	134.00	138.46
17	99.77	104.49	137.51	142.23
18	100.11	104.48	135.12	139.49
19	97.10	102.58	141.02	146.50
20–24	?	?	?	?
25–29	?	?	?	?
30–34	103.67	108.65	143.55	148.53
35–39	103.70	108.90	145.30	150.50
40–44	104.16	109.68	148.32	153.84
45–54	102.47	109.09	155.41	162.03
55–64	106.91	114.22	165.38	172.74

For example, the highest healthy limit for the 20- to 24-year group is obtained as follows:

$$Pr(x \geq ?) = .10$$

$$= Pr\left(\frac{x - 123.9}{13.74} \geq \frac{? - 123.9}{13.74}\right)$$

and from Example 3.5 we have

$$1.28 = \frac{? - 123.9}{13.74}$$

leading to

$$? = 123.9 + (1.28)(13.74)$$

$$= 141.49$$

3.3. PROBABILITY MODELS FOR CONTINUOUS DATA

In Section 3.2 we treated the family of normal curves very informally because it was intended to reach more students and readers for whom mathematical formulas may not be very relevant. This section is aimed to provide some supplement that may be desirable for those who may be more interested in the fundamentals of biostatistical inference.

A class of measurements or a characteristic on which individual observations or measurements are made is called a *variable*. If values of a variable may theoretically lie anywhere on the numerical scale, we have a *continuous variable*; examples include weight, height, and blood pressure, among others. It can be seen from Section 3.2 that each continuous variable is characterized by a smooth *density curve*. Mathematically, a curve can be characterized by an equation of the form

$$y = f(x)$$

called probability density function, which includes one or several parameters. The probability that the variable assumes any value in an interval between two specific points a and b is given by

$$\int_a^b f(x)\, dx$$

The probability density function for the family of normal curves, sometimes referred to as the Gaussian distribution, is given by

$$f(x) = \frac{1}{\sigma\sqrt{2\pi}} \exp\left[-\frac{1}{2}\left(\frac{x-\mu}{\sigma}\right)^2\right] \qquad \text{for } -\infty < x < \infty$$

The meaning and significance of the parameters μ and σ/σ^2 have been discussed in section 3.2; μ is the mean, σ^2 is the variance, and σ is the standard deviation. When $\mu = 1$ and $\sigma^2 = 1$, we have the *standard* normal distribution. The numerical values listed in Appendix B are those given by

$$\int_0^z \frac{1}{\sqrt{2\pi}} \exp\left[-\frac{1}{2}(x)^2\right] dx$$

The normal distribution plays an important role in statistical inference because

1. Many real-life distributions are approximately normal.
2. Many other distributions can be almost normalized by appropriate data transformations (e.g., taking log). When log X has a normal distribution, X is said to have a *lognormal* distribution.
3. As a sample size increases, the means of samples drawn from a population of any distribution will approach the normal distribution. This theorem, when rigorously stated, is known as the Central Limit Theorem (more details in Chapter 4).

In addition to the normal distribution (Appendix B), topics introduced in subsequent chapters will involve three other continuous distributions:

- The t distribution (Appendix C)
- The Chi-square distribution (Appendix D)
- The F distribution (Appendix E)

The t distribution is similar to the standard normal distribution in that it is unimodal, bell-shaped, and symmetrical, it extends infinitely in either direction, and the *mean* is zero. This is a family of curves, each indexed by a number called the *degrees of freedom* (df). Given a sample of continuous data, the degrees of freedom measure the quantity of information available in a data set that can be used for estimating the population variance σ^2—that is, $(n-1)$, the denominator of s^2. The t curves have "thicker" tails as compared to the standard normal curve, and their variance is slightly greater than 1 ($= df/(df-2)$); however, the area under each curve is still equal to unity (or 100%). Areas under a curve from the right tail, shown by the shaded region, are listed in Appendix C; the t distribution for infinite degrees of freedom is precisely equal to the standard normal distribution. This equality is readily seen by examining the column marked with, say, Area $= .025$. The last row (infinite df) shows a value of 1.96, which can be verified using the table in Appendix B.

Unlike the normal and the t distributions, the chi-square and the F distributions are concerned with nonnegative attributes and will be used only for certain "tests" in Chapter 6 (chi-square distribution) and Chapter 7 (F distribution). Similar to the case of the t distribution, the formulas for the probability distribution functions of the chi-square and the F distributions are rather mathematically complex and are not presented here. Each chi-square distribution is indexed by a number called the *degrees of freedom* r. We will refer to it as "the chi-square distribution with r degrees of freedom; its mean and variance are r and $2r$, respectively. An F distribution is indexed by two degrees of freedom (m, n).

3.4. PROBABILITY MODELS FOR DISCRETE DATA

Again, a class of measurements or a characteristic on which individual observations or measurements are made is called a *variable*. If values of a variable may lie only at a few isolated points, we have a *discrete variable*; examples include race, sex, or some sort of artificial grading. Topics introduced in subsequent chapters will involve two of these discrete distributions: the binomial distribution and the Poisson distribution.

3.4.1. The Binomial Distribution

In Chapter 1 we discussed cases with dichotomous outcomes such as Male–Female, Survived–Not survived, Infected–Not infected, White–Nonwhite, or simply Positive-Negative. We have seen that such data can be summarized into proportions, rates, and ratios. In this section, we are concerned with the probability of a compound event: the occurrence of x (positive) outcomes ($0 \leq x \leq n$) in n trials, called a *binomial probability*. For example, if a certain drug is known to cause a side effect 10% of the time and if five patients are given this drug, then what is the probability that four or more experience the side effect?

Let S denote a side-effect outcome and let N an outcome without side effects. The process of determining the chance of x S's in n trials consists of listing all the possible mutually exclusive outcomes, calculating the probability of each outcome using the multiplication rule (where the trials are assumed to be independent), and then combining the probability of all those outcomes that are compatible with the desired results using the addition rule. With five patients there are 32 mutually exclusive outcomes, as shown in the table below.

Because the results for the five patients are independent, the multiplication rule produces the probabilities shown for each combined outcome. For example:

- The probability of obtaining an outcome with 4 S's and 1 N is

$$(.1)(.1)(.1)(.1)(1 - .1) = (.1)^4(.9)$$

- The probability of obtaining all 5 S's is

$$(.1)(.1)(.1)(.1)(.1) = (.1)^5$$

Because the event "all five with side effects" corresponds to only one of the 32 outcomes above and the event "four with side effects and one without" pertains to 5 of the 32 outcomes, each with probability $(.1)^4(.9)$, the addition rule yields a probability

$$(.1)^5 + (5)(.1)^4(.9) = .00046$$

for the compound event that "four or more have side effects." In general, the binomial model applies when each trial of an experiment has two possible outcomes (often referred to as "failure" and "success," or "negative" and "positive"; one has a success when the primary outcome is observed). Let the probabilities of failure and success be, respectively, $1 - \pi$ and π, and we "code" these two outcomes as 0 (zero successes) and 1 (one success). The experiment consists of n repeated trials satisfying these assumptions:

(i) The n trials are all independent;
(ii) The parameter π is the same for each trial.

The model is concerned with the total number of successes in n trials as a random variable, denoted by X. Its probability density function is given by

$$\Pr(X = x) = \binom{n}{x} \pi^x (1 - \pi)^{n-x} \qquad \text{for } x = 0, 1, 2, \ldots, n$$

where $\binom{n}{x}$ is the number of combinations of x objects selected from a set of n objects,

$$\binom{n}{x} = \frac{n!}{x!(n-x)!}$$

Outcome						Number of
First Patient	Second Patient	Third Patient	Fourth Patient	Fifth Patient	Probability	Patients Having Side Effects
S	S	S	S	S	$(.1)^5$	→ 5
S	S	S	S	N	$(.1)^4(.9)$	→ 4
S	S	S	N	S	$(.1)^4(.9)$	→ 4
S	S	S	N	N	$(.1)^3(.9)^2$	3
S	S	N	S	S	$(.1)^4(.9)$	→ 4
S	S	N	S	N	$(.1)^3(.9)^2$	3
S	S	N	N	S	$(.1)^3(.9)^2$	3
S	S	N	N	N	$(.1)^2(.9)^3$	2
S	N	S	S	S	$(.1)^4(.9)$	→ 4
S	N	S	S	N	$(.1)^3(.9)^2$	3
S	N	S	N	S	$(.1)^3(.9)^2$	3
S	N	S	N	N	$(.1)^2(.9)^3$	2
S	N	N	S	S	$(.1)^3(.9)^2$	3
S	N	N	S	N	$(.1)^2(.9)^3$	2
S	N	N	N	S	$(.1)^2(.9)^3$	2
S	N	N	N	N	$(.1)(.9)^4$	1
N	S	S	S	S	$(.1)^4(.9)$	→ 4
N	S	S	S	N	$(.1)^3(.9)^2$	3
N	S	S	N	S	$(.1)^3(.9)^2$	3
N	S	S	N	N	$(.1)^2(.9)^3$	2
N	S	N	S	S	$(.1)^3(.9)^2$	3
N	S	N	S	N	$(.1)^2(.9)^3$	2
N	S	N	N	S	$(.1)^2(.9)^3$	2
N	S	N	N	N	$(.1)(.9)^4$	1
N	N	S	S	S	$(.1)^3(.9)^2$	3
N	N	S	S	N	$(.1)^2(.9)^3$	2
N	N	S	N	S	$(.1)^2(.9)^3$	2
N	N	S	N	N	$(.1)(.9)^4$	1
N	N	N	S	S	$(.1)^2(.9)^3$	2
N	N	N	S	N	$(.1)(.9)^4$	1
N	N	N	N	S	$(.1)(.9)^4$	1
N	N	N	N	N	$(.9)^5$	0

and $n!$ is the product of the first n integers. For example,

$$3! = (1)(2)(3)$$

The mean and variance of the Binomial distribution are

$$\mu = n\pi$$
$$\sigma^2 = n\pi(1 - \pi)$$

and when the number of trials n is from moderate to large ($n > 25$, say), we we approximate the binomial distribution by a normal distribution and answer probability questions by first converting to the standard normal score

$$z = \frac{x - n\pi}{\sqrt{n\pi(1 - \pi)}}$$

where π is the probability of having a positive outcome from a single trial. For example, for $\pi = .1$ and $n = 30$, we have

$$\mu = (30)(.1)$$
$$= 3$$
$$\sigma^2 = (30)(.1)(.9)$$
$$= 2.7$$

so that

$$\Pr(x \geq 7) \cong \Pr\left(z \geq \frac{7 - 3}{\sqrt{2.7}}\right)$$
$$= \Pr(z \geq 2.43)$$
$$= .0075$$

In other words, if the true probability for having the side effect is 10%, then the probability of having 7 or more of 30 patients with the side effect is less than 1% (= .0075).

3.4.2. The Poisson Distribution

The next discrete distribution that we consider is the Poisson distribution, named after a French mathematician. This distribution has been used extensively in health science in order to model the distribution of the number of occurrences x of some random event in an interval of time or space, or some volume of matter. For example, a hospital administrator has been studying daily emergency admissions over a period of several months and has found that admissions have averaged 3 per day. He/she is then interested in finding the probability that no emergency admissions will occur on a particular day. The Poisson distribution is characterized by its probability density function:

$$Pr(X = x) = \frac{\theta^x e^{-\theta}}{x!} \qquad \text{for } x = 0, 1, 2, \ldots$$

It turns out, interestingly enough, that for a Poisson distribution the variance is equal to the mean, the above parameter θ. Therefore, we can answer probability questions by using the above formula for the Poisson density or by converting the number of occurrences x to the standard normal score, provided that $\theta \geq 10$:

$$z = \frac{x - \theta}{\sqrt{\theta}}$$

In other words, we can approximate a Poisson distribution by a normal distribution with mean θ if θ is at least 10.

Here is another example involving the Poisson distribution. The infant mortality rate (IMR) is defined as

$$IMR = \frac{d}{N}$$

for a certain target population during a given year where d is the number of deaths during the first year of life and N is the total number of live births. In the studies of IMRs, N is conventionally assumed as fixed and d is assumed to follow a Poisson distribution.

Example 3.9

For the year 1981 we have the following data for the New England states (Connecticut, Maine, Massachusetts, New Hampshire, Rhode Island, and Vermont):

$$d = 1585$$

$$N = 164,200$$

For the same year, the national infant mortality rate was 11.9 (per 1000 live births). If we apply national IMR to the New England states, then we would have

$$\theta = (11.9)(164.2)$$

$$\cong 1954 \text{ infant deaths}$$

Then the event of having as few as 1585 infant deaths would occur with a probability

$$\Pr(d \le 1{,}585) = \Pr\left(z \le \frac{1585 - 1{,}954}{\sqrt{1954}}\right)$$
$$= \Pr(z \le -8.35)$$
$$\cong 0$$

The conclusion is clear: Either we observed an extremely improbable event, or the infant mortality of New England states is lower than the national average. The observed rate for New England states was 9.7 deaths per 1000 live births.

3.5. NOTES ON COMPUTATIONS

Sections 1.4 and 2.5 covered basic techniques for Microsoft's Excel: How to open/form a spreadsheet, save it, retrieve it, and perform certain descriptive statistical tasks. Topics included data entry steps such as *select and drag*, use of *formula bar*, bar and pie charts, histograms, calculations of descriptive statistics such as mean and standard deviation, and calculation of a coefficient of correlation. This short section covers probability models focusing on the calculation of areas under density curves, especially the normal curves and the *t* curves.

Normal Curves

The first two steps are the same as in obtaining descriptive statistics (but no data are needed now): (1) Click the *paste function icon*, f*, and (2) click *Statistical*. Among functions available, two are related to the *normal curves*: NORMDIST and NORMINV. Excel provides needed information for any normal distribution, not just the standard normal distribution as in Appendix B. Upon selecting either one of the above two function, a box appears asking you to (1) provide the mean μ, (2) provide the standard deviation σ, and (3) in last row, marked with *cumulative*, enter *TRUE* (there is a choice *FALSE*, but you do not need that). The answer will appear in a *preselected* cell.

- NORMDIST gives the *area under the normal curve* (with mean and variance provided) all the way from the far left side (minus infinity) to the value *x that you have to specify*. For example, if you specify $\mu = 0$ and $\sigma = 1$; the return is the area under the standard normal curve up to the specified point (which is the same as the number from Appendix B *plus .5*).
- NORMINV performs the inverse process where *you* provide the area under the normal curve (a number between 0 and 1), together with mean μ and standard deviation σ, and requests the point x on the horizontal axis so that the area under that normal curve from the far left side (minus infinity) to the value x is equal to the provided number between 0 and 1. For example, if you put in $\mu = 0$, $\sigma = 1$, and probability $= .975$, the return is 1.96; unlike Appendix B, if you want some number in right tail of the curve, the input probability should be a number greater than .5.

The "*t*" Curves: Procedures TDIST and TINV

We want to learn how to find the areas under the normal curves so that we can determine the *p values* for statistical tests (a topic starting in Chapter 5). Another popular family in this category is the *t distributions*. Use the same first two steps: (1) Click the *paste function icon*, f*, and (2) click *Statistical*. Among functions available, two are related to the *t distributions*: TDIST and TINV. Similar to the case of NORMDIST and NORMINV, TDIST gives the *area under the t curve* and TINV performs the inverse process where you provide the area under the curve and requests for the point *x* on the horizontal axis. In each case you have to provide the *degrees of freedom*. In addition, in last row, marked with *tails*, enter

- (Tails =) *1* if you want *one-sided* and
- (Tails =) *2* if you want *two-sided*
  (more details on the concepts of one-sided and two-sided areas are in Chapter 5). For example:
- Example 1: If you enter
  (*x* =) *2.73*
  (deg freedom =) *18*, and
  (Tails =) *1*
  you're requesting the area under a "*t*" curve with 18 degrees of freedom and *to the right* of 2.73 (i.e., right tail); the answer is .00687.
- Example 2: If you enter
  (*x* =) *2.73*
  (deg freedom =) *18*, and
  (Tails =) *2*
  you're requesting the area under a "*t*" curve with 18 degrees of freedom and *to the right* of 2.73 and *to the left* of − 2.73 (i.e., both right and left tails); the answer is .01374, which is twice the previous answer of .00687.

EXERCISES

3.1. Although cervical cancer is not a leading cause of death among American women, it has been suggested that virtually all such deaths are preventable (5166 American women died from cervical cancer in 1977). In an effort to find out who is being or not being screened for cervical cancer (Pap testing), the following data were collected from a certain community:

Pap Test	White	Black	Total
No	5,244	785	6,029
Yes	25,117	2348	27,465
Total	30,361	3133	33,494

Is there a statistical relationship here? (Try a few different methods: calculation of odds ratio, comparison of conditional and unconditional probabilities, and comparison of conditional probabilities.)

3.2. In a study of intraobserver variability in assessing cervical smears, 3325 slides were screened for the presence or absence of abnormal squamous cells. Each slide was screened by a particular observer and then re-screened 6 months later by the same observer. The results are as follows:

First Screening	Second Screening		
	Present	Absent	Total
Present	1763	489	2252
Absent	403	670	1073
Total	2166	1159	3325

Is there a statistical relationship between first screening and second screening? (Try a few different methods as in the previous exercise.)

3.3. From the above intraobserver variability study, find

(a) The probability that abnormal squamous cells were found to be absent in both screenings.

(b) The probability of an absence in the second screening given that abnormal cells were found in the first screening.

(c) The probability of an abnormal presence in the second screening given that no abnormal cells were found in the first screening.

(d) The probability that the screenings disagree.

3.4. Given the screening test of Example 1.4, where

$$\text{Sensitivity} = .406$$
$$\text{Specificity} = .985,$$

calculate the positive predictive values when the test is applied to the following populations:

Population A: 80% prevalence

Population B: 25% prevalence

3.5. Consider the following data on the use of X ray as a screening test for tuberculosis.

| | Tuberculosis | |
X ray	No	Yes
Negative	1739	8
Positive	51	22
Total	1790	30

(a) Calculate the sensitivity and specificity.

(b) Find the disease prevalence.

(c) Calculate the positive predictive value both directly and indirectly using Bayes' theorem.

3.6. From the sensitivity and specificity of X rays found in exercise 3.5, compute the positive predictive value corresponding to these prevalences: .2, .4, .6, .7, .8, and .9. Can we find a prevalence when the positive predictive value is preset at .80 or 80%?

3.7. Refer to the standard normal distribution. What is the probability of obtaining a z value of

(a) at least 1.25?

(b) at least $-.84$?

3.8. Refer to the standard normal distribution. What is the probability of obtaining a z value

(a) between -1.96 and 1.96?

(b) between 1.22 and 1.85?

(c) between $-.84$ and 1.28?

3.9. Refer to the standard normal distribution. What is the probability of obtaining z value

(a) less than 1.72?

(b) less than -1.25?

3.10. Refer to the standard normal distribution. Find a z value such that the probability of obtaining a larger z value is

(a) .05;

(b) .025;

(c) .20.

3.11. Verify the numbers in the first two rows of the Table in Example 3.7; for example, show that the lowest healthy systolic blood pressure for 16 year old boys is 102.8.

3.12. Complete the table in Example 3.8 at the question marks.

3.13. Medical research has concluded that individuals experience a common cold roughly two times per year. Assume that the time between colds is normally distributed with a mean of 160 days and a standard deviation of 40 days.

(a) What is the probability of going 200 or more days between colds? Of going 365 or more days?

(b) What is the probability of getting a cold within 80 days of a previous cold?

3.14. Assume that the test scores for a large class are normally distributed with a mean of 74 and a standard deviation of 10.

(a) Suppose you receive a score of 88. What percent of the class received scores higher than yours?

(b) Suppose the teacher wants to limit the number of A grades in the class to no more than 20%. What would be the lowest score for an A?

3.15. Intelligence test scores, referred to as *intelligence quotient* or IQ scores, are based on characteristics such as verbal skills, abstract reasoning power, numerical ability, and spatial visualization. If plotted on a graph, the distribution of IQ scores approximates a normal curve with a mean of about 100. An IQ score above 115 is considered superior. Studies of "intellectually gifted" children have generally defined the lower limit of their IQ scores at 140; approximately 1% of the population have IQ scores above this limit. (Based on "Your Intelligence Quotient" by Tom Biracree in *How You Rate*, New York: Dell Publishing Co. Inc., 1984.)

(a) Find the standard deviation of this distribution.

(b) What percent are in the "superior" range of 115 or above?

(c) What percent of the population have IQ scores of 70 or below?

3.16. IQ scores for college graduates are normally distributed with a mean of 120 (as compared to 100 for the general population) with a standard deviation of 12. What is the probability of randomly selecting a graduate student with an IQ score

(a) between 110 and 130?

(b) above 140?

(c) below 100?

3.17. Suppose it is known that the probability of recovery for a certain disease is .4. If 35 people are stricken with the disease, what is the probability that

(a) 25 or more will recover?

(b) fewer than 5 will recover?

(use the normal approximation)

3.18. A study found that for 60% of the couples who have been married 10 years or less, both spouses work. A sample of 30 couples who have been married 10 years or less are selected from marital records available at a local courthouse. We are interested in the number of couples in this sample in which both spouses work. What is the probability that this number is

(a) 20 or more?

(b) 25 or more?

(c) 10 or fewer?

(use the normal approximation)

3.19. Many samples of water, all the same size, are taken from a river suspected of having been polluted by irresponsible operators at a sewage treatment plant. The number of coliform organisms in each sample was counted; the average number of organisms per sample was 15. Assuming the number of organisms to be Poisson-distributed, find the probability that

(a) The next sample will contain at least 20 organisms.

(b) The next sample will contain no more than 5 organisms.

3.20. For the year 1981 (see Example 3.8), we also have the following data for the South Atlantic states (Delaware, Florida, Georgia, Maryland, North and South Carolina, Virginia, and West Virginia, and the District of Columbia):

$$d = 7,643 \text{ infant deaths}$$

$$N = 550,300 \text{ live births}$$

Find the infant mortality rate, and compare it to the national average using the method of Example 3.9.

3.21. For the t curve with 20 df, find the areas

(a) To the left of 2.086 and of 2.845

(b) To the right of 1.725 and of 2.528

(c) Beyond ± 2.086 and beyond ± 2.845

3.22. For the Chi square distribution with 2 df, find the areas

(a) To the right of 5.991 and of 9.210

(b) To the right of 6.348

(c) Between 5.991 and 9.210

3.23. For the F distribution with 2 numerator dfs and 30 denominator dfs, find the areas

(a) To the right of 3.32 and of 5.39

(b) To the right of 2.61

(c) Between 3.32 and 5.39

3.24. In a study of intraobserver variability in assessing cervical smears, 3325 slides were screened for the presence or absence of abnormal squamous cells. Each slide was screened by a particular observer and then rescreened 6 months later by the same observer. The results are as follows:

First Screening	Second Screening		Total
	Present	Absent	
Present	1763	489	2252
Absent	403	670	1073
Total	2,166	1,159	3,325

Calculate the kappa statistic representing the agreement between the two screenings.

3.25. Ninety-eight heterosexual couples, at least one of whom was HIV-infected, were enrolled in an HIV transmission study and interviewed about sexual behavior. The following table provides a summary of condom use reported by heterosexual partners:

Woman	Man Ever	Man Never	Total
Ever	45	6	51
Never	7	40	47
Total	52	46	98

How strongly do the couples agree?

4

Confidence Estimation

The whole process of statistical design and analysis can be described briefly as follows. The target of a scientist's investigation is a population with a certain characteristic of interest—for example, a man's systolic blood pressure or his cholesterol level, or whether a leukemia patient respond to an investigative drug. A numerical characteristic of a target population is called a *parameter*; for example, the population mean μ (average SBP) or the population proportion π (a drug's response rate). Most of the times it would be too time-consuming or too costly to obtain the totality of population information in order to learn about the parameter(s) of interest. For example, there are millions of men in a target population to survey, and the value of the information may not justify the high cost. Sometimes the population does not even exist. For example, in the case of an investigative drug for leukemia, we are interested in *future* patients as well as present patients. To deal with the problem, the researcher may decide to take a sample or to conduct a small phase II clinical trial. Chapters 1 and 2 provide methods by which we can learn about data from the sample or samples. We learned how to organize data, how to summarize data, and how to present them. The topic of probability in Chapter 3 sets the framework for dealing with uncertainties. By this point, the researcher is ready to draw inferences about the population of his interest based on what he or she learned from his/her sample(s). Depending on the research's objectives, we can classify inferences into two categories: one in which we want to estimate the value of a parameter—for example, the response rate of a leukemia investigative drug—and one where we want to compare the parameters for two subpopulations using statistical tests of significance. For example, we want to know whether men have higher cholesterol level, on the average, than women. This chapter deals with the first category and the statistical procedure called *estimation*. It is extremely useful, one of the most useful procedures of statistics. The word "estimate" actually has a language problem, the opposite of the language problem of statistical "tests" (the topic of Chapter 5). The colloquial meaning of the word "test" makes one think that statistical tests are especially objective, no-nonsense procedures that reveal the truth. Conversely, the colloquial meaning of the word "estimate" is that of guessing, perhaps off the top of the head and uninformed, not to be taken too seriously. It is used by car body repair shops, who "estimate" how much it will cost to fix your car after an accident. The "estimate" in that case is actually a bid of a for-profit business establishment seeking your trade. In our case, the word "estimation" is used in the usual sense that provides a "substitute" for an unknown truth, but it isn't that bad a choice of word, once you understand *how* to do it. But it is important to make it clear that statistical estimation is no less objective than any other formal statistical procedure; statistical estimation requires calculations and tables just as statistical testing does. In addition, it is very important to differentiate formal statistical estimation from ordinary guessing. In formal statistical estimation, we can determine the *amount of uncertainty* (and so the error) in the estimate. How often have you heard of someone making a guess and then giving you a number measuring the "margin of error" of the guess? That's what statistical estimation does. It gives you the best guess and then tells you how "wrong" the guess could be, in quite precise terms. Certain media, sophisticated newspapers in particular, are starting to educate the public about statistical estimation. They do it when they report the results of polls. They say things like, "74% of the voters disagree with the governor's budget proposal," and then go on to say that the margin error is plus or minus 3%. What they are saying is that whoever conducted the poll is claiming to have polled about 1000 people chosen at random and that statistical estimation theory tells us to be 95% certain that if *all* the voters were polled, their disagreement percentage would be discovered to be within 3% of 74%. In other words, it's very unlikely that the 74% is off the mark by more than 3%; the truth is almost certainly between 71% and 77%. In subsequent sections of this chapter, we will introduce the strict interpretation of these so-called *confidence intervals*.

4.1. BASIC CONCEPTS

A class of measurements or a characteristic on which individual observations or measurements are made is called a *variable* or *random variable*. The value of a random variable varies from subject to subject; examples include weight, height, blood pressure, or the presence or absence of a certain habit or practice, such as smoking or use of drugs. The distribution of a random variable is often assumed to belong to a certain family of distributions such as binomial, Poisson, or normal. This assumed family of distributions is specified or indexed by one or several parameters such as a population mean μ or a population proportion π. It is usually either impossible, too costly, or too time-consuming to obtain the entire population data on any variable in order to learn about a parameter involved in its distribution. Decisions in health science are thus often made using a small sample of a population. The problem for a decision maker is to decide on the basis of data the estimated value of a parameter, such as the population mean, as well as to provide certain ideas concerning errors associated with that estimate.

4.1.1. Statistics As Variables

A parameter is a numerical property of a population; examples include population mean μ and population proportion π. The corresponding quantity obtained from a sample is called a *statistic*; examples of statistics include the sample mean $\bar{x}$ and sample proportion p. Statistics help us draw inferences or conclusions about population parameters. After a sample has already been obtained, the value of a statistic—for example, the sample mean $\bar{x}$—is known and fixed; however, if we take a different sample, we almost certainly have a different numerical value for that same statistic. In this repeated sampling context, a statistic is looked upon as a variable that takes different values from sample to sample.

4.1.2. Sampling Distributions

The distribution of values of a statistic obtained from repeated samples of the same size from a given population is called the *sampling distribution* of that statistic.

Example 4.1

Consider a population consisting of six subjects (this small size is impractical, but we need something small enough to use as an illustration here); the following table gives the subject names (for identification) and values of a variable under investigation (for example, 1 for a smoker and 0 for a nonsmoker):

Subject	Value
A	1
B	1
C	1
D	0
E	0
F	0

In this case the population mean μ (also population proportion π for this very special dichotomous variable) is .5 ($= 3/6$). We now consider all *possible* samples, without replacement, of size 3; none or some or all subjects in each sample have value "1," the remaining "0." The following table represents the sampling distribution of the sample mean:

Samples	Number of Samples	Value of Sample Mean $\bar{x}$
(D, E, F)	1	0
(A, D, E), (A, D, F), (A, E, F) (B, D, E), (B, D, F), (B, E, F) (C, D, E), (C, D, F), (C, E, F)	9	1/3
(A, B, D), (A, B, E), (A, B, F) (A, C, D), (A, C, E), (A, C, F) (B, C, D), (B, C, E), (B, C, F)	9	2/3
(A, B, C)	1	1
Total	20	

This sampling distribution gives us a few interesting properties:

(i) Its mean—that is, the mean of *all possible* sample means—is

$$\frac{(1)(0) + (9)(1/3) + (9)(2/3) + (1)(1)}{20} = .5$$

which is the same as the mean of the original distribution. Because of this we say that the sample mean (sample proportion) is an *unbiased estimator* for the population mean (population proportion). In other words, if we use the sample mean (sample proportion) to estimate the population mean (population proportion), we are *correct on the average*.

(ii) If we form a bar graph for this sampling distribution,

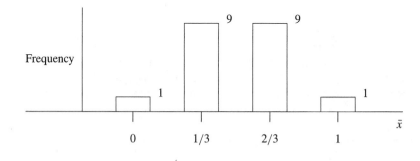

it shows a shape somewhat similar to that of a symmetric, bell-shaped normal curve. This resemblance is much clearer with real populations and larger sample sizes.

We now consider the same population and all possible samples of size $n = 4$. The following table represents the new sampling distribution:

Samples	Number of Samples	Value of Sample Mean $\bar{x}$
(A, D, E, F), (B, D, E, F), (C, D, E, F)	3	.25
(A, B, D, E), (A, B, D, F), (A, B, E, F) (A, C, D, E), (A, C, D, F), (A, C, E, F) (B, C, D, E), (B, C, D, F), (B, C, E, F)	9	.50
(A, B, C, D), (A, B, C, E), (A, B, C, F)	3	.75
Total	15	

It can be seen that we have a different sampling distribution because the sample size is different. However, we still have both above-mentioned properties:

(i) Unbiasedness of the sample mean

$$\frac{(3)(.25) + (9)(.50) + (3)(.75)}{15} = .5$$

(ii) Normal shape of the sampling distribution (bar graph)

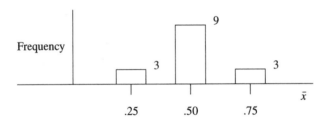

In addition, we can see that

(iii) the variance of the new distribution is smaller. The two faraway values of $\bar{x}$, 0 and 1, are no longer possible; new values—.25 and .75—are closer to the mean .5 and the majority (9 samples) have values that are right at the sampling distribution mean. The major reason for this is that the new sampling distribution is associated with a larger sample size, $n = 4$ as compared to $n = 3$ of the previous sampling distribution.

4.1.3. Introduction to Confidence Estimation

Statistical inference is the procedure whereby inferences about a population are made on the basis of the results obtained from a sample drawn from that population.

Professionals in health science are often interested in a parameter of a certain population. For example, a health professional may be interested in knowing what proportion of a certain type of individual, treated with a particular drug, suffers undesirable side effects. The process of estimation entails calculating, from the data of a sample, some statistic that is offered as an estimate of the corresponding parameter of the population from which the sample was drawn.

A point estimate is a single numerical value used to estimate the corresponding population parameter. For example, the sample mean is a point estimate for the population mean, and the sample proportion is a point estimate for the population proportion. However, having access to the data of a sample and a knowledge of statistical theory, we can do more than just providing a point estimate. The sampling distribution of a statistic—if available—would provide information on

(i) Biasedness/unbiasedness—several statistics, such as $\bar{x}$, p, and s^2 are unbiased
(ii) Variance

Variance is important; a small variance for a sampling distribution indicates that most possible values for the statistic are close to each other so that a particular value is more likely to be reproduced. In other words, the variance of a sampling distribution of a statistic can be used as a measure of precision or reproducibility of that statistic; the smaller this quantity, the better the statistic as an estimate of the corresponding parameter. The square root of this variance is called the *standard error* of the statistic; for example, we will have the standard error of the sample mean, or $SE(\bar{x})$, standard error of the sample proportion, $SE(p)$, and so on. It is the same quantity, but we use the term *standard deviation* for measurements and the term *standard error* when we refer to the standard deviation of a statistic. In the next few sections, we will introduce a process whereby the point estimate and its standard error are combined to form an interval estimate or a *confidence interval*. A confidence interval consists of two numerical values defining an interval which, with a specified degree of confidence, we believe includes the parameter being estimated.

4.2. ESTIMATION OF MEANS

The results of Example 4.1 are not coincidences but are examples of the characteristics of sampling distributions in general. The key tool here is the *central limit theorem*, introduced in Section 3.2.1, which may be summarized as follows:

Given any population with mean μ and variance σ^2, the sampling distribution of $\bar{x}$ will be approximately normal with mean μ and variance σ^2/n when the sample size n is large (of course, the larger the sample size, the better the approximation; in practice, an $n = 25$ or more could be considered adequately large). This means we have the two properties

$$\mu_{\bar{x}} = \mu$$
$$\sigma_{\bar{x}}^2 = \sigma^2/n.$$

as seen in Example 4.1.

The following example will show how good $\bar{x}$ is as an estimate for the population μ even if the sample size is as small as 25 (of course, it is used only as an illustration; in practice, μ and σ^2 are unknown).

Example 4.2

Birth weights obtained from deliveries over a long period of time at a certain hospital show a mean μ of 112 ounces and a standard deviation σ of 20.6 ounces. Let us suppose we want to compute the probability that the mean birth weight from a sample of 25 infants will fall between 107 and 117 ounces (i.e., the estimate is off the mark by no more than 5 ounces).

The Central Limit Theorem is applied, and it indicates that $\bar{x}$ follows a normal distribution with mean

$$\mu_{\bar{x}} = 112$$

and variance

$$\sigma_{\bar{x}}^2 = (20.6)^2/25$$

or standard error

$$\sigma_{\bar{x}} = 4.12.$$

It follows that

$$Pr(107 \le \bar{x} \le 117) = Pr\left(\frac{107 - 112}{4.12} \le z \le \frac{117 - 112}{4.12}\right)$$

$$= Pr(-1.21 \le z \le 1.21)$$

$$= (2)(.3869)$$

$$= .7738$$

In other words, if we use the mean of a sample of size $n = 25$ to estimate the population mean, about 80% of the time we are correct within 5 ounces; this figure would be 98.5% if the sample size is 100.

4.2.1. Confidence Intervals for a Mean

Similar to what was done in Example 4.2 we can write, for example,

$$Pr\left[-1.96 \le \frac{\bar{x} - \mu}{\sigma/\sqrt{n}} \le 1.96\right] = (2)(.475)$$

$$= .95$$

This statement is a consequence of the Central Limit Theorem which indicates that, for a large sample size n, $\bar{x}$ is a random variable (in the context of repeated sampling) with a normal sampling distribution in which

$$\mu_{\bar{x}} = \mu$$
$$\sigma_{\bar{x}}^2 = \sigma^2/n$$

The quantity inside the square bracket of the above equation is equivalent to

$$\bar{x} - 1.96\sigma/\sqrt{n} \le \mu \le \bar{x} + 1.96\sigma/\sqrt{n}$$

All we need to do now is to select a random sample, calculate the numerical value of $\bar{x}$ and its standard error with σ replaced by sample variance s, $s/\sqrt{n}$, and substitute these values to form the endpoints of the interval,

$$\bar{x} \pm 1.96s/\sqrt{n}$$

In a specific numerical case this will produce two numbers,

$$a = \bar{x} - 1.96s/\sqrt{n}$$

and

$$b = \bar{x} + 1.96s/\sqrt{n}$$

and we have the interval

$$a \le \mu \le b$$

But here we run into a logical problem. We are sampling from a fixed population. We are examining values of a random variable obtained by selecting a random sample from that fixed population. The random variable has a distribution with mean μ that we wish to estimate. Because the population and the distribution of the random variable we are investigating are fixed, it follows that the parameter μ is fixed. The quantities μ, a, and b are all fixed (after the sample has been obtained); then we cannot assert the probability that μ lies between a and b is .95. In fact, either μ lies in (a, b) or it does not, and it is not correct to assign a probability to the statement (even the truth remains unknown).

The difficulty here arises at the point of substitution of the observed numerical values for $\bar{x}$ and its standard error. The random variation in $\bar{x}$ is variation from sample to sample in the context of repeated sampling. When we substitute $\bar{x}$ and its standard error $s/\sqrt{n}$ by their numerical values resulting in interval (a, b), it is understood that the repeated sampling process could produce many different intervals of the same form:

$$\bar{x} \pm 1.96\text{SE}(\bar{x})$$

About 95% of these intervals would actually include μ. Because we have only one of these possible intervals, that is the interval (a, b) from our sample, we say we are 95% confident that μ lies between these limits. The interval (a, b) is called a *95% confidence interval* for μ, and the figure "95" is called the *degree of confidence* or *confidence level*.

In forming confidence intervals, the degree of confidence is determined by the investigator of a research project. Different investigators may prefer different confidence intervals; the coefficient to be multiplied with the standard error of the mean should be determined accordingly. Here are a few typical choices; 95% is the most conventional:

Degree of Confidence	Coefficient
99%	2.576
$\longrightarrow$ 95%	1.960
90%	1.645
80%	1.282

Finally, it should be noted that because the standard error is

$$\text{SE}(\bar{x}) = s/\sqrt{n}$$

the width of a confidence interval becomes narrower as sample size increases, and the above process is applicable only to large samples ($n > 25$, say). The next section will show how to handle smaller samples (there is nothing magic about "25"; see note at the end of the Section 4.2.2).

_____

Example 4.3

For the data on percentage saturation of bile for 31 male patients of Example 2.4

40, 86, 111, 86, 106, 66, 123, 90, 112, 52, 88, 137, 88, 88, 65, 79, 87, 56, 110, 106, 110, 78, 80, 47, 74, 58, 88, 73, 118, 67, 57

we have

$$n = 31$$
$$\bar{x} = 84.65$$
$$s = 24.00$$

leading to a standard error

$$\text{SE}(\bar{x}) = 24.00/\sqrt{31}$$
$$= 4.31$$

and a 95% confidence interval for the population mean

$$84.65 \pm (1.96)(4.31) = (76.2, 93.1)$$

(The resulting interval is wide due to a large standard deviation as observed from the sample, $s = 24.0$, reflecting heterogeneity of sample subjects.)

4.2.2. Uses of Small Samples

The procedure in the previous section for confidence intervals is applicable only to large samples (say, $n > 25$). For smaller samples, the results are still valid if the population variance σ^2 is known and the standard error is expressed as $\sigma/\sqrt{n}$. However, σ^2 is almost always unknown. When σ is unknown, we can estimate it by s, but the procedure has to be modified by changing the coefficient to be multiplied by the standard error to accommodate the error in estimating σ by s; how much larger the coefficient is depends on how much information we have in estimating σ (by s), that is, the sample size n.

Therefore, instead of taking coefficients from the standard normal distribution table (numbers such as 2.576, 1.960, 1.645, and 1.282 for degrees of confidence 99%, 95%, 90%, and 80%), we will use corresponding numbers from the t curves where the quantity of information is indexed by the degree of freedom (df $= n - 1$). The figures are listed in Appendix C; the column to read is the one with the correct normal coefficient on the bottom row (marked with df $= \infty$). For example, if the degree of confidence is .95, we have

df	t coefficient (percentile)
5	2.571
10	2.228
15	2.131
20	2.086
24	2.064
$\rightarrow \infty$	1.960

(For better results, it is a good practice to always use the t table regardless of sample size because coefficients such as 1.96 are only for very large sample sizes.)

Example 4.4

In an attempt to assess the physical condition of joggers, a sample of $n = 25$ joggers was selected and maximum volume oxygen (VO_2) uptake was measured with the following results:

$$\bar{x} = 47.5 \text{ ml/kg}$$

$$s = 4.8 \text{ ml/kg}$$

$$SE(\bar{x}) = 4.8/\sqrt{25}$$

$$= .96$$

From Appendix C we find that the t coefficient with 24 df for use with a 95% confidence interval is 2.064, leading to a 95% confidence interval for the population mean μ (this is the population of joggers' VO$_2$ uptake) of

$$47.5 \pm (2.064)(.96) = (45.5, 49.5)$$

_____

_____

Example 4.5

In addition to the data in Example 4.4, we have data from a second sample consisting of 26 nonjoggers which were summarized into these statistics:

$$n_2 = 26$$

$$\bar{x}_2 = 37.5 \text{ ml/kg}$$

$$s_2 = 5.1 \text{ ml/kg}$$

$$SE(\bar{x}) = 5.1/\sqrt{26}$$

$$= 1.0$$

From Appendix C we find that the t coefficient with 25 df for use with a 95% confidence interval is 2.060, leading to a 95% confidence interval for the population mean μ (this is the population of non-joggers' VO$_2$ uptake) of

$$37.5 \pm (2.060)(1.0) = (35.4, 39.6)$$

_____

4.2.3. Evaluation of Interventions

In efforts to determine the effect of a risk factor or an intervention, we may want to estimate the _difference of means_—say, between the population of cases and the population of controls. However, we choose not to present the methodology with much details at this level with one exception, the case of matched design or before-and-after intervention where each experimental unit serves as its own control. This design makes it possible to control for confounding variables that are difficult to measure—for example, environmental exposure—and therefore difficult to adjust at the analysis stage. The main reason to include this method here, however, is because we treat the data as one sample and the aim is still estimating the (population) mean. That is, data from matched or before-and-after experiments should not be considered as coming from two independent samples. The procedure is to reduce the data to a one-sample problem by computing before-and-after (or control-and-case) difference for each subject (or pairs of matched subjects). By doing this with paired observations, we get a set of differences that can be handled as a single sample problem. The mean to be estimated, using the sample of differences, represents the effects of the intervention (or the effects of of the disease) under investigation.

Example 4.6

The systolic blood pressures of 12 women between the ages of 20 and 35 were measured before and after administration of a newly developed oral contraceptive. Given the data in Table 4.1 we have from the column of differences, the d_i's,

$$n = 12$$
$$\sum d_i = 31$$
$$\sum d_i^2 = 185.$$

Table 4.1. Systolic blood pressure in mm Hg

Subject	Before	After	After–Before Difference, d_i	d_i^2
1	122	127	5	25
2	126	128	2	4
3	132	140	8	64
4	120	119	−1	1
5	142	145	3	9
6	130	130	0	0
7	142	148	6	36
8	137	135	−2	4
9	128	129	1	1
10	132	137	5	25
11	128	128	0	0
12	129	133	4	16

leading to

$$\bar{d} = \text{Average difference}$$
$$= 31/12$$

$$= 2.58 \text{ mmHg}$$

$$s^2 = \frac{185 - (31)^2/12}{11}$$

$$= 9.54$$

$$s = 3.09$$

$$\text{SE}(\bar{d}) = 3.09/\sqrt{12}$$

$$= .89$$

With a degree of confidence of .95 the t coefficient from Appendix C is 2.201 for 11 degrees of freedom, so that a 95% confidence interval for the mean difference is

$$2.58 \pm (2.201)(.89) = (.62, 4.54)$$

That means the "after" mean is larger than the "before" mean, an increase of between .62 and 4.54.

In many other interventions, or in studies to determine possible effects of a risk factor, it may not be possible to employ matched design. The comparison of means is based on data from two independent samples. The process of estimating the *difference of means* is briefly summarized as follows:

(i) Data are summarized separately to obtain

$$\begin{array}{ll} \text{Sample 1:} & n_1, \bar{x}_1, s_1^2 \\ \text{Sample 2:} & n_2, \bar{x}_2, s_2^2 \end{array}$$

(ii) Standard error of the difference of means is given by

$$\text{SE}(\bar{x}_1 - \bar{x}_2) = \sqrt{\frac{s_1^2}{n_1} + \frac{s_2^2}{n_2}}$$

(iii) Finally, a 95% confidence interval for the difference of population means, $\mu_1 - \mu_2$, can be calculated from the formula

$$(\bar{x}_1 - \bar{x}_2) \pm (\text{Coefficient})\text{SE}(\bar{x}_1 - \bar{x}_2)$$

where the coefficient is 1.96 if $n_1 + n_2$ is large; otherwise, a t coefficient is used with approximately

$$\text{df} = n_1 + n_2 - 2$$

4.3. ESTIMATION OF PROPORTIONS

The sample proportion is defined as in Chapter 1,

$$p = \frac{x}{n}$$

where x is the number of positive outcomes and n is the sample size. However, it can also be expressed as

$$p = \frac{\sum x_i}{n}$$

where x_i is "1" if the ith outcome is positive and "0" otherwise. In other words, a sample proportion can be viewed as a special case of sample means where data are coded as 0/1; and because of this, the Central Limit Theorem applies: The sampling distribution of p will be approximately normal when the sample size n is large. In this context, that of the proportion viewed as a sample mean $\bar{x}$, its standard error is still derived using the same process:

$$SE(p) = \frac{s}{\sqrt{n}}$$

with a standard deviation s to be determined. First, we can write out s using the following shortcut formula of Chapter 2—but with denominator n instead of $(n-1)$ (this would make little difference because we always deal with *large* samples of binary data):

$$s = \sqrt{\frac{\sum x_i^2 - \frac{(\sum x_i)^2}{n}}{n}}$$

Because x_i is binary, with "1" if the ith outcome is positive and "0" otherwise, we have

$$x_i^2 = x_i$$

and, therefore,

$$s = \sqrt{\frac{\sum x_i - \frac{(\sum x_i)^2}{n}}{n}}$$
$$= \sqrt{\frac{\sum x_i}{n}(1 - \frac{\sum x_i}{n})}$$
$$= \sqrt{p(1-p)}$$

In other words, the standard error of the sample proportion is calculated from

$$SE(p) = \sqrt{p(1-p)/n}.$$

To state it more formally, the Central Limit Theorem implies that the sampling distribution of p will be approximately normal when the sample size n is large; the mean and variance of this sampling distribution are

$$\mu_p = \pi$$

and

$$\sigma_p^2 = \frac{\pi(1 - \pi)}{n}$$

respectively, where π is the population proportion.

Example 4.7

Suppose the true proportion of smokers in a community is known to be in the vicinity of $\pi = .4$, and we want to estimate it using a sample of size $n = 100$.

The Central Limit Theorem indicates that p follows a normal distribution with mean

$$\mu_p = .40$$

and variance

$$\sigma_p^2 = \frac{(.4)(.6)}{100}$$

or standard error

$$\sigma_p = .049$$

Suppose we want our estimate to be correct within $\pm 3\%$; it follows that

$$Pr(.37 \le p \le .43) = Pr\left(\frac{.37 - .40}{.049} \le z \le \frac{.43 - .40}{.049}\right)$$

$$= Pr(-.61 \le z \le .61)$$

$$= (2)(.2291)$$

$$= .4582, \text{ or approximately } 46\%$$

That means if we use the proportion of smokers from a sample of $n = 100$ to estimate the true proportion of smokers, only about 46% of the time we are correct within $\pm 3\%$; this figure would be 95.5% if the sample size is raised to $n = 1000$. What we learn from this example is that, as compared to the case of continuous data in Example 4.2, it may take a much larger sample to have a good estimate of a proportion such as a disease prevalence or a drug side effect.

From this sampling distribution of the sample proportion, in the context of repeated sampling, we have an approximate 95% confidence interval for a population proportion π:

$$p \pm 1.96\text{SE}(p)$$

where, again, the standard error of the sample proportion is calculated from

$$\text{SE}(p) = \sqrt{p(1-p)/n}.$$

There are no easy ways for small samples; this is applicable only to larger samples ($n > 25$, n should be much larger for a narrow intervals; procedures for small samples are rather complicated and are not covered in this book).

Example 4.8

Consider the problem of estimating the prevalence of malignant melanoma in 45 to 54-year-old women in the United States. Suppose a random sample of $n = 5000$ women is selected from this age group and $x = 28$ are found to have the disease. Our point estimate for the prevalence of this disease is

$$p = \frac{28}{5000}$$
$$= .0056$$

Its standard error is

$$\text{SE}(p) = \sqrt{(.0056)(1 - .0056)/5000}$$
$$= .0011$$

Therefore, a 95% confidence interval for the prevalence π of malignant melanoma in 45 to 54-year-old women in the United States is given by

$$.0056 \pm (1.96)(.0011) = (.0034, .0078)$$

Example 4.9

A public health official wishes to know how effective health education efforts are regarding smoking. Of $n_1 = 100$ males sampled in 1965 at the time of the release of the Surgeon General's Report on the health consequences of smoking, $x_1 = 51$ were found to be smokers. In 1980 a second random sample of $n_2 = 100$ males, similarly gathered, indicated that $x_2 = 43$ were smokers. Application of the above method yields the following 95% confidence intervals for the smoking rates:

(i) In 1965, the estimated rate was

$$p_1 = \frac{51}{100}$$
$$= .51$$

with its standard error

$$SE(p_1) = \sqrt{(.51)(1 - .51)/100}$$
$$= .05$$

leading to a 95% confidence interval of

$$.51 \pm (1.96)(.05) = (.41, .61)$$

(ii) In 1980, the estimated rate was

$$p_2 = \frac{43}{100}$$
$$= .43$$

with its standard error

$$SE(p_2) = \sqrt{(.43)(1 - .43)/100}$$
$$= .05$$

leading to a 95% confidence interval of

$$.43 \pm (1.96)(.05) = (.33, .53)$$

It can be seen that the two confidence intervals, one for 1965 and one for 1980, are both quite long and overlapped, even though the estimated rates show a decrease of 8% in smoking rate, because the sample sizes are rather small.

_____

_____

Example 4.10

A study was conducted to look at the effects of oral contraceptives (OC) on heart disease in women 40–44 years of age. It is found that among $n_1 = 5000$ current OC users, 13 develop a myocardial infarction (MI) over a 3-year period, while among $n_2 = 10,000$ non-OC users, 7 develop an MI over a 3-year period. Application of the above method yields the following 95% confidence intervals for the MI rates:

(i) For OC users, the estimated rate was

$$p_1 = \frac{13}{5,000}$$
$$= .0026$$

with its standard error

$$SE(p_2) = \sqrt{(.0026)(1 - .0026)/5000}$$
$$= .0007$$

leading to a 95% confidence interval of

$$.0026 \pm (1.96)(.0007) = (.0012, .0040)$$

(ii) For non-OC users, the estimated rate was

$$p_2 = \frac{7}{10,000}$$
$$= .0007$$

with its standard error

$$SE(p_2) = \sqrt{(.0007)(1 - .0007)/10,000}$$
$$= .0003$$

leading to a 95% confidence interval of

$$.0007 \pm (1.96)(.0003) = (.0002, .0012)$$

It can be seen that the two confidence intervals, one for OC users and one for non-OC users, do not overlap, a strong indication that the two population MI rates are likely not the same.

In many trials for interventions, or in studies to determine possible effects of a risk factor, the comparison of proportions is based on data from two independent samples. However, the process of constructing two confidence intervals separately, one from each sample, as briefly mentioned at the end of the last few examples is not efficient. The reason is that the *overall confidence* level may no longer be, say, 95% as intended because the process involves *two* separate inferences; possible errors may add up. The estimation of the *difference of proportions* should be formed using the following formula (for a 95% confidence interval):

$$(p_1 - p_2) \pm (1.96)\text{SE}(p_1 - p_2)$$

where

$$\text{SE}(p_1 - p_2) = \sqrt{p_1(1 - p_1)/n_1 + p_2(1 - p_2)/n_2}$$

4.4. ESTIMATION OF ODDS RATIOS

So far we have relied heavily on The Central Limit Theorem in forming confidence intervals for the means (Section 4.2) and the proportions (Section 4.3). The Central Limit Theorem stipulates that, as a sample size increases, the means of samples drawn from a population of any distribution will approach the normal distribution, and a proportion can be seen as a special case of the means. Even when the sample sizes are not large, because many real-life distributions are approximately normal, we still can form confidence intervals for the means (see Section 4.2.2 on the uses of small samples).

Besides the mean and the proportion, we have had two other statistics of interest, the *odds ratio* and the (Pearson's) *coefficient of correlation*. However, the method used to form confidence intervals for the means and the proportions does not directly apply to the case of these two new parameters. The sole reason is that they do not have the backing of the Central Limit Theorem. The sampling distributions of the (sample) odds ratio and (sample) coefficient of correlation are positively skewed. Fortunately, these sampling distributions can be almost normalized by an appropriate data transformation—in these cases, by taking the logarithm. Therefore, we will learn to form confidence intervals on the log scale; then taking antilogs of the two endpoints, a method has been used in Chapter 2 in order to obtain the *geometric mean*. In this section, we present in details such a method for the calculation of confidence intervals for odds ratios.

Data from a case–control study, for example, may be summarized in a 2 × 2 table:

Exposure	Cases	Controls
Exposed	a	c
Unexposed	b	d

We have:

(i) The odds that a case was exposed is

$$\text{Odds for cases} = \frac{a}{b}$$

(ii) The odds that a control was exposed is

$$\text{Odds for controls} = \frac{c}{d}$$

Therefore, the (observed) odds ratio from the samples is

$$\text{OR} = \frac{\frac{a}{b}}{\frac{c}{d}}$$

$$= \frac{ad}{bc}$$

Confidence intervals are derived from the normal approximation to the sampling distribution of $\ln(\text{OR})$ with variance:

$$\text{Variance}[\ln(\text{OR})] \cong \frac{1}{a} + \frac{1}{b} + \frac{1}{c} + \frac{1}{d}$$

Consequently, an approximate 95% confidence interval, on the log scale, for odds ratio is given by

$$\ln\frac{ad}{bc} \pm 1.96\sqrt{\frac{1}{a} + \frac{1}{b} + \frac{1}{c} + \frac{1}{d}}$$

(again, "ln" is logarithm to base e, also called the "natural" logarithm.) A 95% confidence interval for the odds ratio under investigation is obtained by *exponentiating* (the reverse log operation or antilog) the two endpoints:

$$\ln\frac{ad}{bc} - 1.96\sqrt{\frac{1}{a} + \frac{1}{b} + \frac{1}{c} + \frac{1}{d}}$$

and

$$\ln\frac{ad}{bc} + 1.96\sqrt{\frac{1}{a} + \frac{1}{b} + \frac{1}{c} + \frac{1}{d}}$$

Example 4.11

The role of smoking in pancreatitis has been recognized for many years; the following are data from a case–control study carried out in Eastern Massachusetts and Rhode Island (1975–1979; see Example 1.10).

Use of Cigarettes	Cases	Controls
Current smokers	38	81
Ex-smokers	13	80
Never	2	56

We have

(i) For ex-smokers, compared to those who never smoked,

$$OR = \frac{(13)(56)}{(80)(2)}$$
$$= 4.55$$

and a 95% confidence interval for the population odds ratio on the log scale is from

$$\ln 4.55 - 1.96\sqrt{\frac{1}{13} + \frac{1}{56} + \frac{1}{80} + \frac{1}{2}} = -.01$$

to

$$\ln 4.55 + 1.96\sqrt{\frac{1}{13} + \frac{1}{56} + \frac{1}{80} + \frac{1}{2}} = 3.04$$

and, hence, the corresponding 95% confidence interval for the population odds ratio is $(.99, 20.96)$.

(ii) For current smokers, compared to those who never smoked,

$$OR = \frac{(38)(56)}{(81)(2)}$$
$$= 13.14$$

and a 95% confidence interval for the population odds ratio on the log scale is from

$$\ln 13.14 - 1.96\sqrt{\frac{1}{38} + \frac{1}{56} + \frac{1}{81} + \frac{1}{2}} = 1.11$$

to

$$\ln 13.14 + 1.96\sqrt{\frac{1}{38} + \frac{1}{56} + \frac{1}{81} + \frac{1}{2}} = 4.04$$

and, hence, the corresponding 95% confidence interval for the population odds ratio is $(3.04, 56.70)$.

Example 4.12

Toxic shock syndrom (TSS) is a disease first recognized in the 1980s, characterized by sudden onset of high fever (> 102°), vomiting, diarrhea, rapid progression to hypotension, and, in most cases, shock. Because of the striking association with menses, several studies have been undertaken to look at various practices associated with the menstrual cycle. In a study by the Center for Disease Control, 30 of 40 TSS cases and 30 of 114 controls who used a single brand of tampons used "Rely" brand. Data are presented in a 2-by-2 table as follows:

Brand	Cases	Controls
Rely	30	30
Others	10	84
Total	40	114

We have

$$OR = \frac{(30)(84)}{(10)(30)}$$
$$= 8.4$$

and a 95% confidence interval for the population odds ratio on the log scale is from

$$\ln 8.4 - 1.96\sqrt{\frac{1}{30} + \frac{1}{10} + \frac{1}{30} + \frac{1}{84}} = 1.30$$

to

$$\ln 8.4 + 1.96\sqrt{\frac{1}{30} + \frac{1}{10} + \frac{1}{30} + \frac{1}{84}} = 2.96$$

and, hence, the corresponding 95% confidence interval for the population odds ratio is (3.67, 19.30), indicating a very high risk elevation for Rely users.

4.5. ESTIMATION OF CORRELATION COEFFICIENTS

Similar to the case of the odds ratio, the sampling distribution of the (Pearson's) coefficient of correlation is also positively skewed. After completing our descriptive analysis (Section 2.4 of Chapter 2), information about a possible relationship between two continuous factors are sufficiently contained in two statistics: the number of pairs of data n (sample size) and the (Pearson's) coefficient of correlation r (which is a number between 0 and 1).

Confidence intervals are then derived from the normal approximation to the sampling distribution of

$$z = \frac{1}{2} \ln \left\{ \frac{(1+r)}{(1-r)} \right\}$$

with variance of approximately

$$\text{Variance}(z) = \frac{1}{n-3}$$

Consequently, an approximate 95% confidence for correlation coefficient interval, on this newly transformed scale, for the Pearson's correlation coefficient is given by

$$z \pm 1.96 \sqrt{\frac{1}{n-3}}$$

(again, "ln" is logarithm to base e, also called the "natural" logarithm.) A 95% confidence interval (r_l, r_u) for the coefficient of correlation under investigation is obtained by transforming the two endpoints

$$z_l = z - 1.96 \sqrt{\frac{1}{n-3}}$$

and

$$z_u = z + 1.96 \sqrt{\frac{1}{n-3}}$$

as follows to obtain the lower endpoint

$$r_l = \frac{[\exp(2z_l) - 1]}{[\exp(2z_l) + 1]}$$

and the upper endpoint of the confidence interval for the population coefficient of correlation

$$r_u = \frac{[\exp(2z_u) - 1]}{[\exp(2z_u) + 1]}$$

(in these formulas, "exp" is the exponentiation, or anti-natural log, operation).

Example 4.13

The following data represent systolic blood pressure readings on 15 women:

Age (x)	SBP (y)	Age (x)	SBP (y)
42	130	85	162
46	115	72	158
42	148	64	155
71	100	81	160
80	156	41	125
74	162	61	150
70	151	75	165
80	156		

The descriptive analysis in Example 2.12 yields $r = .566$, and we have

$$z = \frac{1}{2} \ln \left\{ \frac{(1 + .566)}{(1 - .566)} \right\}$$

$$= .642$$

$$z_l = .642 - 1.96\sqrt{\frac{1}{12}}$$

$$= .076$$

$$z_u = .642 + 1.96\sqrt{\frac{1}{12}}$$

$$= 1.207$$

$$r_l = \frac{[\exp(.152) - 1]}{[\exp(.152) + 1]}$$

$$= .076$$

$$r_u = \frac{[\exp(2.414) - 1]}{[\exp(2.414) + 1]}$$

$$= .836$$

or a 95% confidence interval for the population coefficient of correlation of $(.076, .836)$, indicating a positive association between a woman's age and her systolic blood pressure; that is, older women are likely to have higher systolic blood pressure (it is just a coincidence that $z_l = r_l$).

Example 4.14

The following tables give the values for the birth weight (x) and the increase in weight between the 70th and 100th days of life, expressed as a percentage of the birth weight (y)

for 12 infants:

x (oz)	y (%)
112	63
111	66
107	72
119	52
92	75
80	118
81	120
84	114
118	42
106	72
103	90
94	91

The descriptive analysis in Example 2.11 yields $r = -.946$ and we have

$$z = \frac{1}{2}\ln\left\{\frac{(1-.946)}{(1+.946)}\right\}$$

$$= -1.792$$

$$z_l = .014 - 1.96\sqrt{\frac{1}{9}}$$

$$= -2.446$$

$$z_u = .014 + 1.96\sqrt{\frac{1}{9}}$$

$$= -1.139$$

$$r_l = \frac{[\exp(-4.892) - 1]}{[\exp(-4.892) + 1]}$$

$$= -.985$$

$$r_u = \frac{[\exp(-2.278) - 1]}{[\exp(-2.278) + 1]}$$

$$= -.814$$

or a 95% confidence interval for the population coefficient of correlation of $(-.985, -.814)$, indicating a very strong negative association between a baby's birth weight and his or her increase in weight between the 70th and 100th days of life; that is, smaller babies are likely to growth faster during that period (that may be why, at 3 months, most babies look the same size).

4.6. NOTES ON COMPUTATIONS

All the computations for confidence intervals can be put together using a calculator, even though some are quite tedious—especially the confidence intervals for odds ratios and coefficients of correlation. Descriptive statistics, such as mean $\bar{x}$ and standard deviation s, can be obtained with the help of Excel (see Section 2.5). Standard normal and "t" coefficients can be obtained with the help of Excel too (see Section 3.5). If you try the first two usual steps—that is, (1) click the *paste function icon*, f*, and (2) click *Statistical*—among the functions available you will find CONFIDENCE, which is intended for forming confidence intervals. But it is not worth the effort: The process is only for 95% confidence intervals of the mean using a large sample with coefficient 1.96, and you still need to enter sample mean, standard deviation, and sample size.

EXERCISES

4.1. Consider a population consisting of four subjects—A, B, C, and D—with the following values for a random variable X under investigation:

Subject	Value
A	1
B	1
C	0
D	0

Form the sampling distribution for the sample mean of size $n = 2$ and verify that

$$\mu_{\bar{x}} = \mu$$

Then repeat the process with sample size of $n = 3$.

4.2. The body mass index (kg/m^2) is calculated by dividing a person's weight by the square of his/her height and is used as a measure of the extent to which the individual is overweight. Suppose the distribution of the body mass index for men has a standard deviation of $\sigma = 3 \, kg/m^2$, and we wish to estimate the mean μ using a sample of size $n = 49$. Find the probability that we would be correct within $1 \, kg/m^2$.

4.3. Self-reported injuries among left-handed and right-handed people were compared in a survey of 1896 college students in British Columbia, Canada. 93 of the 180 left-handed students reported at least one injury and 619 of the 1716 right-handed students reported at least one injury in the same period. Calculate the 95% confidence interval for the proportion of students with at least one injury for each of the two subpopulations, left-handed students and right-handed students.

4.4. A study was conducted in order to evaluate the hypothesis that tea consumption and premenstrual syndrome are associated. One hundred eighty-eight nursing students and 64 tea factory workers were given questionnaires. The prevalence of premenstrual syndrome was 39% among the nursing students and 77% among the tea factory workers. Calculate the 95% confidence interval for the prevalence of premenstrual syndrome for each of the two populations, nursing students and tea factory workers.

4.5. A study was conducted to investigate drinking problems among college students. In 1983, a group of students were asked whether they had ever driven an automobile while drinking. In 1987, after the legal drinking age was raised, a different group of college students were asked the same question. The results are as follows:

Drove While Drinking	Year		Total
	1983	1987	
Yes	1250	991	2241
No	1387	1666	3053
Total	2637	2657	5294

Calculate, separately for 1983 and 1987, the 95% confidence interval for the proportion of students who had driven an automobile while drinking.

4.6. In August 1976, tuberculosis was diagnosed in a high school student (INDEX CASE) in Corinth, Mississippi. Subsequently, laboratory studies revealed that the student's disease was caused by drug-resistant tubercule bacilli. An epidemiologic investigation was conducted at the high school.

The following table gives the rates of positive tuberculin reaction, determined for various groups of students according to degree of exposure to the index case.

Exposure level	Number Tested	Number Positive
High	129	63
Low	325	36

Calculate the 95% confidence interval for the rate of positive tuberculin reaction separately for each of the two subpopulations, those with high exposure and those with low exposure.

4.7. The prevalence rates of hypertension among adult (ages 18–74) white and black Americans were measured in the second National Health and Nutrition Examination Survey, 1976–1980. Prevalence estimates (and their standard errors) for women are given below:

Race	$p(\%)$	$SE(p)$
Whites	25.3	0.9
Blacks	38.6	1.8

Calculate and compare the 95% confidence intervals for the proportions of the two groups, blacks and whites, and draw an appropriate conclusion. Do you need the sample sizes to do your calculations? Why or why not?

4.8. Consider the following data:

| | Tuberculosis | | |
X Ray	No	Yes	Total
Negative	1739	8	1747
Positive	51	22	73
Total	1790	30	1820

Calculate the 95% confidence intervals for the sensitivity and specificity of X ray as a screening test for tuberculosis.

4.9. Sera from a T-lyphotropic virus type (HTLV-I) risk group (prostitute women) were tested with two commercial "research" enzyme-linked immunoabsorbent assays (EIA) for HTLV-I antibodies. These results were compared with a gold standard, and outcomes are shown below.

| | Dupont's EIA | | | Cellular Product's EIA | |
TRUE	Positive	Negative	TRUE	Positive	Negative
Positive	15	1	Positive	16	0
Negative	2	164	Negative	7	179

Calculate the 95% confidence intervals for the sensitivity and specificity separately for the two EIAs.

4.10. In a seroepidemiologic survey of health workers representing a spectrum of exposure to blood and patients with hepatitis B virus (HBV), it was found that infection increased as a function of contact. The following table provides data for hospital workers with uniform socioeconomic status at an urban teaching hospital in Boston, Massachusetts.

Personnel	Exposure	n	HBV Positive
Physicians	Frequent	81	17
	Infrequent	89	7
Nurses	Frequent	104	22
	Infrequent	126	11

Calculate the 95% confidence intervals for the proportions of HBV positive workers in each subpopulation.

4.11. Consider the data taken from a study that attempts to determine whether the use of electronic fetal monitoring (EFM) during labor affects the frequency of caesarean section deliveries. Of the 5,824 infants included in the study, 2850 were electronically monitored and 2974 were not. The outcomes are as follows:

Caesarean Delivery	EFM Exposure		
	Yes	No	Total
Yes	358	229	587
No	2492	2745	5237
Total	2850	2974	5824

(a) Use the data from the group without EFM exposure, calculate the 95% confidence interval for the proportion of caesarean delivery.

(b) Calculate the 95% confidence interval for the odds ratio representing the relationship between EFM exposure and caesarean delivery.

4.12. A study was conducted to investigate the effectiveness of bicycle safety helmets in preventing head injury. The data consist of a random sample of 793 individuals who were involved in bicycle accidents during a one-year period.

Head Injury	Wearing Helmet		
	Yes	No	Total
Yes	17	218	235
No	130	428	558
Total	147	646	793

(a) Using the data from the group without helmets, calculate the 95% confidence interval for the proportion of head injury.

(b) Calculate the 95% confidence interval for the odds ratio representing the relationship between use (or not use) of helmet and head injury.

4.13. A case–control study was conducted in Auckland, New Zealand to investigate the effects of alcohol consumption on both nonfatal myocardial infarction and coronary death in the 24 hours after drinking, among regular drinkers. Data were tabulated separately for men and women.

(a) Men

Drink in the Last 24 hr	Myocardial Infarction		Coronary Death	
	Controls	Cases	Controls	Cases
No	197	142	135	103
Yes	201	136	159	69

(b) Women

Drink in the Last 24 hr	Myocardial Infarction		Coronary Death	
	Controls	Cases	Controls	Cases
No	144	41	89	12
Yes	122	19	76	4

(a) Refer to myocardial infarction (table on the left) and calculate the 95% confidence interval for the odds ratio associated with drinking, separately for men and women.

(b) Refer to coronary deaths (table on the right) and calculate the 95% confidence interval for the odds ratio associated with drinking, separately for men and women.

(c) From the results in (a) and/or (b), is there any indication that *gender* may act as an effect modifier?

4.14. Adult male residents of 13 counties of western Washington state in whom testicular cancer had been diagnosed during 1977–1983 were interviewed over the telephone regarding their history of genital tract conditions, including vasectomy. For comparison, the same interview was given to a sample of men selected from the population of these counties by dialing telephone numbers at random. The following data are tabulated by religious background.

Religion	Vasectomy	Cases	Controls
Protestant	Yes	24	56
	No	205	239
Catholic	Yes	10	6
	No	32	90
Others	Yes	18	39
	No	56	96

Calculate the 95% confidence interval for the odds ratio associated with vasectomy for each religious group. Is there any evidence of an effect modification?

4.15. A case–control study was conducted relating to the epidemiology of breast cancer and the possible involvement of dietary fats, along with other vitamins and nutrients. It included 2024 breast cancer cases who were admitted to Roswell Park Memorial

Institute, Erie County, New York, from 1958 to 1965. A control group of 1463 was chosen from the patients having no neoplasms and no pathology of gastrointestinal or reproductive systems. The primary factors being investigated were vitamins A and E (measured in international units per month). The following are data for 1500 women over 54 years of age.

Vitamin A (IU/mo)	Cases	Controls
≤ 150,500	893	392
> 150,500	132	83
Total	1025	475

(a) Calculate the 95% confidence interval for the proportion among the controls who consumed at least 150,500 international units of vitamin A per month.

(b) Calculate the 95% confidence interval for the odds ratio associated with vitamin A deficiency.

4.16. A study was undertaken to investigate the roles of blood-borne environmental exposures on ovarian cancer from assessment of consumption of coffee, tobacco, and alcohol. Study subjects consist of 188 women in the San Francisco Bay area with epithelial ovarian cancers diagnosed in 1983–1985, along with 539 control women. Of the 539 controls, 280 were hospitalized women without overt cancer, and 259 were chosen from the general population by random telephone dialing. Data for coffee consumption are summarized as follows:

Coffee Drinkers	Cases	Hospital Controls	Population Controls
No	11	31	26
Yes	177	249	233

Calculate the odds ratio and its 95% confidence interval for

(a) Cases versus hospital controls

(b) Cases versus population controls

4.17. Postneonatal mortality due to respiratory illnesses is known to be inversely related to maternal age, but the role of young motherhood as a risk factor for respiratory morbidity in infants has not been thoroughly explored. A study was conducted in Tucson, Arizona aimed at the incidence of lower respiratory tract illnesses during the first year of life. In this study, over 1200 infants were enrolled at birth between 1980 and 1984 and the following data are concerned with wheezing lower respiratory tract illnesses (wheezing LRI): No/Yes.

Maternal Age	Boys		Girls	
(years)	No	Yes	No	Yes
< 21	19	8	20	7
21–25	98	40	128	36
26–30	160	45	148	42
> 30	110	20	116	25

Using "> 30" as the baseline, calculate the odds ratio and its 95% confidence interval for each other maternal age group; do it separately for boys and girls.

4.18. Data were collected from 2197 white ovarian cancer patients and 8893 white controls in 12 different U.S. case–control studies conducted by various investigators in the period 1956–1986. These were used to evaluate the relationship of invasive epithelial ovarian cancer to reproductive and menstrual characteristics, exogenous estrogen use, and prior pelvic surgeries. The following are parts of the data:

(a)

Duration of Unprotected Intercourse (years)	Cases	Controls
< 2	237	477
2–9	166	354
10–14	47	91
≥ 15	133	174

Using "< 2" as the baseline, calculate the odds ratio and its 95% confidence interval for each other level of exposure.

(b)

History of Infertility	Cases	Controls
No	526	966
Yes		
No drug use	76	124
Drug use	20	11

Using "no history of infertility" as the baseline, calculate the odds ratio and its 95% confidence interval for each group with a history of infertility.

4.19. Consider this data taken from a study that examines the response to ozone and sulfur dioxide among adolescents suffering from asthma. The following are measurements of forced expiratory volume (liters) for 10 subjects:

{3.50, 2.60, 2.75, 2.82, 4.05, 2.25, 2.68, 3.00, 4.02, 2.85}

Calculate the 95% confidence interval for the (population) mean of forced expiratory volume (liters).

4.20. The percentage of ideal body weight was determined for 18 randomly selected insulin-dependent diabetics. The outcomes (%) are:

107	119	99	114	120	104	124	88	114
116	101	121	152	125	100	114	95	117

Calculate the 95% confidence interval for the (population) mean of the percentage of ideal body weight.

4.21. A study on birthweight provided the following data (in ounces) on 12 newborns:

$$\{112, 111, 107, 119, 92, 80, 81, 84, 118, 106, 103, 94\}$$

Calculate the 95% confidence interval for the (population) mean of the birthweight.

4.22. The ages (in days) at time of death for samples of 11 girls and 16 boys who died of sudden infant death syndrome are shown below:

Females	Males	
53	46	115
56	52	133
60	58	134
60	59	175
78	77	175
87	78	
102	80	
117	81	
134	84	
160	103	
277	114	

Calculate, separately for boys and girls, the 95% confidence interval for the (population) mean of age (in days) at time of death.

4.23. A study was conducted to investigate whether oat bran cereal helps to lower serum cholesterol in men with high cholesterol levels. Fourteen men were randomly placed on a diet which included either oat bran or corn flakes; after 2 weeks, their low-density lipoprotein cholesterol levels were recorded. Each man was then switched to the alternative diet. After a second 2-week period, the LDL cholesterol level of each individual was again recorded. The data were:

	LDL (mmol/liter)	
Subject	Corn Flakes	Oat Bran
1	4.61	3.84
2	6.42	5.57
3	5.40	5.85
4	4.54	4.80
5	3.98	3.68
6	3.82	2.96
7	5.01	4.41
8	4.34	3.72
9	3.80	3.49
10	4.56	3.84
11	5.35	5.26
12	3.89	3.73
13	2.25	1.84
14	4.24	4.14

Calculate the 95% confidence interval for the (population) mean difference of the low-density lipoprotein cholesterol level LDL (mmol/liter; Cornflake − Oat bran).

4.24. An experiment was conducted at the University of California at Berkeley to study the psychological environment effect on the anatomy of the brain. A group of 19 rats was randomly divided into two groups. Twelve animals in the treatment group lived together in a large cage, furnished with playthings that were changed daily, while animals in the control group lived in isolation with no toys. After a month, the experimental animals were killed and dissected. The following table gives the cortex weights (the thinking part of the brain) in milligrams:

Treatment	Control
707	669
740	650
745	651
652	627
649	656
676	642
699	698
696	
712	
708	
749	
690	

Calculate, separately for each treatment, the 95% confidence interval for the (population) mean of the cortex weight. How do the means compare?

4.25. The systolic blood pressures (in mmHg) of 12 women between the ages of 20 and 35 were measured before and after administration of a newly developed oral contraceptive.

Subject	Before	After	After–Before Difference, d_i
1	122	127	5
2	126	128	2
3	132	140	8
4	120	119	−1
5	142	145	3
6	130	130	0
7	142	148	6
8	137	135	−2
9	128	129	1
10	132	137	5
11	128	128	0
12	129	133	4

(a) Calculate the 95% confidence interval for the mean systolic blood pressure *change*. Does the oral contraceptive seem to change the mean systolic blood pressure?

(b) Calculate a 95% confidence interval for the Pearson's correlation coefficient representing a possible relationship between systolic blood pressures measured before and after the administration of oral contraceptive. What does it mean that these measurements are correlated (if confirmed)?

4.26. Suppose that we are interested in studying patients with systemic cancer who subsequently develop a brain metastasis; our ultimate goal is to prolong their lives by controlling the disease. A sample of 23 such patients, all of whom were treated with radiotherapy, were followed from the first day of their treatment until recurrence of the original tumor. Recurrence is defined as the reappearance of a metastasis in exactly the same site, or, in the case of patients whose tumor never completely disappeared, enlargement of the original lesion. Times to recurrence (in weeks) for the 23 patients were: 2, 2, 2, 3, 4, 5, 5, 6, 7, 8, 9, 10, 14, 14, 18, 19, 20, 22, 22, 31, 33, 39, 195. First, calculate the 95% confidence interval for the mean time to recurrence on the log scale, then convert the endpoints to *week*.

4.27. An experimental study was conducted with 136 5-year-old children in four Quebec schools to investigate the impact of simulation games designed to teach children to obey certain traffic safety rules. The transfer of learning was measured by observing children's reactions to a quasi-real-life model of traffic risks. The scores on the transfer of learning for the control and attitude/behavior simulation game groups are summarized below:

Summarized Data	Control	Simulation Game
n	30	33
$\bar{x}$	7.9	10.1
s	3.7	2.3

Find and compare the 95% confidence intervals for the means of the two groups, and draw an appropriate conclusion.

4.28. The body mass index is calculated by dividing a person's weight by the square of his/her height (it is used as a measure of the extent to which the individual is over-weight). A sample of 58 men, selected (retrospectively) from a large group of middle-aged men who later developed diabetes mellitus, yields $\bar{x} = 25.0\,\mathrm{kg/m^2}$ and $s = 2.7\,\mathrm{kg/m^2}$.

(a) Calculate a 95% confidence interval for the mean of this sub-population.

(b) If it is known that the average body mass index for middle-aged men who do not develop diabetes is $24.0\,\mathrm{kg/m^2}$, what can you say about the relationship between body mass index and diabetes in middle-aged men?

4.29. A study was undertaken in order to clarify the relationship between heart disease and occupational carbon disulfide exposure along with another important factor, elevated diastolic blood pressure (DBP), in a data set obtained from a 10-year prospective follow-up of two cohorts of over 340 male industrial workers in Finland. Carbon disulfide is an industrial solvent that is used all over the world in the production of viscose rayon fibers. The following table gives the mean and standard deviation (SD) of serum cholesterol (mg/100 ml) among exposed and nonexposed cohorts, by diastolic blood pressure (DBP).

DBP	Exposed			Nonexposed		
(mmHg)	n	Mean	SD	n	Mean	SD
< 95	205	220	50	271	221	42
95–100	92	227	57	53	236	46
≥ 100	20	233	41	10	216	48

Compare serum cholesterol levels between exposed and nonexposed cohorts at each level of DBP by calculating the two 95% confidence intervals for the means (exposed and nonexposed groups).

4.30. Refer to the data on cancer of the prostate in Exercise 2.39, and calculate the 95% confidence interval for the (Pearson's) correlation between age and the level of serum acid phosphatase.

4.31. The following data give the net food supply (x, the number of calories per person per day) and the infant mortality rate (y, number of infant deaths per 1000 live births) for certain selected countries before World War I:

Country	x	y	Country	x	y
Argentina	2730	98.8	Iceland	3160	42.4
Australia	3300	39.1	India	1970	161.6
Austria	2990	87.4	Ireland	3390	69.6
Belgium	3000	83.1	Italy	2510	102.7
Burma	1080	202.1	Japan	2180	60.6
Canada	3070	67.4	New Zealand	3260	32.2
Chile	2240	240.8	Netherlands	3010	37.4
Cuba	2610	116.8	Sweden	3210	43.3
Egypt	2450	162.9	England	3100	55.3
France	2880	66.1	USA	3150	53.2
Germany	2960	63.3	Uruguay	2380	94.1

Calculate the 95% confidence interval for the (Pearson's) correlation coefficient between the net food supply and the infant mortality rate.

4.32. In an assay of heparin, a standard preparation is compared with a test preparation by observing the log clotting times (y, in seconds) of blood containing different doses of heparin (x is log dose, replicate readings are made at each dose level):

Log Clotting Times				
Standard		Test		Log Dose
1.806	1.756	1.799	1.763	0.72
1.851	1.785	1.826	1.832	0.87
1.954	1.929	1.898	1.875	1.02
2.124	1.996	1.973	1.982	1.17
2.262	2.161	2.140	2.100	1.32

Calculate, separately for the standard preparation and the test preparation, the 95% confidence interval for the (Pearson's) correlation coefficient between the log clotting times and log dose.

4.33. There have been times that the city of London experienced periods of dense fog. The following table shows such data for a 15-day very severe period that include the number of deaths in each day (y), the mean atmospheric smoke (x_1, in mg/m^3), and the mean atmospheric sulfur dioxide content (x_2, in parts/million):

Number of Deaths	Smoke	Sulfur Dioxide
112	0.30	0.09
140	0.49	0.16
143	0.61	0.22
120	0.49	0.14
196	2.64	0.75
294	3.45	0.86
513	4.46	1.34
518	4.46	1.34
430	1.22	0.47
274	1.22	0.47
255	0.32	0.22
236	0.29	0.23
256	0.50	0.26
222	0.32	0.16
213	0.32	0.16

Calculate the 95% confidence interval for the (Pearson's) correlation coefficient between the number of deaths (y) and the mean atmospheric smoke (x_1, in mg/m^3), and between the number of deaths (y) and the mean atmospheric sulfur dioxide content (x_2), respectively.

4.34. The following are the heights (measured to the nearest 2 cm) and the weights (measured to the nearest kg) of 10 men and 10 women.

Men:

Height:	162	168	174	176	180	180	182	184	186	186
Weight:	65	65	84	63	75	76	82	65	80	81

Women:

Height:	152	156	158	160	162	162	164	164	166	166
Weight:	52	50	47	48	52	55	55	56	60	60

Calculate, separately for men and women, the 95% confidence interval for the (Pearson's) correlation coefficient between height and weight. Is there any indication of an effect modification?

4.35. Data are shown below for two groups of patients who died of acute myelogenous leukemia. Patients were classified into the two groups according to the presence or absence of a morphologic characteristic of white cells. Patients termed "AG positive" were identified by the presence of Auer rods and/or significant granulature of the leukemic cells in the bone marrow at diagnosis. For the AG-negative patients these factors were absent. Leukemia is a cancer characterized by an overproliferation of white blood cells; the higher the white blood count (WBC), the more severe the disease.

(AG Positive) $N = 17$		(AG Negative) $N = 16$	
White Blood Count (WBC)	Survival Time (weeks)	White Blood Count (WBC)	Survival Time (weeks)
2,300	65	4,400	56
750	156	3,000	65
4,300	100	4,000	17
2,600	134	1,500	7
6,000	16	9,000	16
10,500	108	5,300	22
10,000	121	10,000	3
17,000	4	19,000	4
5,400	39	27,000	2
7,000	143	28,000	3
9,400	56	31,000	8
32,000	26	26,000	4
35,000	22	21,000	3
100,000	1	79,000	30
100,000	1	100,000	4
52,000	5	100,000	43
100,000	65		

Calculate, separately for the AG-positive patients and AG-negative patients, the 95% confidence interval for the Pearson's correlation coefficient between survival time and white blood count (both on log scale). Is there any indication of an effect modification?

5

Introduction to Hypothesis Testing or Statistical Tests

This chapter covers the most used and yet most misunderstood statistical procedures, called *tests* or *tests of significance*. The reason for the misunderstanding is simple: language. The colloquial meaning of the word "test" is one of no-nonsense objectivity. Students take tests in school, hospitals draw blood to be sent to laboratories for tests, and automobiles are tested by the manufacturer for performance and safety. It is thus natural to think that statistical tests are the "objective" procedures to use on data. The truth is that statistical tests are no more or less objective than any other statistical procedure such as confidence estimation of Chapter 4.

Statisticians have made the problem worse by using the word "significance." Significance is another word that has a powerful meaning in ordinary, colloquial language: *importance.* Statistical tests that result in "significance" are naturally misunderstood by the public to mean that the findings or results are important. That's not what statisticians mean; it only means that, for example, the difference they hypothesized was *real*.

Statistical tests are commonly and seriously misinterpreted by nonstatisticians, but the misinterpretations are very natural. It is very natural to look at data and ask whether there is "anything going on," or whether it is just a bunch of meaningless numbers that can't be interpreted. Statistical tests appeal to investigators and readers of research for a reason in addition to the aforementioned reasons of language confusion. Statistical tests are appealing because they seem to make a *decision*; they are attractive because they say "yes" or "no." There is comfort in using a procedure that gives definitive *answers* from confusing data.

One way of explaining statistical tests is to use criminal court procedures as a metaphor. In criminal court, the accused is "presumed innocent" until "proven guilty beyond all reasonable doubt." This framework of presumed innocence has nothing whatsoever to do with anyone's personal belief as to the innocence or guilt of the defendant. Sometimes everybody in their right mind, including the jury, the judge, and even the defendant's attorney, thinks the defendant is guilty as sin. The rules and procedures of criminal court, however, must be followed. There may be a mistrial or a hung jury, or the arresting officer may have forgotten to read the defendant his or her rights. Any number of things can happen to save the guilty from a conviction. On the other hand, an innocent defendant is sometimes convicted by overwhelming circumstantial evidence. Criminal courts occasionally make mistakes, sometimes releasing the guilty and sometimes convicting the innocent. Statistical tests are like that. Sometimes statistical significance is attained when nothing is going on, and sometimes no statistical significance is attained when something very important is going on.

Just as in the court room, everyone would like statistical tests to make mistakes as infrequently as possible. Actually, the mistake rate of one of two possible mistakes made by statistical tests has usually been (arbitrarily) chosen to be 5% or 1%. The kind of mistake referred to here is the mistake of attaining statistical significance when there is actually nothing going on, analogous to the mistake of convicting the innocent in a trial by jury. This mistake is called a Type I mistake or *Type I error*. Statistical tests are often constructed so that Type I errors occur 5% or 1% of the time. There is no custom regarding the rate of *Type II errors*, however. A Type II error is the mistake of not getting statistical significance when there is something going on, analogous to the mistake of releasing the guilty in a trial by jury. The rate of Type II mistakes is dependent on several factors. One of the factors is *how much* is going on, analogous to the severity of the crime in a trial by jury. If there is a lot going on, one is less likely to make Type II errors. Another factor is the amount of variability ("noise") there is in the data, analogous to the quality of collected evidence in a trial by jury. A lot of variability makes Type II errors more likely. Yet another factor is the size of the study, just as the amount of collected evidence in a trial by jury. There are more Type II errors in small studies than there are in big ones. Type II errors are rare in really huge studies, but quite common in small studies.

There is a very important, subtle aspect of statistical tests, based on the aforementioned three things that make Type II errors very improbable. Because really huge studies virtually guarantee getting statistical significance if there is even the slightest amount going on, such studies result in statistical significance when the *amount* that is going on is of no practical importance. In this case, statistical significance is attained in the face of no practical significance. On the other hand, small studies can result in statistical *non*-significance when something of great practical importance is going on. The conclusion is that the attainment of statistical significance in a study is just as affected by extraneous factors as it is by practical importance. It is essential to learn that statistical significance is not synonymous with practical importance.

5.1. BASIC CONCEPTS

From the introduction of sampling distributions in Chapter 4, it was clear that the value of a sample mean is influenced by

(i) The population μ, because

$$\mu_{\bar{x}} = \mu$$

(ii) Chance; $\bar{x}$ and μ are almost never identical. The variance of the sampling distribution is

$$\sigma_{\bar{x}}^2 = \frac{\sigma^2}{n}$$

a combined effect of natural variation in the population (σ^2) and sample size (n).

Therefore, when an observed value $\bar{x}$ is far from a hypothesized value of μ (e.g., mean high blood pressures for a group of oral contraceptive users as compared to a typical average for women in the same age group), a natural question would be "Was it just due to chance, or something else?" To deal with questions such as this, statisticians have invented the concept of *hypothesis tests*, and these tests have become widely used statistical techniques in the health sciences. In fact, it is almost impossible to read a research article in public health or medical sciences without running across hypothesis tests!

5.1.1. Hypothesis Tests

When a health investigator seeks to understand or explain something—for example, the effect of a toxin or a drug—he or she usually formulates his or her research question in the form of a *hypothesis*. In the statistical context, a hypothesis is a statement about a distribution (e.g., "the distribution is normal") or its underlying parameter(s) (e.g., "$\mu = 10$"), or a statement about the relationship between probability distributions (e.g., "there is no statistical relationship") or its parameters (e.g., "$\mu_1 = \mu_2$"—equality of population means). The hypothesis to be tested is called the *null hypothesis* and will be denoted by H_0; it is usually stated in the "null" form, indicating no difference or no relationship between distributions or parameters, analogous to the constitutional guarantee that the accused is presumed innocent until proven guilty. In other words, under the null hypothesis, an observed difference (like the one between sample means $\bar{x}_1$ and $\bar{x}_2$ for Sample 1 and Sample 2, respectively) just reflects chance variation. A *hypothesis test* is a decision-making process that examines a set or sets of data and, on the basis of expectation under H_0, leads to a decision on whether or not to reject H_0. An *alternative hypothesis*, which we denote by H_A, is a hypothesis that in some sense contradicts the null hypothesis H_0, analogous to the *charge* by the prosecution in a trial by jury. Under H_A, the observed difference is real (e.g., $\bar{x}_1 \neq \bar{x}_2$ not by chance but because $\mu_1 \neq \mu_2$). A null hypothesis is rejected if and only if there is sufficiently strong evidence from the data to support its alternative; the names are somewhat unsettling, because the "alternative hypothesis" is, for a health investigator, the one he or she usually wants to prove (the null hypothesis is just a dull explanation of the findings—in terms of chance variation!). However, these are entrenched statistical terms and will be used as standard terms for the rest of this book.

Why is hypothesis testing important? Because in many circumstances we merely wish to know whether a certain proposition is true or false. The process of hypothesis tests provides a framework for making decisions on an *objective* basis, by weighing the relative merits of different hypotheses, rather than a *subjective* basis by simply looking at the numbers. Different people can form different opinions by looking at data (confounded by chance variation or sampling errors), but a hypothesis test provides a standardized decision-making process that will be consistent for all people. The mechanics of the tests vary with the hypotheses and measurement scales (Chapters 6, 7, and 8), but the general philosophy and foundation is common and will be discussed with some details in this chapter.

5.1.2. Statistical Evidence

A null hypothesis is often concerned with a parameter or parameters of population(s). However, it is often either impossible or too costly or time-consuming to obtain the entire population data on any variable in order to see whether or not a null hypothesis is true. Decisions are thus made using sample data. Sample data are summarized into a statistic or statistics that are used to estimate the parameter(s) involved in the null hypothesis. For example, if a null hypothesis is about μ (e.g., $H_0 : \mu = 10$), then a good place to look for information about μ is $\bar{x}$. In that context, the statistic $\bar{x}$ is called a *test statistic*; a test statistic can be used to measure the difference between the data (i.e., the numerical value of $\bar{x}$ obtained from the sample) and what is expected if the null hypothesis is true (i.e., "$\mu = 10$"). However, this evidence is statistical evidence; it varies from sample to sample (in the context of repeated sampling). It is a variable with a specific sampling distribution. The observed value is thus usually converted to a standard unit: the number of standard errors away from a hypothesized value. At this point, the logic of the test can be seen more clearly. It is an argument by contradiction, designed to show that the null hypothesis will lead to a less acceptable conclusion (an almost impossible event—some event that occurs with near zero probability) and must therefore be rejected. In other words, the difference between the data and what is expected on the null hypothesis would be very difficult—even absurd—to explain as a chance variation; it makes you want to abandon (or reject) the null hypothesis and believe in the alternative hypothesis because it is more plausible.

5.1.3. Errors

Because a null hypothesis H_0 may be true or false and our possible decisions are whether to reject or not to reject it, there are four possible outcomes or combinations. Two of the four outcomes are correct decisions:

(i) Not rejecting a true H_0
(ii) Rejecting a false H_0

but there are also two possible ways to commit an error:

(i) *Type I*: A true H_0 is rejected.
(ii) *Type II*: A false H_0 is not rejected.

These possibilities are shown as follows:

	Decision	
Truth	H_0 is not rejected	H_0 is rejected
H_0 is true	Correct decision	Type I error
H_0 is false	Type II error	Correct decision

The general aim in hypothesis testing is to keep α and β, the probabilities (in the context of repeated sampling) of Types I and II, respectively, as small as possible. However, if resources are limited, this goal requires a compromise because these actions are contradictory; for example, a decision to decrease the size of α will increase the size of β, and vice versa. Conventionally, we fix α at some specific conventional level—say .05 or .01—and β is controlled through the use of sample size(s). The value of $(1-\beta)$ is called the (statistical) power of the test.

Example 5.1

Suppose the national smoking rate among men is 25% and we want to study the smoking rate among men in the New England states. Let π be the proportion of New England men who smoke. The null hypothesis that the smoking prevalence in New England is the same as the national rate is expressed as

$$H_0 : \pi = .25$$

Suppose we plan to take a sample of size $n = 100$ and use this decision-making rule:

"If $p \leq .20$, H_0 is rejected"

where p is the proportion obtained from the sample.

(i) Alpha (α) is defined as the probability of wrongly rejecting a true null hypothesis, that is,

$$\alpha = \Pr(p \leq .20, \text{ given that } \pi = .25)$$

Because $n = 100$ is large enough for the Central Limit Theorem to apply, the sampling distribution of p is approximately normal with mean and variance, under H_0, given by

$$\mu_p = \pi$$
$$= .25$$
$$\sigma_p^2 = \frac{\pi(1-\pi)}{n}$$
$$= (.043)^2$$

respectively. Therefore, for this decision-making rule,

$$\alpha = \Pr\left(z \leq \frac{.20 - .25}{.043}\right)$$
$$= \Pr(z \leq -1.16)$$
$$= .123 \text{ or } 12.3\%$$

Of course, we can make this smaller (as small as we wish) by changing the decision-making rule; however, that action will increase the value of β (or the probability of a Type II error).

(ii) Suppose that the truth is

$$H_A : \pi = .15$$

Beta (β) is defined as the probability of not rejecting a false H_0, that is,

$$\beta = \Pr(p > .20; \text{ knowing that } \pi = .15)$$

Again, an application of the Central Limit Theorem indicates that the sampling distribution of p is approximately normal with mean

$$\mu_p = .15$$

and variance

$$\sigma_p^2 = \frac{(.15)(.85)}{100}$$
$$= (.036)^2$$

Therefore

$$\beta = \Pr\left(z \geq \frac{.20 - .15}{.036}\right)$$
$$= \Pr(z \geq 1.39)$$
$$= .082 \text{ or } 8.2\%$$

The above results can be represented graphically as follows:

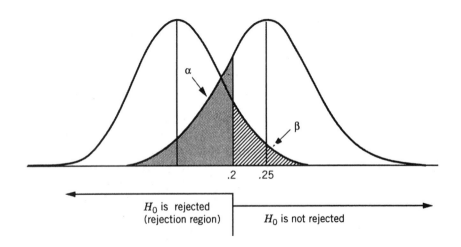

It can be seen that β depends on a specific alternative (e.g., β is larger for $H_A : \pi = .17$ or any alternative hypothesis that specifies a value of π that is nearer to .25); and, from the above graph, if we change the decision-making rule by using a smaller "cut point" then we would decrease α but increase β.

5.2. ANALOGIES

To reinforce some of the definitions or terms we have encountered, we consider in this section two analogies: trials by jury and medical screening tests.

5.2.1. Trials by Jury

Statisticians and statistics users may find a lot in common between a court trial and a statistical test of significance. In a criminal court, the jury's duty is to evaluate the evidence of the prosecution and the defense to determine whether a defendant is guilty or innocent. By use of the judge's instructions, which provide guidelines for their reaching a decision, the members of the jury can arrive at one of two verdicts: guilty or not guilty. Their decision may be correct or they could make one of two possible errors: Convict an innocent person or free a criminal. The analogy between statistics and trials by jury goes as follows:

Test of significance $\leftrightarrow$ Court trial

Null hypothesis $\leftrightarrow$ "Every defendant is innocent until proven guilty"

Research design $\leftrightarrow$ Police investigation

Data/test statistics $\leftrightarrow$ Evidence/exhibits

Statistical principles $\leftrightarrow$ Judge's instruction

Statistical decision $\leftrightarrow$ Verdict

Type I error $\leftrightarrow$ Conviction of an innocent defendant

Type II error $\leftrightarrow$ Acquittal of a criminal

This analogy clarifies a very important concept: When a null hypothesis is not rejected, it does not necessarily lead to its acceptance, because a "not guilty" verdict is just an indication of "lack of evidence" and "innocence" is one of the possibilities. That is, when a difference is not statistically significant, there are still two possibilities:

(i) The null hypothesis is true.

(ii) The null hypothesis is false, but there is not enough evidence from sample data to support its rejection (i.e., sample size is too small).

5.2.2. Medical Screening Tests

Another analogy of hypothesis testing can be found in the application of screening tests or diagnostic procedures. Following these procedures, clinical observations or laboratory techniques, individuals are classified as healthy or as having a disease. Of course, these tests are imperfect: Healthy individuals will occasionally be classified wrongly as being ill, whereas some individuals who are ill may fail to be detected. The analogy between statistical tests and screening tests goes briefly as follows:

$$\text{Type I error} \leftrightarrow \text{False positives}$$

$$\text{Type II error} \leftrightarrow \text{False negatives}$$

so that

$$\alpha = 1 - \text{specificity}$$

$$\beta = 1 - \text{sensitivity}.$$

5.2.3. Common Expectations

The medical care system, with its high visibility and remarkable history of achievements, has been perceived somewhat naively by the general public as a perfect remedy factory. Medical tests are expected to correctly diagnose any disease (and physicians are expected to effectively treat and cure all diseases!). Another common misconception is the assumption that all tests, regardless of the disease being tested for, are equally accurate. People are shocked to learn that a test result is wrong (of course, the psychological effects could be devastating). Another analogy between tests of significance and screening tests exists here: Statistical tests are also expected to provide a correct decision!

In some medical cases such as infections, the presence or absence of bacteria and viruses are easier to confirm correctly. In other cases, such as the diagnosis of diabetes by a blood sugar test, the story is different. One very simple model for these situations would be to assume that the variable X (e.g., sugar level in blood) on which the test is based is distributed with different means for the healthy and diseased subpopulations:

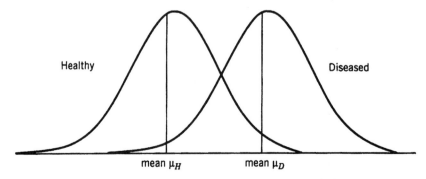

Difference between healthy and diseased subpopulations.

It can be seen from the figure that errors are unavoidable, especially when the two means μ_H and μ_D are close. The same is true for statistical tests of significance; when the null hypothesis H_0 is not true, it could be wrong a little or it could be very wrong. For example, for

$$H_0 : \mu = 10$$

the truth could be "$\mu = 12$" or "$\mu = 50$." If $\mu = 50$, Type II errors would be less likely, and if $\mu = 12$, Type II errors are more likely.

5.3. SUMMARIES AND CONCLUSIONS

To perform an hypothesis test we take the following steps to:

1. Formulate a null hypothesis and an alternative hypothesis. (This would follow our research question, providing an explanation of what we want to prove in terms of chance variation; the statement resulting from our research question forms our alternative hypothesis.)
2. Design the experiment and obtain data.
3. Choose a test statistic. (This choice depends on the null hypothesis as well as measurement scale.)
4. Summarize findings and state appropriate conclusions.

This section involves the last step of the above process.

5.3.1. Rejection Region

The most common approach is the formation of a "Decision Rule." All possible values of the chosen test statistic (in the repeated sampling context) are divided into two regions. The region consisting of values of the test statistic for which the null hypothesis H_0 is rejected is called the *rejection region*. The values of the test statistic comprising the rejection region are those values that are less likely to occur if the null hypothesis is true, and the decision rule tells us to reject H_0 if the value of the test statistic that we calculate from our sample(s) is one of the values in this region. For example, if a null hypothesis is about μ, say

$$H_0 : \mu = 10$$

then a good place to look for a test statistic for H_0 is $\bar{x}$, and it is obvious that H_0 should be rejected if $\bar{x}$ is far away from "10," the hypothesized value of μ. Before we proceed, a number of related concepts should be made clear:

One-sided Versus Two-sided Tests

In the above example, a vital question is, "Are we interested in the deviation of $\bar{x}$ from 10 in one or both directions?" If we are interested in determining whether μ is significantly *different* from 10, we would perform a two-sided test and the rejection region would be as follows:

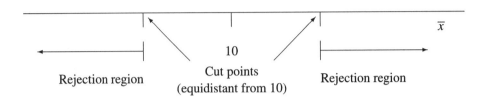

On the other hand, if we are interested in whether μ is significantly *larger* than 10, we would perform a one-sided test and the rejection region would be as follows:

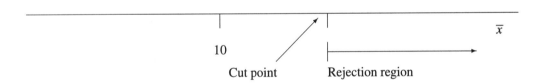

A one-sided test is indicated for research questions like these: Is a new drug *superior* to a standard drug? Does the air pollution *exceed* safe limits? Has the death rate been *reduced* for those who quit smoking? A two-sided test is indicated for research questions like these: Is there a *difference* between cholesterol levels of men and women? Does the mean age of a target population *differ* from that of the general population?

Level of Significance

The decision as to which values of the test statistic go into the rejection region, or where is the cut point, is made on the basis of the desired level of Type I error α (also called the *size* of the test). A calculated value of the test statistic that falls in the rejection region is said to be *statistically significant*. Common choices for α, the level of significance, are .01, .05, and .10; the .05 or 5% level is especially popular.

Reproducibility

Here we aim to clarify another misconception about hypothesis tests. A very simple and common situation for hypothesis tests is that the test statistic—for example, the sample mean $\bar{x}$—is normally distributed with different means under the null hypothesis H_0 and alternative hypothesis H_A. A one-tailed test could be graphically represented as follows:

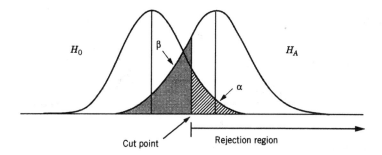

It should now be clear that a statistical conclusion is not guaranteed to be reproducible. For example, if the alternative hypothesis is true and the mean of the distribution of the test statistic (see graph above) is right at the cut point then the probability would be 50% to obtain a test statistic inside the rejection region.

5.3.2. *p*-Values

Instead of saying that an observed value of the test statistic is significant (i.e., falling into the rejection region for a given choice of α) or is not significant, many writers in the research literature prefer to report findings in terms of *p-values*. The *p*-value is the probability of getting values of the test statistic as extreme as, or more extreme than, that observed if the null hypothesis is true. For the above example of

$$H_0 : \mu = 10$$

if the test is a one-sided test, we would have

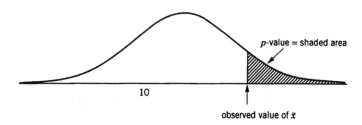

and if the test is a two-sided test, then we have

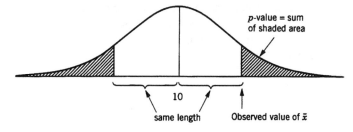

The curve in these graphs represents the sampling distribution of $\bar{x}$ if H_0 is true.

As compared to the approach of choosing a level of significance and formulating a decision rule, the use of the p-value criterion would be as follows:

(i) If $p < \alpha$, H_0 is rejected.
(ii) If $p \geq \alpha$, H_0 is not rejected.

However, the reporting of p-values as part of the results of an investigation is more informative to the readers than such statements as "the null hypothesis is rejected at the .05 level of significance" or "the results were not significant at the .05 level." Reporting the p-value associated with a test lets the reader know how common or how rare is the computed value of the test statistic given that H_0 is true. In other words, the p-value can be used as a *measure* of the compatibility between the data (reality) and a null hypothesis (theory); the smaller the p-value, the less compatible the theory and the reality. A compromise between the two approaches would be to report both in statements such as "the difference is statistically significant ($p < .05$)." In doing so, researchers generally agree on the following conventional terms:

p-Value	Interpretation
$p > .10$	Result is not significant.
$.05 < p < .10$	Result is marginally significant.
$.01 < p < .05$	Result is significant.
$p < .01$	Result is highly significant.

Finally, it should be noted that the difference, between means for example, although statistically significant may be so small that it has little health consequence. In other words, the result may be *statistically significant* but may **not** be *practically significant*.

Example 5.2

Suppose the national smoking rate among men is 25% and we want to study the smoking rate among men in the New England states. The null hypothesis under investigation is

$$H_0 : \pi = .25$$

Of $n = 100$ males sampled, $x = 15$ were found to be smokers. Does the proportion π of smokers in New England states *differ* from that of the nation?

Because $n = 100$ is large enough for the Central Limit Theorem to apply, it indicates that the sampling distribution of the sample proportion p is approximately normal with mean and variance under H_0:

$$\mu_p = .25$$
$$\sigma_p^2 = \frac{(.25)(1 - .25)}{100}$$
$$= (.043)^2$$

The observed value of proportion p from our sample is

$$\frac{15}{100} = .15$$

representing a difference of .10 from the hypothesized value of .25. The p-value is defined as the probability of getting a value of the test statistic as extreme as, or more extreme than, that observed if the null hypothesis is true. This is represented graphically as follows:

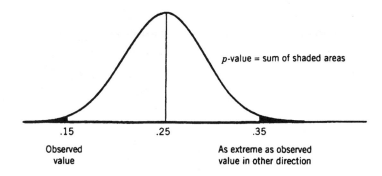

Therefore

$$p\text{-value} = \Pr(p \leq .15 \text{ or } p \geq .35)$$
$$= 2 \times \Pr(p \geq .35)$$
$$= 2 \times \Pr\left(z \geq \frac{.35 - .25}{.043}\right)$$
$$= 2 \times \Pr(z \geq 2.33)$$
$$= (2)(.5 - .4901)$$
$$\cong .02$$

In other words, with the data given, the difference between the national smoking rate and the smoking rate of New England states is statistically significant ($p < .05$).

5.3.3. Relationship to Confidence Intervals

Suppose we consider a hypothesis of the form

$$H_0 : \mu = \mu_0$$

where μ_0 is a known hypothesized value. A two-sided hypothesis test for H_0 is related to confidence intervals as follows:

1. If μ_0 is not included in the 95% confidence interval for μ, H_0 should be rejected at the .05 level. This is represented graphically as follows:

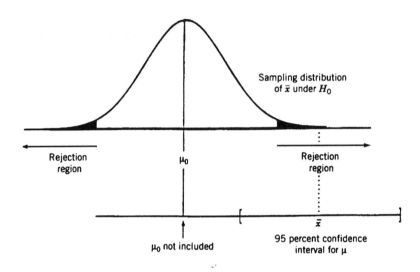

2. If μ_0 is included in the 95% confidence interval for μ, H_0 should not be rejected at the .05 level:

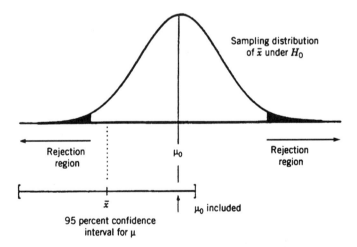

Example 5.3

Consider the hypothetical data set in Example 5.2. Our point estimate of smoking prevalence in New England is

$$p = \frac{15}{100}$$
$$= .15$$

Its standard error is

$$SE(p) = \sqrt{(.15)(1 - .15)/100}$$
$$= .036$$

Therefore, a 95% confidence interval for the New England states smoking rate π is given by

$$.15 \pm (1.96)(.036) = (.079, .221)$$

It is noted that the national rate of .25 is *not included* in that confidence interval.

EXERCISES

5.1. For each part, state the null (H_0) and alternative (H_A) hypotheses:
   (a) Has the average community level of suspended particulates for the month of August exceeded $30\,\mu/m^3$?
   (b) Does mean age of onset of a certain acute disease for school children differ from 11.5?
   (c) A psychologist claims that the average IQ of a sample of 60 children is significantly above the normal IQ of 100.
   (d) Is the average cross-sectional area of the lumen of coronary arteries for men, ages 40 to 59, less than 31.5% of the total arterial cross section?
   (e) Is the mean hemoglobin level of a group of high-altitude workers different from $16\,g/ml$?
   (f) Does the average speed of 50 cars as checked by radar on a particular highway differ from 55 mph?

5.2. The distribution of diastolic blood pressures for the population of female diabetics between the ages of 30 and 34 has an unknown mean μ and a standard deviation of $\sigma = 9$ mmHg. It may be useful to physicians to know whether the mean μ of this population is equal to the mean diastolic blood pressure of the general population of females of this age group, which is 74.5 mmHg. What is the null hypothesis and what is the alternative hypothesis for this test?

5.3. *E. canis* infection is a tick-borne disease of dogs that is sometimes contracted by humans. Among infected humans, the distribution of white blood cell counts has an unknown mean μ and a standard deviation σ. In the general population the mean white blood count is $7250/mm^3$. It is believed that persons infected with *E. canis* must on average have a lower white blood cell count. What is the null hypothesis for the test? Is this a one-sided or two-sided alternative?

5.4. It is feared that the smoking rate in young females has increased in the last several years. In 1985, 38% of the females in the 17- to 24-year age group were smokers. An experiment is to be conducted to gain evidence to support the increase contention. Set up the appropriate null and alternative hypotheses. Explain in a practical sense what, if anything, has occurred if a Type I or Type II error has been committed.

5.5. A group of investigators wishes to explore the relationship between the use of hair dyes and the development of breast cancer in females. A group of 1000 beauticians 40–49 years of age is identified and followed for 5 years. After 5 years, 20 new cases of breast cancer have occurred. Assume that breast cancer incidence over this time period for average American women in this age group is $\frac{7}{1,000}$. We wish to test the hypothesis that using hair dyes increases the risk of breast cancer. Is a one-sided or a two-sided test appropriate here? Compute the p-value for your choice.

5.6. Height and weight are often used in epidemiological studies as possible predictors of disease outcomes. If the people in the study are assessed in a clinic, then heights and weights are usually measured directly. However, if the people are interviewed at home or by mail, then a person's self-reported height and weight are often used instead. Suppose we conduct a study on 10 people to test the comparability of these two methods. Data from these 10 people were obtained using both methods on each person. What is the criterion for the comparison? What is the null hypothesis? Should a two-sided or a one-sided test be used here?

5.7. Suppose that 28 cancer deaths are noted among 5000 workers exposed to asbestos in a building materials plant from 1981 to 1985. Only 20.5 cancer deaths are expected from statewide mortality rates. Suppose we want to know if there is a significant excess of cancer deaths among these workers. What is the null hypothesis? Is a one-sided or two-sided test appropriate here?

5.8. A food frequency questionnaire was mailed to 20 subjects to assess the intake of various food groups. The sample standard deviation of vitamin C intake over the 20 subjects was 15 (exclusive of vitamin C supplements). Suppose we know from using an in-person diet interview method in a large previous study that the standard deviation is 20. Formulate the null and alternative hypotheses if we want to test for any differences between the standard deviations of the two methods.

5.9. In Example 5.1, it was assumed that the national smoking rate among men is 25%. A study is to be conducted for New England states using a sample size $n = 100$ and the decision rule

"If $p \leq .20$, H_0 is rejected"

where H_0 is

$$H_0 : \pi = .25$$

where π and p are population and sample proportions, respectively, for New England states. Is this a one-tailed or two-tailed test?

5.10. In Example 5.1, with the rule

"If $p \leq .20$, H_0 is rejected"

it was found that the probabilities of Type I and Type II errors are

$$\alpha = .123$$
$$\beta = .082$$

for $H_A : \pi = .15$. Find α and β if the rule is changed to

"If $p \leq .18$, H_0 is rejected"

How does this change affect α and β values?

5.11. Answer the questions in Exercise 5.10 above for the decision rule

"If $p \leq .22$, H_0 is rejected"

5.12. Recalculate the p-value in Example 5.2 if it was found that 18 (instead of 15) men in a sample of $n = 100$ are smokers.

5.13. Calculate the 95% confidence interval for π using the sample in Exercise 5.12 above and compare the findings to the testing results of Exercise 5.9.

5.14. Plasma glucose levels are used to determine the presence of diabetes. Suppose the mean log plasma glucose concentration (mg/dl) in 35- to 44-year-olds is 4.86 with standard deviation .54. A study of 100 sedentary persons in this age group is planned to test whether they have higher levels of plasma glucose than the general population.
   (a) Set up the null and alternative hypotheses.
   (b) If the real increase is .1 log units, then what is the power of such a study if a two-sided test is to be used with $\alpha = .05$?

5.15. Suppose we are interested in investigating the effect of race on level of blood pressure. The mean and standard deviation of systolic blood pressure among 25- to 34-year-old white males were reported as 128.6 mmHg and 11.1 mmHg, respectively, based on a very large sample. Suppose the actual mean for black males in the same age group is 135 mmHg. What is the power of the test (two-sided, $\alpha = .05$) if $n = 100$ and we assume that the variances for whites and blacks are the same?

6

Analysis of Categorical Data

This chapter presents basic inferential methods for categorical data, especially the analysis of two-way contingency tables. Let X_1 and X_2 denote two categorical variables, X_1 having I levels and X_2 having J levels; there are IJ combinations of classifications. We display the data in a rectangular table having I rows for the categories of X_1 and J columns for the categories of X_2; the IJ cells represent the IJ combinations of outcomes. When the cells contain frequencies of outcomes, the table is called a contingency table or cross-classified table, also referred to as I-by-J or I × J table.

Most topics in this chapter are devoted to the analyses of these two-way tables; however, before we can get there, let's first start with the most simple case of the one-sample problem with binary data.

6.1. ONE-SAMPLE PROBLEM WITH BINARY DATA

In this type of problem, we have a sample of binary data (n, x) with n being an adequately large sample size and x the number of positive outcomes among the n observations, and we consider the null hypothesis

$$H_0 : \pi = \pi_0$$

where π_0 is a fixed and known number between 0 and 1—for example,

$$H_0 : \pi = .25$$

π_0 is often a standardized or referenced figure—for example, the effect of a standardized drug or therapy, or the national smoking rate (where the national sample is often large enough so as to produce negligible sampling error in π_0). Or, we could be concerned with a research question like "Does the side effect (of a certain drug) exceed regulated limit π_0?" In Exercise 5.2, we tried to compare the incidence of breast cancer among female beauticians (who are frequently exposed to the use of hair dyes) versus a standard level of 7/1000 (for 5 years) for "average American women." The figure 7/1000 is π_0 for that example.

In a typical situation, the null hypothesis of a statistical test is concerned with a parameter; the parameter in this case is the proportion π. Sample data are summarized into a statistic which is used to estimate the parameter under investigation. Because the parameter under investigation is the proportion π, our focus in this case is the sample proportion p. In general, a statistic is itself a variable with a specific sampling distribution (in the context of repeated sampling). Our statistic in this case is the sample proportion p, and the corresponding sampling distribution is easily obtained by invoking the *Central Limit Theorem*. With large sample size and assuming that the null hypothesis H_0 is true, it is the normal distribution with mean and variance given by

$$\mu_p = \pi_0$$

$$\sigma_p^2 = \frac{\pi_0(1 - \pi_0)}{n}$$

respectively. From this sampling distribution, the observed value of the sample proportion can be converted to standard unit: the number of standard errors away from the hypothesized value of π_0. In other words, to perform a test of significance for H_0, we proceed with the following steps:

1. Decide whether a one-sided or a two-sided test is appropriate.
2. Choose a level of significance α, a common choice being .05.
3. Calculate the z-score

$$z = \frac{p - \pi_0}{\sqrt{\frac{\pi_0(1-\pi_0)}{n}}}$$

4. From the table for the standard normal distribution (Appendix B) and the choice of α (e.g. $\alpha = .05$), the rejection region is determined by the following:

- For a one-sided test,

$$z \leq -1.65 \quad \text{for } H_A : \pi < \pi_0$$

$$z \geq \quad 1.65 \quad \text{for } H_A : \pi > \pi_0$$

- For a two-sided test or $H_A : \pi \neq \pi_0$,

$$z \leq -1.96 \quad \text{or} \quad z \geq 1.96.$$

Example 6.1

A group of investigators wish to explore the relationship between the use of hair dyes and the development of breast cancer in women. A sample of $n = 1000$ female beauticians 40–49 years of age is identified and followed for 5 years. After 5 years, $x = 20$ new cases of breast cancer have occurred. It is known that breast cancer incidence over this time period for average American women in this age group is $\pi_0 = 7/1000$. We wish to test the hypothesis that using hair dyes *increases* the risk of breast cancer (a one-sided alternative). We have the following:

1. A one-sided test with

$$H_A : \pi > 7/1000$$

2. Using the conventional choice of $\alpha = .05$ leads to the rejection region: $z > 1.65$.
3. From the data,

$$p = \frac{20}{1000}$$
$$= .02$$

an observed sample proportion leading to z-score

$$z = \frac{.02 - .007}{\sqrt{\frac{(.007)(.993)}{1000}}}$$
$$= 4.93$$

that is, the observed proportion p is 4.93 standard errors away from the hypothesized value of $\pi_0 = .007$.

4. Because the computed z-score falls into the rejection region ($4.93 > 1.65$), the null hypothesis is rejected at the chosen .05 level. In fact, the difference is very highly significant ($p < .001$).

6.2. ANALYSIS OF PAIR-MATCHED DATA

The method presented in this section applies to cases where each subject or member of a group is observed twice for the presence or absence of certain characteristics (e.g., at admission to and discharge from a hospital), or matched pairs are observed for the presence or absence of the same characteristic. A popular application is an epidemiological design called a *pair-matched case–control study*. In case–control studies, cases of a specific disease are ascertained as they arise from population-based registers or lists of hospital admissions, and controls are sampled either as disease-free individuals from the population at risk or as hospitalized patients having a diagnosis other than the one under investigation. As a technique to control confounding factors, individual cases are matched, often one-to-one, to controls chosen to have similar values for confounding variables such as age, sex, race, and so on.

For pair-matched data with a single binary exposure (e.g., smoking versus nonsmoking), data can be represented by a 2×2 table, where $(+, -)$ denotes the (exposed, nonexposed) outcome, as follows:

Control

		+	−
Case	+	a	b
	−	c	d

In this 2×2 table, "a" denotes the number of pairs with two exposed members, "b" denotes the number of pairs where the case is exposed but the matched control is unexposed, "c" denotes the number of pairs where the case is unexposed but the matched control is exposed, and "d" denotes the number of pairs with two unexposed members. The analysis of pair-matched data with a single binary exposure can be seen, heuristically, as follows. What we really want to do is to compare the incidence of exposure among the cases versus the controls; the parts of the data showing no difference, the number "a" of pairs with two exposed members and the number "d" of pairs with two unexposed members, would contribute nothing as evidence in such a comparision. The comparision, therefore, relies soly on two other frequencies, "b" and "c"; under the null hypothesis that the exposure has nothing to do with the disease, we *expect $b = c$ or $(b)/(b + c) = .5$*. In other words, the analysis of pair-matched data with a single binary exposure can be seen as a special case of the one-sample problem with binary of Section 6.1 with $n = b + c$, $x = b$, and $\pi_0 = .5$. Recall the form of the test statistic of the previous section, we have

$$z = \frac{p - \pi_0}{\sqrt{\frac{\pi_0(1-\pi_0)}{b+c}}}$$

$$= \frac{\frac{b}{b+c} - \frac{1}{2}}{\sqrt{\frac{(\frac{1}{2})(1-\frac{1}{2})}{b+c}}}$$

$$= \frac{b - c}{\sqrt{b + c}}$$

The decision is based on the standardized z-score and referring to the percentiles of the standard normal distribution or, in the two-sided form, the square of the above statistic, denoted by

$$X^2 = \frac{(b-c)^2}{b+c}$$

and the test is known as the *McNemar's chi-square*. If the test is one-sided, z is used and the null hypothesis is rejected at the .05 level when

$$z \geq 1.65$$

If the test is two-sided, X^2 is used and the null hypothesis is rejected at the .05 level when

$$X^2 \geq 3.84$$

[It should be noted that $3.84 = (1.96)^2$, so that $X^2 \geq 3.84$ is equivalent to $z \leq -1.96$ or $z \geq 1.96$.]

Example 6.2

It has been noted that metal workers have an increased risk for cancer of the internal nose and paranasal sinuses, perhaps as a result of exposure to cutting oils. Therefore, a study was conducted to see whether this particular exposure also increases the risk for squamous cell carcinoma of the scrotum.

Cases included all 45 squamous cell carcinomas of the scrotum diagnosed in Connecticut residents from 1955 to 1973, as obtained from the Connecticut Tumor Registry. Matched controls were selected for each case based on the age at death (within 8 years), year of death (within 3 years), and number of jobs as obtained from combined death certificate and Directory sources. An occupational indicator of metal worker (yes/no) was evaluated as the possible risk factor in this study; results are as follows:

		Controls	
		Yes	No
Cases	Yes	2	26
	No	5	12

We have, for a one-tailed test,

$$z = \frac{26-5}{\sqrt{26+5}}$$
$$= 3.77$$

indicating a very highly significant increase of risk associated with the exposure ($p < .001$).

Example 6.3

A study in Maryland identified 4032 white persons, enumerated in a nonofficial 1963 census, who became widowed between 1963 and 1974. These people were matched, one-to-one, to married persons on the basis of race, sex, year of birth, and geography of residence. The matched pairs were followed to a second census in 1975, and we have the following overall male mortality:

		Married Men	
		Died	Alive
Widowed	Died	2	292
Men	Alive	210	700

An application of the McNemar's chi-square test (two-sided) yields

$$X^2 = \frac{(292 - 210)^2}{292 + 210}$$
$$= 13.39$$

It can be seen that the null hypothesis of equal mortality should be rejected at the .05 level ($13.39 > 3.84$).

6.3. COMPARISON OF TWO PROPORTIONS

Perhaps the most common problem involving categorical data is the comparison of two proportions. In this type of problem, we have two independent samples of binary data (n_1, x_1) and (n_2, x_2), where the n's are adequately large sample sizes that may or may not be equal, the x's are the numbers of "positive" outcomes in the two samples, and we consider the null hypothesis

$$H_0 : \pi_1 = \pi_2$$

expressing the equality of the two population proportions.

To perform a test of significance for H_0, we proceed with the following steps:

1. Decide whether a one-sided test, say

$$H_A : \pi_2 > \pi_1$$

or a two-sided test,

$$H_A : \pi_1 \neq \pi_2$$

is appropriate.

2. Choose a significance level α, a common choice being .05.
3. Calculate the z-score

$$z = \frac{p_2 - p_1}{\sqrt{p(1-p)\left(\frac{1}{n_1} + \frac{1}{n_2}\right)}}$$

where p is the "pooled proportion" defined by

$$p = \frac{x_1 + x_2}{n_1 + n_2}$$

an estimate of the common proportion under H_0.

4. Refer to the table for standard normal distribution (Appendix B) for selecting a cut point. For example, if the choice of α is .05, then the rejection region is determined by the following:

- For the one-sided alternative $H_A : \pi_2 > \pi_1, z \geq 1.65$.
- For the one-sided alternative $H_A : \pi_2 < \pi_1, z \leq -1.65$.
- For the two-sided alternative $H_A : \pi_1 \neq \pi_2, z \leq -1.96$ or $z \geq 1.96$.

What we are doing here follows the same format used in the previous sections.

- The basic term of $p_2 - p_1$ *measures the difference* between the two samples.
- Its expected hypothesized value (i.e. under H_0) is zero.
- The denominator of z is the standard error of $p_2 - p_1$, a measure of how good $p_2 - p_1$ is as an estimate of $\pi_2 - \pi_1$.
- Therefore, z measures the number of standard errors that $p_2 - p_1$, *the* evidence, is away from its hypothesized value.

In the two-sided form, the square of the z-score, denoted X^2, is more often used. The test is referred to as the *chi-square test*. The test statistic can also be obtained using the shortcut formula

$$X^2 = \frac{(n_1 + n_2)[x_1(n_2 - x_2) - x_2(n_1 - x_1)]^2}{n_1 n_2 (x_1 + x_2)(n_1 + n_2 - x_1 - x_2)}$$

and the null hypothesis is rejected at the .05 level when

$$X^2 \geq 3.84$$

It should be noted that, in the general case, with data in a 2 × 2 table of the form:

Factor	Sample 1	Sample 2	Total
Present	a	c	$a+c$
Absent	b	d	$b+d$
Sample size	$n_1 = a+b$	$n_2 = c+d$	$N = a+b+c+d$

The above chi-square statistic is simply

$$X^2 = \frac{(a+b+c+d)(ad-bc)^2}{(a+c)(b+d)(a+b)(c+d)}$$

with its denominator being the product of the four marginal totals.

Example 6.4

A study was conducted to see whether an important public health intervention would significantly reduce the smoking rate among men. Of $n_1 = 100$ males sampled in 1965 at the time of the release of the Surgeon General's report on the health consequences of smoking, $x_1 = 51$ were found to be smokers. In 1980 a second random sample of $n_2 = 100$ males, similarly gathered, indicated that $x_2 = 43$ were smokers.

An application of the above method yields

$$p = \frac{51+43}{100+100}$$

$$= .47$$

$$z = \frac{.51 - .43}{\sqrt{(.47)(.53)\left(\frac{1}{100} + \frac{1}{100}\right)}}$$

$$= 1.13$$

It can be seen that the observed rate was reduced from 51% to 43%, but the reduction is not statistically significant at the .05 level ($z = 1.13 < 1.65$).

Example 6.5

An investigation was made into fatal poisonings of children by two drugs which were among the leading causes of such deaths. In each case, an inquiry was made as to how the child had received the fatal overdose and responsibility for the accident was assessed. Results were as follows:

	Drug A	Drug B
Child responsible	8	12
Child not responsible	31	19

We have the proportions of cases for which the child is responsible,

$$p_A = \frac{8}{8+31}$$
$$= .205 \text{ or } 20.5\%$$
$$p_B = \frac{12}{12+19}$$
$$= .387 \text{ or } 38.7\%$$

suggesting that they are not the same and that a child seems more prone to taking B than A. However, the chi-square statistic

$$X^2 = \frac{(39+31)[(8)(19)-(31)(12)]^2}{(39)(31)(20)(50)}$$
$$= 2.80 (< 3.84; \alpha = .05)$$

shows that the difference is not statistically significant at the .05 level.

_____

_____

Example 6.6

In Example 1.2, a case–control study was conducted to identify reasons for the exceptionally high rate of lung cancer among male residents of coastal Georgia. The primary risk factor under investigation was employment in shipyards during World War II, and the following table provides data for nonsmokers:

Shipbuilding	Cases	Controls
Yes	11	35
No	50	203

We have for the cases

$$p_2 = 11/61$$
$$= .180$$

and for the controls

$$p_1 = 35/238$$
$$= .147$$

An application of the procedure yields a pooled proportion of

$$p = \frac{11 + 35}{61 + 238}$$
$$= .154$$

leading to

$$z = \frac{.180 - .147}{\sqrt{(.154)(.846)\left(\frac{1}{61} + \frac{1}{238}\right)}}$$
$$= .64$$

It can be seen that the rate of employment for the cases (18.0%) was higher than that for the controls (14.7%), but the difference is not statistically significant at the .05 level ($z = .64 < 1.65$).

―――――

―――――

Example 6.7

The role of smoking in the etiology of pancreatitis has been recognized for many years. In order to provide estimates of the quantitative significance of these factors, a hospital-based study was carried out in eastern Massachusetts and Rhode Island between 1975 and 1979. Ninety-eight patients who had a hospital discharge diagnosis of pancreatitis were included in this unmatched case–control study. The control group consisted of 451 patients admitted for diseases other than those of the pancreas and biliary tract. Risk factor information was obtained from a standardized interview with each subject, conducted by a trained interviewer.

The following are some data for the males:

Use of Cigarettes	Cases	Controls
Current smokers	38	81
Never or ex-smokers	15	136
Total	53	217

With currently smoking being the exposure, we have for the cases

$$p_2 = 38/53$$
$$= .717$$

and for the controls

$$p_1 = 81/217$$
$$= .373$$

An application of the procedure yields a pooled proportion of

$$p = \frac{38 + 81}{53 + 217}$$
$$= .441$$

leading to

$$z = \frac{.717 - .373}{\sqrt{(.441)(.559)\left(\frac{1}{53} + \frac{1}{217}\right)}}$$
$$= 4.52$$

It can be seen that the proportion of smokers among the cases (71.7%) was higher than that for the controls (37.7%), and the difference is highly statistically significant ($p < .001$).

6.4. THE MANTEL–HAENSZEL METHOD

We are often interested only in investigating the relationship between two binary variables—for example, a disease and an exposure; however, we have to control for confounders. A confounding variable is a variable that may be associated with either the disease or exposure or both. For example, in Example 1.2 a case–control study was undertaken to investigate the relationship between lung cancer and employment in shipyards during World War II among male residents of coastal Georgia. In this case, smoking is a possible confounder; it has been found to be associated with lung cancer, and it may be associated with employment because construction workers are likely to be smokers. Specifically, we want to know:

 (i) Among smokers, whether or not shipbuilding and lung cancer are related, and
(ii) Among nonsmokers, whether or not shipbuilding and lung cancer are related.

The underlying question is the question concerning conditional independence between lung cancer and shipbuilding; however, we do not want to reach separate conclusions, one at each level of smoking. Assuming that the confounder, smoking, is not an effect modifier (i.e. smoking does not alter the relationship between lung cancer and shipbuilding), we want to pool data for a combined decision. When both the disease and the exposure are binary, a popular method to achieve this task is the Mantel–Haenszel method. The process can be summarized as follows:

(i) We form 2×2 tables, one at each level of the confounder.

(ii) At a level of the confounder, we have

	Disease Classification		
Exposure	$+$	$-$	Total
$+$	a	b	r_1
$-$	c	d	r_2
Total	c_1	c_2	n

Under the null hypothesis and fixed marginal totals, cell $(1, 1)$ frequency "a" is distributed with mean and variance:

$$E_0(a) = \frac{r_1 c_1}{n}$$

$$Var_0(a) = \frac{r_1 r_2 c_1 c_2}{n^2(n-1)}$$

and the Mantel–Haenszel test is based on the z statistic

$$z = \frac{\sum a - \sum \frac{r_1 c_1}{n}}{\sqrt{\sum \frac{r_1 r_2 c_1 c_2}{n^2(n-1)}}}$$

where the summation $(\sum)$ is across levels of the confounder. Of course, one can use the square of the z-score, a *chi-square test* at one degree of freedom, for two-sided alternatives.

When the above test is statistically significant, the association between the disease and the exposure is *real*. Because we assume that the counfounder is not an effect modifier, the odds ratio is constant accross its levels. The odds ratio at each level is estimated by ad/bc; the Mantel–Haenszel procedure pools data accross levels of the confounder to obtain a combined estimate:

$$OR_{MH} = \frac{\sum \frac{ad}{n}}{\sum \frac{bc}{n}}$$

Example 6.8

A case–control study was conducted to identify reasons for the exceptionally high rate of lung cancer among male residents of coastal Georgia. The primary risk factor under investigation was employment in shipyards during World War II, and data are tabulated separately for three levels of smoking as follows:

Smoking	Shipbuilding	Cases	Controls
No	Yes	11	3 5
	No	50	203
Moderate	Yes	70	42
	No	217	220
Heavy	Yes	14	3
	No	96	50

There are three 2×2 tables, one for each level of smoking; in Example 1.1, the last two tables were combined and presented together for simplicity.

We begin with the 2×2 table for nonsmokers:

Shipbuilding	Cases	Controls	Total
Yes	11(a)	35(b)	46(r_1)
No	50(c)	203(d)	253(r_2)
Total	61(c_1)	238(c_2)	299(n)

We have, for the nonsmokers,

$$a = 11$$

$$\frac{r_1 c_1}{n} = \frac{(46)(61)}{299}$$

$$= 9.38$$

$$\frac{r_1 r_2 c_1 c_2}{n^2(n-1)} = \frac{(46)(253)(61)(238)}{(299)^2(298)}$$

$$= 6.34$$

$$\frac{ad}{n} = \frac{(11)(203)}{299}$$

$$= 7.47$$

$$\frac{bc}{n} = \frac{(35)(50)}{299}$$

$$= 5.85$$

The process is repeated for each of the other two smoking levels. For moderate smokers

$$a = 70$$

$$\frac{r_1 c_1}{n} = \frac{(112)(287)}{549}$$

$$= 58.55$$

$$\frac{r_1 r_2 c_1 c_2}{n^2(n-1)} = \frac{(112)(437)(287)(262)}{(549)^2(548)}$$

$$= 22.28$$

$$\frac{ad}{n} = \frac{(70)(220)}{549}$$

$$= 28.05$$

$$\frac{bc}{n} = \frac{(42)(217)}{549}$$

$$= 16.60$$

and for heavy smokers

$$a = 14$$

$$\frac{r_1 c_1}{n} = \frac{(17)(110)}{163}$$

$$= 11.47$$

$$\frac{r_1 r_2 c_1 c_2}{n^2(n-1)} = \frac{(17)(146)(110)(53)}{(163)^2(162)}$$

$$= 3.36$$

$$\frac{ad}{n} = \frac{(14)(50)}{163}$$

$$= 4.29,$$

$$\frac{bc}{n} = \frac{(3)(96)}{163}$$

$$= 1.77$$

These results are combined to obtain the z-score

$$z = \frac{(11 - 9.38) + (70 - 58.55) + (14 - 11.47)}{\sqrt{6.34 + 22.28 + 3.36}}$$

$$= 2.76$$

and a z-score of 2.76 yields a one-tailed p-value of .0029, which is beyond the 1% level. This result is stronger than those for tests at each level because it is based on more information where all data at all three smoking levels are used. The combined odds ratio estimate is

$$OR_{MH} = \frac{7.47 + 28.05 + 4.29}{5.85 + 16.60 + 1.77}$$

$$= 1.64$$

representing an approximate increase of 64% in lung cancer risk for those employed in the shipbuilding industry.

Note: a SAS program would include these instructions:

```
DATA;
INPUT SMOKE SHIP CANCER COUNT;
CARDS;
1 1 1 11
1 1 2 35
1 2 1 50
1 2 2 203
2 1 1 70
2 1 2 42
2 2 1 217
2 2 2 220
3 1 1 14
3 1 2 3
3 2 1 96
3 2 2 50;
PROC FREQ;
WEIGHT COUNT;
TABLES SMOKE*SHIP*CANCER/CMH;
```

The result is given in a chi-square form ($X^2 = 7.601, p = .006$); CMH stands for Cochran–Mantel–Haenszel statistic.

Example 6.9

A case–control study was conducted to investigate the relationship between myocardial infarction (MI) and oral contraceptive use (OC). The data, stratified by cigarette smoking, were as follows

Smoking	OC Use	Cases	Controls
No	Yes	4	52
	No	34	754
Yes	Yes	25	83
	No	171	853

An application of the Mantel–Haenszel procedure yields the following:

	Smoking	
	No	Yes
a	4	25
$\dfrac{r_1 c_1}{n}$	2.52	18.70
$\dfrac{r_1 r_2 c_1 c_2}{n^2(n-1)}$	2.25	14.00
$\dfrac{ad}{n}$	3.57	18.84
$\dfrac{bc}{n}$	2.09	12.54

The combined z-score is

$$z = \frac{(4 - 2.52) + (25 - 18.70)}{\sqrt{2.25 + 14.00}}$$

$$= 1.93$$

which is significant at the 5% level (one-sided). The combined odds ratio estimate is:

$$OR_{MH} = \frac{3.57 + 18.84}{2.09 + 12.54}$$

$$= 1.53$$

representing an approximate increase of 53% in myocardial infarction for oral contraceptive users.

6.5. INFERENCES FOR GENERAL TWO-WAY TABLES

Data forming two-way contingency tables do not necessarily come from two binomial samples. There may be more than two binomial samples to compare. They may come from two independent samples, but the endpoint may have more than two categories. They may come from a survey (i.e., *one* sample), but data are cross-tabulated based on two binary factors of interest (so we still have a 2 × 2 table as in the comparison of two proportions).

Consider the general case of an I × J table, say resulting from a survey of size n. Let X_1 and X_2 denote two categorical variables, X_1 having I levels and X_2 having J levels; there are IJ combinations of classifications. The IJ cells represent the IJ combinations of classifications; their probabilities are $\{\pi_{ij}\}$, where π_{ij} denotes the probability that the outcome (X_1, X_2) falls in the cell in row i and column j. When two categorical variables forming the two-way table are independent, all $\pi_{ij} = \pi_{i+}\pi_{+j}$. This is the *Multiplication Rule* for probabilities of independence events introduced in Chapter 3; here π_{i+} and π_{+j} are the two marginal or univariate probabilities. The estimate of π_{ij} under this condition is

$$\widehat{\pi_{ij}} = \widehat{\pi_{i+}}\widehat{\pi_{+j}}$$

$$= p_{i+}p_{+j}$$

$$= \left(\frac{x_{i+}}{n}\right)\left(\frac{x_{+j}}{n}\right)$$

$$= \frac{x_{i+}x_{+j}}{n^2}$$

where the x's are the observed frequencies. Under the assumption of independence, we would have in cell (i, j)

$$e_{ij} = n\widehat{\pi_{ij}}$$

$$= \frac{x_{i+}x_{+j}}{n}$$

$$= \frac{(\text{Row total})(\text{Column total})}{\text{Sample size}}$$

The $\{e_{ij}\}$ are called estimated expected frequencies, the frequencies we expect to have under the null hypothesis of independence. They have the same marginal totals as do the observed data. In this problem we do not compare proportions (because we have only one sample), what we really want to see is if the two factors or variables X_1 and X_2 are *related*. The task we perform is a *test for independence*. We achieve that by comparing the observed frequencies, the x's, versus those expected under the null hypothesis of independence, the expected frequencies e's. This needed comparison is done through the Pearson's chi-quare statistic:

$$\chi^2 = \sum_{i,j} \frac{(x_{ij} - e_{ij})^2}{e_{ij}}$$

For large samples, X^2 has approximately a chi-squared distribution with degrees of freedom (*df*) under the null hypothesis of independence,

$$df = (I - 1)(J - 1)$$

with greater values lead to a rejection of H_0.

_____

Example 6.10

In 1979 the U.S. Veterans Administration conducted a health survey of 11,230 veterans. The advantages of this survey are that it includes a large random sample with a high interview response rate, and it was done before the recent public controversy surrounding the issue of the health effects of possible exposure to Agent Orange. The following are data relating Vietnam service to having sleep problems among the 1787 veterans who entered the military service between 1965 and 1975.

Sleep Problems	Service in Vietnam		
	Yes	No	Total
Yes	173	160	333
No	599	851	1450
Total	772	1011	1783

We have

$$e_{11} = \frac{(333)(772)}{1783}$$

$$= 144.18$$

$$e_{12} = 333 - 144.18$$

$$= 188.82$$

$$e_{21} = 772 - 144.18$$

$$= 627.82$$

$$e_{22} = 1011 - 188.82$$

$$= 822.18$$

leading to

$$X^2 = \frac{(173 - 144.18)^2}{144.18} + \frac{(160 - 188.82)^2}{188.82} + \frac{(599 - 627.82)^2}{627.82} + \frac{(851 - 822.18)^2}{822.18}$$

$$= 12.49$$

This statistic, at 1 df, indicates a significant correlation ($p < .001$) relating Vietnam service to having sleep problems among the veterans. It is interesting to note that we needed to calculate only *one* expected frequency, e_{11}; this explains the *one* degree of freedom we used.

Example 6.11

The following table shows the results of a survey, each subject of a sample of 300 adults was asked to indicate which of three policies they favored with respect to smoking in public places. The numbers in parentheses are expected frequencies.

Highest Education Level	Policy Favored				
	No Restrictions on Smoking	Smoking Allowed in Designated Areas Only	No Smoking at All	No Opinion	Total
College graduate	44(46)	23(13.25)	3(4.5)	75	
High school	15(17.5)	100(92)	30(26.5)	5(9)	150
Grade school	15(8.75)	40(46)	10(13.25)	10(4.5)	75
Total	35	184	63	18	300

An application of the Pearson's chi-quare test, at six degrees of freedom, yields

$$X^2 = \frac{(5-8.75)^2}{8.75} + \frac{(44-46)^2}{46} + \cdots + \frac{(10-4.5)^2}{4.5}$$
$$= 25.50$$

The result indicates a high correlation between education levels and preferences about smoking in public places ($p = .001$).

Note: An SAS program would include these instructions:
```
DATA;
INPUT EDUCAT POLICY COUNT;
CARDS;
1 1 5
1 2 44
1 3 23
1 4 3
2 1 15
2 2 100
2 3 30
2 4 5
3 1 15
3 2 40
3 3 10
3 4 10;
PROC FREQ;
WEIGHT COUNT;
TABLES EDUCAT*POLICY/CHISQ;
```

Statistical decisions based on the Pearson's chi-square statistic make use of the percentiles of the chi-square distribution. Because chi-square is a continuous distribution and categorical data are discrete, some statisticians use a version of the Pearson's statistic with a *continuity correction*, called Yates corrected chi-square test, which can be expressed as

$$X_c^2 = \sum_{i,j} \frac{(|x_{ij} - e_{ij}| - 0.5)^2}{e_{ij}}$$

Statisticians still disagree about whether or not a continuity correction is needed. Generally, the corrected version is more conservative and more widely used in applied literature.

So far, the test for the comparison of two proportions and the test for independence have been presented in very different way; fortunately, they are not that different. For example, if we apply the test of independence to a 2×2 table where data came from two binomial samples, say a case–control study, we get the same chi-square statistic as if we applied the chi-square test to compare the two proportions against a two-sided alternative. In other words, the chi-square test—presented as a comparison of observed versus expected frequencies —applies regardless of the sampling mechanism. For example, we can use the chi square test to compare several proportions *simultaneously* using data from several binomial samples (see Example 6.13). [In this type of problem, we have k independent samples of binary data $(n_1, x_1), (n_2, x_2), \ldots, (n_k, x_k)$, where the n's are sample sizes and the x's are the numbers of positive outcomes in the k samples. For these k independent binomial samples, we consider the null hypothesis

$$H_0 : \pi_1 = \pi_2 = \cdots = \pi_k$$

expressing the equality of the k population proportions.]

Example 6.12

Referring to the case–control study was conducted to identify reasons for the exceptionally high rate of lung cancer among male residents of coastal Georgia of Example 6.6:

Shipbuilding	Cases	Controls	Total
Yes	11	35	46
No	50	203	253
Total	61	238	299

We have

$$e_{11} = \frac{(46)(61)}{299}$$
$$= 9.38$$
$$e_{12} = 46 - 9.38$$
$$= 36.62$$
$$e_{21} = 61 - 9.38$$

$$= 51.62$$

$$e_{22} = 253 - 51.62$$

$$= 201.38$$

leading to

$$X^2 = \frac{(11 - 9.38)^2}{9.38} + \frac{(35 - 36.62)^2}{36.62} + \frac{(50 - 51.62)^2}{51.62} + \frac{(203 - 201.38)^2}{201.38}$$

$$= .42$$

This result, a chi-square value, is identical to that from Example 6.6 where we obtained a z-score of .64 [*note:* $(.64)^2 = .42$].

Example 6.13

A study was undertaken to investigate the roles of blood-borne environmental exposures on ovarian cancer from assessment of consumption of coffee, tobacco, and alcohol. Study subjects consist of 188 women in the San Francisco Bay area with epithelial ovarian cancers diagnosed in 1983–1985, along with 539 control women. Of the 539 controls, 280 were hospitalized women without overt cancer, and 259 were chosen from the general population by random telephone dialing. Data for coffee consumption are summarized as follows:

Coffee Drinkers	Cases	Hospital Controls	Population Controls	Total
Yes	177(170.42)	249(253.81)	233(234.77)	659
No	11(17.58)	31(26.19)	26(24.23)	68
Total	188	280	259	727

(the numbers in parentheses are expected frequencies). In this example, we want to *compare* the three proportions of coffee drinkers, but we still can apply the same chi-square test:

$$X^2 = \frac{(177 - 170.42)^2}{170.42} + \cdots + \frac{(26 - 24.23)^2}{24.23}$$

$$= 3.83$$

The result indicates that the difference between the three groups is not significant at the 5% level (the cutpoint at 5% level for a chi-square with 2 degrees of freedom is 5.99). In other words, there are enough evidence to implicate coffee consumption in this study of epithelial ovarian cancer. It is important to note that in solving the above problem, a comparison of several proportions, one may be tempted to compare all possible pairs of proportions and do many chi-square tests. What is the matter with this approach of doing many chi-square tests, one for each pair of samples? As the number of groups increases, so does the number of tests to perform; for example, we would have to do 45 tests if we have 10 groups to compare. Obviously, the amount of work is greater, but that should not be the critical problem—especially with technological aids such as the use of calculators and computers. So, what is the problem? The answer is that performing many tests increases the probability that one or more of the comparisons will result in a Type I error (i.e., a significant test result when the null hypothesis is true). This statement should make sense intuitively. For example, suppose the null hypothesis is true and we perform 100 tests— each has a 0.05 probability of resulting in a Type I error; then 5 of these 100 tests would be statistically significant as the results of Type I errors. Of course, we usually do not need to do that many tests; however, every time we do more than one, then the probability that at least one will result in a Type I error exceeds 0.05, indicating a falsely significant difference! What is needed is a method of *simultaneously* comparing these proportions in one step. And the above chi-square test for a general two-way table, in this case a two-by-three table, achieves just that.

6.6. FISHER'S EXACT TEST

Even with a continuity correction, the *goodness-of-fit* test statistic such as Pearson's X^2 is not suitable when the sample is small. Generally, statisticians suggest to use them only if no expected frequency in the table is less than 5. For studies with small samples, we will introduce a method known as *Fisher's exact test*. For tables in which the use of the chi-square test X^2 is appropriate, the two tests give very similar results.

Our purpose is to find the exact significance level associated with an observed table. The central idea is to enumerate all possible outcomes consistent with a given set of marginal totals and add up the probabilities of those tables more extreme than the one observed. Conditional on the margins, a 2×2 table is a one-dimensional random variable having a known distribution so the exact test is relatively easy to implement. The probability of observing a table with cells a, b, c, and d (with total n) is

$$\Pr(a, b, c, d) = \frac{(a+b)!(c+d)!(a+c)!(b+d)!}{n!a!b!c!d!}$$

The process for doing hand calculations would be as follows:

1. Rearrange the rows and columns of the observed table so that the smaller total is in the first row and the smaller column total is in the first column.
2. Start with the table having 0 in the (1, 1) cell (top left cell). The other cells in this table are determined automatically from the fixed row margins and column margins.

3. Construct the next table by increasing the (1, 1) cell from 0 to 1 and decreasing all other cells accordingly.
4. Continue to increase the (1, 1) cell by 1 until one of the other cells become 0. At that point we have enumerated all possible tables.
5. Calculate and add up the probabilities of those tables with cell (1, 1) having values from 0 to the observed frequency (left tail for a one-tailed test); double the smaller tail for a two-tailed test.

In practice, the calculations are often tedious and should be left to a computer program to implement.

Example 6.14

A study on deaths of men aged over 50 yields the following data; numbers in parentheses are expected frequencies:

	Type of diet		
Cause of Death	High Salt	Low Salt	Total
Non-CVD	2(2.92)	23(22.08)	25
CVD	5(4.08)	30(30.92)	35
Total	7	53	60

An application of the Fisher's exact test yields a one-tailed p-value of .375 or a two-tailed p-value of .688; we cannot say, on the basis of this limited amount of data, that there is a significant association between salt intake and cause of death even though the proportions of CVD deaths are different (71.4% versus 56.6%). For implementing hand calculations, we would focus on the tables where cell (1, 1) equals 0, 1, and 2 (observed value); the probabilities for these tables are 0.017, 0.105, and 0.252, respectively.

Note: a SAS program would include these instructions:
```
DATA;
INPUT CVM DIET COUNT;
CARDS;
1 1 2
1 2 23
2 1 5
2 2 30;
PROC FREQ;
WEIGHT COUNT;
TABLES CVD*DIET/CHISQ;
```
The output also includes Pearson's test ($X^2 = 0.559$; $p = 0.455$) as well.

6.7. ORDERED 2 x *k* CONTINGENCY TABLES

This section presents an efficient method for use with ordered 2 × *k* contingency tables—that is, tables with 2 rows and with *k* columns having a certain natural ordering. We first introduce it in Chapter 1 so as to provide a descriptive statistic, the *generalized odds*.

In general, consider an ordered 2 × *k* table with frequencies:

	Column Level				
Row	1	2	$\cdots$	*k*	Total
1	a_1	a_2	$\cdots$	a_k	A
2	b_1	b_2	$\cdots$	b_k	B
Total	n_1	n_2	$\cdots$	n_k	N

The number of "concordances" is calculated by

$$C = a_1(b_2 + \cdots + b_k) + a_2(b_3 + \cdots + b_k) + \cdots + a_{k-1}b_k$$

The number of "discordances" is

$$D = b_1(a_2 + \cdots + a_k) + b_2(a_3 + \cdots + a_k) + \cdots + b_{k-1}a_k$$

In order to perform the test, we calculate the statistic

$$S = C - D$$

then standardize it to obtain

$$z = \frac{S - \mu_S}{\sigma_D}$$

where $\mu_S = 0$ is the mean of S under the null hypothesis and

$$\sigma_S = \left\{ \frac{AB}{3N(N-1)} \left[N^3 - n_1^3 - n_2^3 - \cdots - n_k^3 \right] \right\}^{1/2}$$

The standardized z-score is distributed as standard normal if the null hypothesis is true. For a one-sided alternative, which is a natural choice for this type of tests, the null hypothesis is rejected at the 5% level if $z > 1.65$ (or $z < -1.65$ if the terms "concordance" and "discordance" are switched).

Example 6.15

Consider an example concerning the use of seat belts in automobiles. Each accident in this example is classified according to whether a seat belt was used and the severity of injuries received: none, minor, major, or death. The data were as follows:

	Extent of Injury Received				
Seat Belt	None	Minor	Major	Death	Total
Yes	75	160	100	15	350
No	65	175	135	25	390
Total	130	335	235	40	740

For this study on the use of seat belts in automobiles, an application of the above method yields

$$C = 75(175 + 135 + 25) + 160(135 + 25) + (100)(25)$$
$$= 53,225$$
$$D = 65(160 + 100 + 15) + 175(100 + 15) + (135)(15)$$
$$= 40,025$$

In addition, we have

$$A = 350$$
$$B = 390$$
$$n_1 = 130$$
$$n_2 = 335$$
$$n_3 = 235$$
$$n_4 = 40$$
$$N = 740$$

Substituting these values into the equations of the test statistic, we have

$$S = 53,225 - 40,025$$
$$= 13,200$$
$$\sigma_S = \left\{ \frac{(350)(390)}{(3)(740)(739)} \left[740^3 - 130^3 - 335^3 - 235^3 - 40^3 \right] \right\}^{1/2}$$
$$= 5414.76$$

leading to

$$z = 13{,}200/5414.76$$

$$= 2.44$$

which shows a high degree of significance (one-sided p-value $= 0.0073$). It is interesting to note that in order to compare the extent of injury in those who used seat belts and those who did not, we can perform a chi-square test as presented in the previous section. Such an application of the chi-square test yields

$$X^2 = 9.26$$

with 3 degrees of freedom ($0.01 \leq p \leq 0.05$). Therefore, the difference between the two groups is significant at the 5% level but not at the 1% level, a lower degree of significance (as compared to the above p-value of 0.0073). This is because the usual chi-square calculation takes no account of the fact that the extent of injury has a natural ordering: none < minor < major < death. In addition, the percent of seat belt users in each injury group decreases from level "none" to level "death":

$$
\begin{aligned}
&\text{None :} & 75/(75 + 65) &= 54\% \\
&\text{Minor :} & 160/(160 + 175) &= 48\% \\
&\text{Major :} & 100/(100 + 135) &= 43\% \\
&\text{Death :} & 15/(15 + 25) &= 38\%
\end{aligned}
$$

The new method of this section seems particularly ideal for the evaluation of ordinal risk factors in case–control studies.

Example 6.16

Prematurity, which ranks as the major cause of neonatal morbidity and mortality, has traditionally been defined on the basis of a birth weight under 2500 g. But this definition encompasses two distinct types of infants: infants who are small because they are born early, and infants who are born at or near term but are small because their growth was retarded. "Prematurity" has now been replaced by

 (i) "Low birth weight" to describe the second type
(ii) "Preterm" to characterize the first type (babies born before 37 weeks of gestation)

A case-control study of the epidemiology of pre-term delivery was undertaken at Yale–New Haven Hospital in Connecticut during 1977. The study population consisted of 175 mothers of singleton preterm infants and 303 mothers of singleton full-term infants. The following tables give the distribution of age of the mother.

Age	Cases	Controls	Total
14–17	15	16	31
18–19	22	25	47
20–24	47	62	109
25–29	56	122	178
≥ 30	35	78	113
Total	175	303	

We have

$$C = 15(25 + 62 + 122 + 78) + 22(62 + 122 + 78) + 47(122 + 78) + (56)(78)$$
$$= 20{,}911$$
$$D = 16(22 + 47 + 56 + 35) + 25(47 + 56 + 35) + (62)(56 + 35) + (122)(35)$$
$$= 15{,}922$$
$$S = 20{,}911 - 15{,}922$$
$$= 4989$$
$$\sigma_S = \left\{ \frac{(175)(303)}{(3)(478)(477)} \left[478^3 - 31^3 - 47^3 - 109^3 - 178^3 - 113^3 \right] \right\}^{1/2}$$
$$= 2794.02$$

leading to

$$z = 4989/27.94.02$$
$$= 1.79$$

which shows a significant association between the mother's age and preterm delivery (one-sided p-value $= 0.0367$); the younger the mother, the more likely the preterm delivery.

6.8. NOTES ON COMPUTATIONS

Samples of SAS program instructions were provided for complicated procedures, at the end of Examples 6.8 and 6.14. Other computations can be implemented easily using a calculator *provided* that data have summarized into the form of a two-way table. Read Section 1.4 on how to use Excel's *Pivot Table* procedure to form a 2 × 2 table from a raw data file. After value of a statistic has been obtained, you can use NORMDIST (Section 3.5) to obtain an exact p-value associated with a z-score and CHIDIST to obtain an exact p-value associated with a chi-square statistic; CHIDIST procedure can be used similar to the case of a one-tailed TDIST (Section 3.5). For the method of Section 6.5, and instead of writing an SAS program, one can calculate expected frequencies (using *formula* and *drag and fill*, Section 1.4), then input into the CHITEST procedure of Excel.

EXERCISES

6.1. Consider a sample of $n = 110$ women drawn randomly from the membership list of the National Organization for Women (NOW), $x = 25$ of whom were found to smoke. Use the result of this sample to test whether the rate found is significantly *different* from the U.S. proportion of .30 for women.

6.2. In a case–control study, 317 patients suffering from endometrial carcinoma were individually matched with 317 other cancer patients in a hospital and the use of estrogen in the 6 months prior to diagnosis was determined. The results were as follows:

	Controls	
Cases	Estrogen	No Estrogen
Estrogen	39	113
No estrogen	15	150

Use McNemar's chi-square test to investigate the significance of the association between estrogen use and endometrial carcinoma; state your null and alternative hypotheses.

6.3. A study in Maryland identified 4032 white persons, enumerated in a nonofficial 1963 census, who became widowed between 1963 and 1974. These people were matched, one-to-one, to married persons on the basis of race, sex, year of birth, and geography of residence. The matched pairs were followed to a second census in 1975, and in Example 6.3 we have analyzed the data for men so as to compare the mortality of widowed men versus married men. The data for 2828 matched pairs of women were as follows:

Widowed	Married Women	
Women	Died	Alive
Died	1	264
Alive	249	2314

Test to compare the mortality of widowed women versus married women; state your null and alternative hypotheses.

6.4. It has been noted that metal workers have an increased risk for cancer of the internal nose and paranasal sinuses, perhaps as a result of exposure to cutting oils. Therefore, a study was conducted to see whether this particular exposure also increases the risk for squamous cell carcinoma of the scrotum. Cases included all 45 squamous cell carcinomas of the scrotum diagnosed in Connecticut residents from 1955 to 1973, as obtained from the Connecticut Tumor Registry. Matched controls were selected for each case based on the age at death (within 8 years), year of death (within 3 years), and number of jobs as obtained from combined death certificate and Directory sources. An occupational indicator of metal worker (yes/no) was evaluated as the possible risk factor in this study; results are as follows:

	Controls	
Cases	Yes	No
Yes	2	26
No	5	12

Test to compare the cases versus the controls using McNemar's chi-square test; state clearly your null and alternative hypotheses, and state your choice of the test size.

6.5. A matched case–control study on endometrial cancer, where the exposure was "ever having taken any estrogen," yields the following data:

	Matching Controls	
Cases	Exposed	Nonexposed
Exposed	27	29
Nonexposed	3	4

Test to compare the cases versus the controls; state clearly your null and alternative hypotheses, and state your choice of the test size.

6.6. Ninety-eight heterosexual couples, at least one of whom was HIV-infected, were enrolled in an HIV transmission study and interviewed about sexual behavior. The following table provides a summary of condom use reported by heterosexual partners:

	Man	
Woman	Ever	Never
Ever	45	6
Never	7	40

Test to compare the men versus the women; state clearly your null and alternative hypotheses, and state your choice of the test size.

6.7. A matched case–control study was conducted in order to evaluate the cumulative effects of acrylate and methacrylate vapors on olfactory function. Cases were defined as scoring at or below the 10th percentile on the UPSIT (University of Pennsylvania Smell Identification Test).

	Cases	
Controls	Exposed	Unexposed
Exposed	25	22
Unexposed	9	21

Test to compare the cases versus the controls; state clearly your null and alternative hypotheses, and state your choice of the test size.

6.8. Self-reported injuries among left-handed and right-handed people were compared in a survey of 1896 college students in British Columbia, Canada. Ninety-three of the 180 left-handed students reported at least one injury, and 619 of the 1716 right-handed students reported at least one injury in the same period. Test to compare the proportions of students with injury, left-handed versus right-handed; state clearly your null and alternative hypotheses, and state your choice of the test size.

6.9. A study was conducted in order to evaluate the hypothesis that tea consumption and premenstrual syndrome are associated. One hundred eighty-eight nursing students and 64 tea factory workers were given questionnaires. The prevalence of premenstrual syndrome was 39% among the nursing students and 77% among the tea factory workers. Test to compare the prevalences of premenstrual syndrome, tea factory workers versus nursing students; state clearly your null and alternative hypotheses, and state your choice of the test size.

6.10. A study was conducted to investigate drinking problems among college students. In 1983, a group of students were asked whether they had ever driven an automobile while drinking. In 1987, after the legal drinking age was raised, a different group of college students were asked the same question. The results are as follows:

Drove While	Year	
Drinking	1983	1987
Yes	1250	991
No	1387	1666
Total	2637	2657

Test to compare the proportions of students with drinking problem, 1987 versus 1983; state clearly your null and alternative hypotheses, and state your choice of the test size.

6.11. In August 1976, tuberculosis was diagnosed in a high school student (INDEX CASE) in Corinth, Mississippi. Subsequently, laboratory studies revealed that the student's disease was caused by drug-resistant tubercule bacilli. An epidemiologic investigation was conducted at the high school.

The following table gives the rates of positive tuberculin reaction, determined for various groups of students according to degree of exposure to the index case.

Exposure Level	Number Tested	Number Positive
High	129	63
Low	325	36

Test to compare the proportions of students with infection, high exposure versus low exposure; state clearly your null and alternative hypotheses, and state your choice of the test size.

6.12. Epidemic keratoconjunctivitis (EKC) or "shipyard eye" is an acute infectious disease of the eye. A case of EKC is defined as an illness

- consisting of redness, tearing, and pain in one or both eyes for more than 3 days' duration,
- diagnosed as EKC by an ophthalmologist.

In late October 1977, one (Physician A) of the two ophthalmologists providing the majority of specialized eye care to the residents of a central Georgia county (population 45,000) saw a 27-year-old nurse who had returned from a vacation in Korea with severe EKC. She received symptomatic therapy and was warned that her eye infection could spread to others; nevertheless, numerous cases of an illness similar to hers soon occurred in the patients and staff of the nursing home (Nursing Home A) where she worked (these individuals came to Physician A for diagnosis and treatment). The following table provides exposure history of 22 persons with EKC between October 27, 1977 and January 13, 1978 (when the outbreak stopped after proper control techniques were initiated). Nursing Home B, included in this table, is the only other area chronic-care facility.

Exposure Cohort	Number Exposed	Number of Cases
Nursing Home A	64	16
Nursing Home B	238	6

Using an appropriate test, compare the proportions of cases from the two nursing homes.

6.13. Consider the data taken from a study that attempts to determine whether the use of electronic fetal monitoring (EFM) during labor affects the frequency of caesarean section deliveries. Of the 5824 infants included in the study, 2850 were electronically monitored and 2974 were not. The outcomes are as follows:

| Caesarean | EFM Exposure | |
Delivery	Yes	No
Yes	358	229
No	2492	2745
Total	2850	2974

Test to compare the rates of caesarean section delivery, EFM-exposed versus Nonexposed; state clearly your null and alternative hypotheses, and your choice of the test size.

6.14. A study was conducted to investigate the effectiveness of bicycle safety helmets in preventing head injury. The data consist of a random sample of 793 individuals who were involved in bicycle accidents during a 1-year period.

| | Wearing Helmet | |
Head Injury	Yes	No
Yes	17	218
No	130	428
Total	147	646

Test to compare the proportions with head injury, those with helmets versus those without; state clearly your null and alternative hypotheses, and state your choice of the test size.

6.15. A case–control study was conducted relating to the epidemiology of breast cancer and the possible involvement of dietary fats, along with other vitamins and nutrients. It included 2024 breast cancer cases who were admitted to Roswell Park Memorial Institute, Erie County, New York, from 1958 to 1965. A control group of 1463 was chosen from the patients having no neoplasms and no pathology of gastrointestinal or reproductive systems. The primary factors being investigated were vitamins A and E (measured in international units per month). The following are data for 1500 women over 54 years of age.

Vitamin A (IU/mo)	Cases	Controls
$\leq 150,500$	893	392
$> 150,500$	132	83
Total	1025	475

Test to compare the proportions of subjects who consumed less vitamin A ($\leq 150,500$ IU/mo), cases versus controls; state clearly your null and alternative hypotheses, and your choice of the test size.

6.16. In a randomized trial, 111 pregnant women had elective induction of labor between 39 and 40 weeks and 117 controls were managed expectantly until 41 weeks. The results were as follows:

	Induction Group	Control Group
Number on patients	111	117
Number with meconium staining	1	13

Use Fisher's exact test to verify the alternative that patients with elective induction have less meconium staining in labor than the control patients.

6.17. A research report states that: "A comparison of the 90 normal patients with the 10 patients with hypotension shows that only 3.3% of the former group died as compared to 30% of the latter." Put the data into a 2×2 contingency table and test the significance of blood pressure as a prognostic sign using:

(a) Pearson's chi-square test,

(b) Pearson's chi-square test with Yates' continuity correction, and

(c) Fisher's exact test.

6.18. In a trial of diabetic therapy, patients were treated either with Phenformin or a placebo. The numbers of patients and deaths from cardiovascular causes were as follows:

Result	Phenformin	Placebo	Total
Cardiovascular deaths	26	2	28
Not deaths	178	62	240
Total	204	64	268

Use Fisher's exact test to investigate the difference in cardiovascular mortality between the Phenformin and Placebo groups; state your null and alternative hypotheses.

6.19. In a seroepidemiologic survey of health workers representing a spectrum of exposure to blood and patients with hepatitis B virus (HBV), it was found that infection increased as a function of contact. The following table provides data for hospital workers with uniform socioeconomic status at an urban teaching hospital in Boston, Massachusetts.

Personnel	Exposure	n	HBV Positive
Physicians	Frequent	81	17
	Infrequent	89	7
Nurses	Frequent	104	22
	Infrequent	126	11

Test to compare the proportions of HBV infection between the four groups (physicians with frequent exposure, physicians with infrequent exposure, nurses with frequent exposure, and nurses with infrequent exposure. State clearly your null and alternative hypotheses, and your choice of the test size.

6.20. It has been hypothesized that dietary fiber decreases the risk of colon cancer, whereas meats and fats are thought to increase this risk. A large study was undertaken to confirm these hypotheses (Graham et al., 1988). Fiber and fat consumptions are classified as "low" or "high," and data are tabulated separately for males and females as follows ("low" means below median):

Diet	Males		Females	
	Cases	Controls	Cases	Controls
Low fat, high fiber	27	38	23	39
Low fat, low fiber	64	78	82	81
High fat, high fiber	78	61	83	76
High fat, low fiber	36	28	35	27

Test to investigate the relationship between the disease (two categories: cases and controls) and the diet (four categories: low fat and high fiber, low fat and low fiber, high fat and high fiber, high fat and low fiber). State clearly your null and alternative hypotheses, and state your choice of the test size. Perform your investigation separately for males and females.

6.21. A case–control study was conducted in Auckland, New Zealand to investigate the effects of alcohol consumption on both nonfatal myocardial infarction and coronary death in the 24 hours after drinking, among regular drinkers. Data were tabulated separately for men and women.

(i) For Men

Drink in the Last 24 Hours	Myocardial Infarction		Coronary Death	
	Controls	Cases	Controls	Cases
No	197	142	135	103
Yes	201	136	159	69

(ii) For Women

Drink in the Last 24 Hours	Myocardial Infarction		Coronary Death	
	Controls	Cases	Controls	Cases
No	144	41	89	12
Yes	122	19	76	4

For each group, men and women, and for each type of event, myocardial infarction and coronary death, test to compare cases versus controls. State, in each analysis, your null and alternative hypotheses, and state your choice of the test size.

6.22. Refer to the data in Exercise 6.21 but assume that Gender (male/female) may be a confounder but not an effect modifier. For each type of event, myocardial infarction and coronary death, use the Mantel–Haenszel method to investigate the effects of alcohol consumption. State, in each analysis, your null and alternative hypotheses, and state your choice of the test size.

6.23. Because incidence rates of most cancers rise with age, this must always be considered a confounder. The following are stratified data for an unmatched case–control study. The disease was esophageal cancer among men, and the risk factor was alcohol consumption.

Age		Daily Alcohol Consumption	
		80+ g	0–79 g
25–44	Cases	5	5
	Controls	35	270
45–64	Cases	67	55
	Controls	56	277
65+	Cases	24	44
	Controls	18	129

Use the Mantel–Haenszel procedure to compare the cases versus the controls. State your null hypothesis and your choice of the test size.

6.24. Postmenopausal women who develop endometrial cancer are on the whole heavier than women who do not develop the disease. One possible explanation is that heavy women are more exposed to endogenous estrogens which are produced in postmenopausal women by conversion of steroid precursors to active estrogens in peripheral fat. In the face of varying levels of endogenous estrogen production, one might ask whether the carcinogenic potential of exogenous estrogens would be the same in all women. A study has been conducted to examine the relation between weight, replacement estrogen therapy, and endometrial cancer in a case–control study.

Weight (kg)		Estrogen Replacement	
		Yes	No
< 57	Cases	20	12
	Controls	61	183
57–75	Cases	37	45
	Controls	113	378
> 75	Cases	9	42
	Controls	23	140

Use the Mantel–Haenszel procedure to compare the cases versus the controls. State your null hypothesis and your choice of the test size.

6.25. Risk factors of gallstone disease were investigated in male self-defense officials who received, between October 1986 and December 1990, a retirement health examination at the Self-Defense Forces Fukuoka Hospital, Fukuoka, Japan. The following are parts of the data:

| | Number of Men Surveyed | |
Factor	Total	Number with Gallstones
Smoking		
Never	621	11
Past	776	17
Current	1342	33
Alcohol		
Never	447	11
Past	113	3
Current	2179	47
Body mass index (kg/m²)		
< 22.5	719	13
22.5–24.9	1301	30
≥ 25.0	719	18

For each of the three criteria (smoking, alcohol, and body mass index), test (at the 5% level) for the trend of men with gallstones.

6.26. Prematurity, which ranks as the major cause of neonatal morbidity and mortality, has traditionally been defined on the basis of a birth weight under 2500 g. But this definition encompasses two distinct types of infants: infants who are small because they are born early, and infants who are born at or near term but are small because their growth was retarded. "Prematurity" has now been replaced by

(i) "low birth weight" to describe the second type

(ii) "preterm" to characterize the first type (babies born before 37 weeks of gestation)

A case–control study of the epidemiology of preterm delivery was undertaken at Yale–New Haven Hospital in Connecticut during 1977. The study population consisted of 175 mothers of singleton preterm infants and 303 mothers of singleton full-term infants. In Example 6.16, we have analyzed and found a significant association between the mother's age and preterm delivery—that is, the younger the mother, the more likely the preterm delivery. The following table gives the distribution of socioeconomic status:

Socioeconomic Level	Cases	Controls
Upper	11	40
Upper middle	14	45
Middle	33	64
Lower middle	59	91
Lower	53	58
Unknown	5	5

Test to prove that there is a significant association between the mother's status and preterm delivery—that is, the poorer the mother, the more likely the preterm delivery (the "unknown" category can be deleted). State your null hypothesis and your choice of the test size.

6.27. Postneonatal mortality due to respiratory illnesses is known to be inversely related to maternal age, but the role of young motherhood as a risk factor for respiratory morbidity in infants has not been thoroughly explored. A study was conducted in Tucson, Arizona aimed at the incidence of lower respiratory tract illnesses during the first year of life. In this study, over 1200 infants were enrolled at birth between 1980 and 1984, and the following data are concerned with wheezing lower respiratory tract illnesses (wheezing LRI): No/Yes.

Maternal Age	Boys		Girls	
(years)	No	Yes	No	Yes
< 21	19	8	20	7
21–25	98	40	128	36
26–30	160	45	148	42
> 30	110	20	116	25

For each of the two groups, boys and girls, test to investigate the relationship between maternal age and respiratory illness. State clearly your null and alternative hypotheses, and state your choice of the test size.

6.28. Data were collected from 2197 white ovarian cancer patients and 8893 white controls in 12 different U.S. case–control studies conducted by various investigators in the period 1956–1986. These were used to evaluate the relationship of invasive epithelial ovarian cancer to reproductive and menstrual characteristics, exogenous estrogen use, and prior pelvic surgeries. The following are parts of the data:

(i)

Duration of Unprotected Intercourse (years)	Cases	Controls
< 2	237	477
2–9	166	354
10–14	47	91
≥ 15	133	174

(ii)

History of Infertility	Cases	Controls
No	526	966
Yes		
No drug use	76	124
Drug use	20	11

For each of the two criteria, duration of unprotected intercourse and history of infertility, test to investigate the relationship between that criterion and ovarian cancer. State clearly your null and alternative hypotheses, and state your choice of the test size.

6.29. The following table compiles data from different studies designed to investigate the accuracy of death certificates. The results of 5373 autopsies were compared to the causes of death listed on the certificates. The results are as follows:

Date of Study	Accurate Certificate		Total
	Yes	No	
1955–1965	2040	694	2,734
1970–1971	437	203	640
1975–1978	1128	599	1727
1980	121	151	272

Test to confirm the downward trend of accuracy over time. State clearly your null and alternative hypotheses, and state your choice of the test size.

6.30. A study was conducted to ascertain factors that influence a physician's decision to transfuse a patient. A sample of 49 attending physicians was selected. Each physician was asked a question concerning the frequency with which an unnecessary transfusion was give because another physician suggested it. The same question was asked of a sample of 71 residents. The data were as follows:

Type of Physician	Frequency of Unnecessary Transfusion				
	Very frequent (1 per week)	Frequent (1 per 2 weeks)	Occasionally (1 per month)	Rarely (1 per 2 months)	Never
Attending	1	1	3	31	13
Resident	2	13	28	23	5

Test the null hypothesis of no association, with attention to the natural ordering of the columns. State clearly your alternative hypothesis and your choice of the test size.

7

Comparison of Population Means

If each element of a data set may lie only at a few isolated points, we have a *discrete* or *categorical* data set; examples include sex, race, or some sort of artificial grading used as outcomes. If each element of a data set may lie anywhere on the numerical scale, we have a *continuous* data set; examples include blood pressure, cholesterol level, or time to a certain event.

The previous chapter deals with the analysis of categorical data—for example, the comparison of two proportions. This chapter is focused on continuous measurements, especially the comparisons of population means. We will follow the same layout, starting with the most simple case, the one-sample problem.

7.1. ONE-SAMPLE PROBLEM WITH CONTINUOUS DATA

In this type of problem, we have a sample of continuous measurements of size n and we consider the null hypothesis

$$H_0 : \mu = \mu_0$$

where μ_0 is a fixed and known number. It is often a standardized or referenced figure—for example, the average blood pressure of men in certain age group (this figure may come from a sample itself, but a referenced sample is often large enough so as to produce negligible sampling error in μ_0). Or, we could be concerned with a question like "Is the average birthweight for boys for this particular sub-population below normal average μ_0—say 7.5 lb?" In Exercise 7.1, we'd try to decide whether air quality on certain given day in a particular city exceeds a regulated limit μ_0 set by a federal agency.

In a typical situation, the null hypothesis of a statistical test is concerned with a parameter; the parameter in this case, with continuous data, is the mean μ. Sample data are summarized into a statistic that is used to estimate the parameter under investigation. Because the parameter under investigation is the proportion μ, our focus in this case is the sample mean $\bar{x}$. In general, a statistic is itself a variable with a specific sampling distribution (in the context of repeated sampling). Our statistic in this case is the sample mean $\bar{x}$, the corresponding sampling distribution is easily obtained by invoking the *Central Limit Theorem*. With large sample size and assuming that the null hypothesis H_0 is true, it is the normal distribution with mean and variance given by

$$\mu_{\bar{x}} = \mu_0$$

$$\sigma_{\bar{x}}^2 = \frac{\sigma^2}{n}$$

respectively. The extra needed parameter, the population variance σ^2, has to be estimated from our data by the sample variance s^2. From this sampling distribution, the observed value of the sample mean can be converted to a standard unit: the number of standard errors away from the hypothesized value of μ_0. In other words, to perform a test of significance for H_0, we proceed with the following steps:

1. Decide whether a one-tailed or a two-sided test is appropriate; this decision depends on the research question.
2. Choose a level of significance; a common choice is .05.
3. Calculate the t-statistic

$$t = \frac{\bar{x} - \mu_0}{SE(\bar{x})}$$

$$= \frac{\bar{x} - \mu_0}{\frac{s}{\sqrt{n}}}$$

4. From the table for t distribution (Appendix C) with $(n-1)$ degrees of freedom and the choice of α (e.g., $\alpha = .05$), the rejection region is determined by the following

   - For a one-sided test, use the column corresponding to the "upper tail area" of .05:

$$t \leq -\text{tabulated value for } H_A : \mu < \mu_0$$

$$t \geq \text{tabulated value for } H_A : \mu > \mu_0$$

   - For a two-sided test or $H_A : \mu \neq \mu_0$, use the column corresponding to the "upper tail area" of .025

$$z \leq -\text{tabulated value or } z \geq \text{tabulated value}$$

This test is referred to as the *one-sample t test*.

Example 7.1

Boys of a certain age have a mean weight of 85 lb. An observation was made that in a city neighborhood, children were underfed. As evidence, all 25 boys in the neighborhood of that age were weighed and found to have a mean $\bar{x}$ of 80.94 lb and a standard deviation s of 11.60 lb. An application of the above procedure yields

$$SE(\bar{x}) = \frac{s}{\sqrt{n}}$$
$$= \frac{11.60}{\sqrt{25}}$$
$$= 2.32$$

leading to

$$t = \frac{80.94 - 85}{2.32}$$
$$= -1.75$$

The underfeeding complaint corresponds to the one-sided alternative

$$H_A : \mu < 85$$

so that we would reject the null hypothesis if

$$t \leq -\text{tabulated value}$$

From Appendix C and with 24 degrees of freedom $(n - 1)$, we find

$$\text{tabulated value} = 1.71$$

under the column corresponding to .05 upper tail area; the null hypothesis is rejected at the .05 level. In other words, there is enough evidence to support the underfeeding complaint.

7.2. ANALYSIS OF PAIR-MATCHED DATA

The method presented in this section applies to cases where each subject or member of a group is observed twice (for example, before and after certain intervention), or matched pairs are measured for the same continuous characteristic. In the study reported in Example 7.2, blood pressure was measured from a group of women before and after each of them took an oral contraceptive. In Exercise 7.2, blood level of insulin was measured from dogs before and after some kind of nerve stimulation. In another exercise, we compared self-reported versus measured height. A popular application is an epidemiological design called a *pair-matched case–control study*. In case–control studies, cases of a specific disease are ascertained as they arise from population-based registers or lists of hospital admissions, and controls are sampled either as disease-free individuals from the population at risk or as hospitalized patients having a diagnosis other than the one under investigation. As a technique to control confounding factors, individual cases are matched, often one-to-one, to controls chosen to have similar values for confounding variables such as age, sex, race, and so on.

Data from matched or before-and-after experiments should never be considered as coming from two independent samples. The procedure is to reduce the data to a one-sample problem by computing before-and-after (or case-and-control) difference for each subject or pairs of matched subjects. By doing this with paired observations, we get a set of differences, each of which is independent of the characteristics of the individual from which measurements were made. The analysis of pair-matched data with a continuous measurent can be seen as follows. What we really want to do is to compare the means, before versus after or cases versus controls; the use of the sample of differences $\{d_i\}$, one for each subject, helps to achieve that. With large sample size and assuming that the null hypothesis H_0 of *no difference* is true, the mean $\bar{d}$ of theses differences is distributed as *normal* with mean and variance given by

$$\mu_{\bar{d}} = 0$$

$$\sigma_{\bar{d}}^2 = \frac{\sigma_d^2}{n}$$

respectively. The extra needed parameter, the variance σ_d^2, has to be estimated from our data by the sample variance s_d^2. In other words, the analysis of pair-matched data with a continuous measurement can be seen as a special case of the one-sample problem of Section 7.1 with $\mu_0 = 0$. Recall the form of the test statistic of the previous section, we have

$$t = \frac{\bar{d} - 0}{\frac{s_d}{\sqrt{n}}}$$

and the rejection region is determined using the t distribution at $(n-1)$ degrees of freedom. This test is referred to as the *one-sample t test*, the same one-sample t test as in the previous section.

Example 7.2

Trace metals in drinking water affect the flavor of the water, and unusually high concentration can pose a health hazard. Table 7.1 shows trace-metal concentrations (zinc, in mg/liter) for both surface water and bottom water at six different river locations (the difference is bottom-surface).

Table 7.1. Zinc Concentration (mg/liter)

Location	Bottom	Surface	Difference, d_i	d_i^2
1	.430	.415	.015	.000225
2	.266	.238	.028	.000784
3	.567	.390	.177	.030276
4	.531	.410	.121	.014641
5	.707	.605	.102	.010404
6	.716	.609	.107	.011449
Total			.550	.068832

The necessary summarized figures are

$$\bar{d} = \text{Average difference}$$

$$= .550/6$$

$$= .0917 \text{ mg/liter}$$

$$s_d^2 = \frac{.068832 - (.550)^2/6}{5}$$

$$= .00368$$

$$s_d = .061$$

$$\text{SE}(\bar{d}) = .061/\sqrt{6}$$

$$= .0249$$

$$t = \frac{.0917}{.0249}$$

$$= 3.68$$

Using the column corresponding to the upper tail area of .025 in Appendix C, we have a tabulated value of 2.571 for 5 degrees of freedom. Because

$$t = 3.68 > 2.571$$

we conclude that the null hypothesis of *no difference* should be rejected at the .05 level; there is enough evidence to support the hypothesis of *different* mean zinc concentrations (two-sided alternative).

Note: A SAS program would include these instructions:
```
DATA;
INPUT BZINC SZINC;
DIFF = BZINC - SZINC;
DATALINES;
.430 .415
.266 .238
```

```
.567 .390
.531 .410
.707 .605
.716 .609;
PROC MEANS N MEAN STDERR T PRT;
```
for which we'll get sample size (N), sample mean (MEAN), standard error (STDERR), t statistic (T), and *p*-value (PRT).

Example 7.3

The systolic blood pressures of $n = 12$ women between the ages of 20 and 35 were measured before and after administration of a newly developed oral contraceptive. Data were shown in Table 7.2 (the difference is after–before).

Table 7.2. Systolic Blood Pressure (mmHg)

Subject	Before	After	Difference, d_i	d_i^2
1	122	127	5	25
2	126	128	2	4
3	132	140	8	64
4	120	119	−1	1
5	142	145	3	9
6	130	130	0	0
7	142	148	6	36
8	137	135	−2	4
9	128	129	1	1
10	132	137	5	25
11	128	128	0	0
12	129	133	4	16
			31	185

The necessary summarized figures are

$$\bar{d} = \text{Average difference}$$
$$= 31/12$$
$$= 2.58 \text{ mmHg}$$
$$s_d^2 = \frac{185 - (31)^2/12}{11}$$
$$= 9.54$$
$$s_d = 3.09$$

$$SE(\bar{d}) = 3.09/\sqrt{12}$$

$$= .89$$

$$t = \frac{2.58}{.89}$$

$$= 2.90$$

Using the column corresponding to the upper tail area of .05 in Appendix C, we have a tabulated value of 1.796 for 11 degrees of freedom. Because

$$t = 2.90 > 2.201$$

we conclude that the null hypothesis of no blood pressure change should be rejected at the .05 level; there is enough evidence to support the hypothesis of *increased* systolic blood pressure (one-sided alternative).

_____

_____

Example 7.4

Data in epidemiologic studies are sometimes self-reported. Screening data from the hypertension detection and follow-up program in Minneapolis, Minnesota (1973–1974) provided an opportunity to evaluate the accuracy of self-reported height and weight. The following table gives the percent discrepancy between self-reported and measured height:

$$x = \frac{\text{Self-reported height} - \text{Measured height}}{\text{Measured height}} \times 100\%.$$

Education	Men			Women		
	n	Mean	SD	n	Mean	SD
$\leq$ High school	476	1.38	1.53	323	.66	1.53
$\geq$ College	192	1.04	1.31	62	.41	1.46

Let's focus on the sample of men with high school education; investigations of other groups and the differences between them can be found in the exercises at the end of this chapter. An application of the one-sample t test yields

$$\bar{x} = 1.38$$

$$s_x = 1.53$$

$$SE(\bar{x}) = 1.53/\sqrt{476}$$

$$= .07$$

$$t = \frac{1.38}{.07}$$
$$= 19.71$$

It can be easily seen that the difference between self-reported height and measured height is highly statistically significant ($p < .01$; comparing 19.71 versus the cutpoint of 2.58 for large sample).

7.3. COMPARISON OF TWO MEANS

Perhaps one of the most common problems in statistical inference is the comparison of two population means using data from two independent samples; the sample sizes may or may not be equal. In this type of problem, we have two sets of continuous measurements, one of size n_1 and one of size n_2, and we consider the null hypothesis

$$H_0 : \mu_1 = \mu_2$$

expressing the equality of the two population means.

To perform a test of significance for H_0, we proceed with the following steps:

1. Decide whether a one-sided test, say

$$H_A : \mu_2 > \mu_1$$

or a two-sided test,

$$H_A : \mu_1 \neq \mu_2$$

is appropriate.
2. Choose a significance level α, a common choice being .05.
3. Calculate the t statistic:

$$t = \frac{\bar{x}_1 - \bar{x}_2}{SE(\bar{x}_1 - \bar{x}_2)}$$

where

$$SE(\bar{x}_1 - \bar{x}_2) = s_p \sqrt{\frac{1}{n_1} + \frac{1}{n_2}}$$

$$s_p^2 = \frac{(n_1 - 1)s_1^2 + (n_2 - 1)s_2^2}{n_1 + n_2 - 2}$$

This test is referred to as the *two-sample t test,* and its rejection region is determined using the t distribution at $(n_1 + n_2 - 2)$ degrees of freedom:

- For a one-tailed test, use the column corresponding to the "upper tail area" of .05, and $\mathcal{H}_0$ is rejected if

$$t \leq - \text{ tabulated value for } \mathcal{H}_A : \mu_1 < \mu_2$$

or

$$t \geq \text{ tabulated value for } \mathcal{H}_A : \mu_1 > \mu_2$$

- For a two-tailed test or $\mathcal{H}_A : \mu_1 \neq \mu_2$, use the column corresponding to the "upper tail area" of .025, and $\mathcal{H}_0$ is rejected if

$$t \leq -\text{tabulated value or } t \geq \text{tabulated value}$$

_____

Example 7.5

In an attempt to assess the physical condition of joggers, a sample of $n_1 = 25$ joggers was selected and their maximum volume of oxygen uptake (VO_2) was measured with the following results:

$$\bar{x}_1 = 47.5 \text{ ml/kg}, \qquad s_1 = 4.8 \text{ ml/kg}$$

Results for a sample of $n_2 = 26$ non-joggers were

$$\bar{x}_2 = 37.5 \text{ ml/kg}, \qquad s_2 = 5.1 \text{ ml/kg}$$

To proceed with the two-tailed, two-sample t test, we have

$$s_p^2 = \frac{(24)(4.8)^2 + (25)(5.1)^2}{49}$$

$$= 24.56$$

$$\text{or } s_p = 4.96$$

$$SE(\bar{x}_1 - \bar{x}_2) = 4.96\sqrt{\frac{1}{25} + \frac{1}{26}}$$

$$= 1.39.$$

It follows that

$$t = \frac{47.5 - 37.5}{1.39}$$

$$= 7.19$$

indicating a significant difference between the joggers and the nonjoggers (at 49 degrees of freedom and $\alpha = .01$, the tabulated "t" value—with upper tail area of .025—is about 2.0).

Example 7.6

Vision, or more specially visual acuity, depends on a number of factors. A study was undertaken in Australia to determine the effect of one of these factors: racial variation. Visual acuity of recognition as assessed in clinical practice has a defined normal value of 20/20 (or zero in log scale). The following summarized data on monocular visual acuity (expressed in log scale) were obtained from two groups:

1. Australian males of European origin

$$n_1 = 89$$

$$\bar{x}_1 = -.20$$

$$s_1 = .18$$

2. Australian males of Aboriginal origin

$$n_2 = 107$$

$$\bar{x}_2 = -.26$$

$$s_2 = .13$$

To proceed with a two-sample t test we have

$$s_p^2 = \frac{(88)(.18)^2 + (106)(.13)^2}{194}$$

$$= (.155)^2$$

$$SE(\bar{x}_1 - \bar{x}_2) = (.155)\sqrt{\frac{1}{89} + \frac{1}{107}}$$

$$= .022$$

$$t = \frac{(-.20) - (-.26)}{.022}$$

$$= 2.73$$

The result indicates that the difference is statistically significant beyond the .01 level (at $\alpha = .01$ and for a two-sided test the cutpoint is 2.58 for large degrees of freedom).

_____

_____

Example 7.7

The extend to which an infant's health is affected by parental smoking is an important public health concern. The following data give the urinary concentrations of cotinine (a metabolite of nicotine); measurements were taken both from a sample of infants who had been exposed to household smoke and from a sample of unexposed infants.

Unexposed ($n_1 = 7$):	8	11	12	14	20	43	111	
Exposed ($n_2 = 8$):	35	56	83	92	128	150	176	208

The statistics needed for our two-sample t test are as follows:

1. For unexposed infants:

$$n_1 = 7$$
$$\bar{x}_1 = 31.29$$
$$s_1 = 37.07$$

2. For exposed infants:

$$n_2 = 8$$
$$\bar{x}_2 = 116.00$$
$$s_2 = 59.99$$

To proceed with a two-sample t test we have

$$s_p^2 = \frac{(6)(37.07)^2 + (7)(59.99)^2}{13}$$

$$= (50.72)^2$$

$$SE(\bar{x}_1 - \bar{x}_2) = (50.72)\sqrt{\frac{1}{7} + \frac{1}{8}}$$

$$= 26.25$$

$$t = \frac{(116.00) - (31.29)}{26.25}$$

$$= 3.23.$$

The result indicates that the difference is statistically significant beyond the .01 level (at $\alpha = .01$ and for a two-sided test the cutpoint is 3.012 for 13 degrees of freedom).

Note: A SAS program would include these instructions:

```
DATA;
INPUT GROUP $ COTININE;
DATALINES;
U 8
...
U 111
E 35
...
E 208;
PROC TTEST;
CLASS GROUP;
VAR COTININE;
```

in which an independent variable name or group follows CLASS and dependent variable name follows VAR.

7.4. NONPARAMETRIC METHODS

In the previous sections, we have seen how to apply the t tests, one-sample t test and two-sample t test, to compare the population means. However, these methods depend on certain assumptions about the distributions in the population; for example, its derivation assumes the population(s) is (are) normally distributed. It has been proven that these procedures are robust; that is, they are relatively insensitive to departures from the assumptions made. In other words, departures from those assumptions have only very little effect on the results, provided that samples are large enough. But the procedures are all sensitive to extreme observations, a few very small or very large—perhaps erroneous—data values. In this section we will learn some nonparametric procedures, or distribution-free methods, where no assumptions about population distributions are made. The results of these nonparametric tests are much less affected by extreme observations.

7.4.1. The Wilcoxon Rank-Sum Test

This is perhaps the most popular nonparametric procedure. The Wilcoxon test is a nonparametric counterpart of the two-sample t test; it is used to compare two samples that have been drawn from independent populations. But unlike the t test, the Wilcoxon test does not assume that the underlying populations are normally distributed, and it is less affected by extreme observations. The Wilcoxon rank sum test evaluates the null hypothesis that the medians of the two populations are identical (for a normally distributed population, the population median is also the population mean).

For example, a study was designed to test the question of whether cigarette smoking is associated with reduced serum-testosterone levels. To carry out this research objective, two samples (each of size 10) are independently selected. The first sample consists of 10 non-smokers who have never smoked whereas the second sample consists of 10 heavy smokers, defined as those who smoke 30 or more cigarettes per day. To perform the Wilcoxon rank sum test, we combine the two samples into one large sample (of size 20), arrange the observations from smallest to largest, and assign a rank, from 1 to 20, to each one. If there are tied observations, then we assign an average rank to all measurements with the same value. For example, if the two observations next to the third smallest are equal, we assign an average rank of $(4 + 5)/(2) = 4.5$ to each one. The next step is to find the sum of the ranks corresponding to each of the original samples. Let n_1 and n_2 be the two sample sizes, and let R be the sum of the ranks from the sample with size n_1.

Under the null hypothesis that the two underlying populations have identical medians, we would expect the averages of ranks to be approximately equal. We test this hypothesis by calculating the statistic

$$z = \frac{R - \mu_R}{\sigma_R}$$

where

$$\mu_R = \frac{n_1(n_1 + n_2 + 1)}{2}$$

is the mean and

$$\sigma_R = \sqrt{\frac{n_1 n_2(n_1 + n_2 + 1)}{12}}$$

is the standard deviation of R. It does not make any difference which rank sum we use. For relatively large values of n_1 and n_2 (say, both greater than or equal to 10), the sampling distribution of this statistic is approximately standard normal. The null hypothesis is rejected at the 5% level, against a two-sided alternative, if

$$z < -1.96 \quad \text{or} \quad z > 1.96$$

Example 7.8

For the above study on cigarette smoking, the following table shows the raw data, where testosterone levels were measured in $\mu g/dl$ and the ranks were as follows:

Nonsmokers		Heavy Smokers	
Measurement	Rank	Measurement	Rank
.44	8.5	.45	10
.44	8.5	.25	1
.43	7	.40	6
.56	14	.27	2
.85	17	.34	4
.68	15	.62	13
.96	20	.47	11
.72	16	.30	3
.92	19	.35	5
.87	18	.54	12

The sum of the ranks for group 1 (nonsmokers) is

$$R = 143$$

In addition,

$$\mu_R = \frac{10(10 + 10 + 1)}{2}$$
$$= 105$$

and

$$\sigma_R = \sqrt{\frac{(10)(10)(10 + 10 + 1)}{12}}$$
$$= 13.23$$

Substituting these values into the equation for the test statistic, we have

$$z = \frac{R - \mu_R}{\sigma_R}$$
$$= \frac{143 - 105}{13.23}$$
$$= 2.87$$

Because $z > 1.96$, we reject the null hypothesis at the 5% level. (In fact, because $z > 2.58$ we reject the null hypothesis at the 1% level.) Note that if we use the sum of the ranks for the other group (heavy smokers), the sum of the ranks is 67 leading to a z score of

$$\frac{67 - 105}{13.23} = -2.87$$

and we would come to the same decision.

Example 7.9

Refer to the nicotine data of Example 7.6, where measurements were taken both from a sample of infants who had been exposed to household smoke and from a sample of unexposed infants:

Unexposed ($n_1 = 7$):	8	11	12	14	20	43	111	
Rank:	1	2	3	4	5	7	11	
Exposed ($n_2 = 8$):	35	56	83	92	128	150	176	208
Rank:	6	8	9	10	12	13	14	15

The sum of the ranks for the group of exposed infants is

$$R = 87$$

In addition,

$$\mu_R = \frac{8(8+7+1)}{2}$$
$$= 64$$

and

$$\sigma_R = \sqrt{\frac{(8)(7)(8+7+1)}{12}}$$
$$= 8.64$$

Substituting these values into the equation for the Wilcoxon test, we have

$$z = \frac{R - \mu_R}{\sigma_R}$$
$$= \frac{87 - 64}{8.64}$$
$$= 2.66$$

Because $z > 1.96$, we reject the null hypothesis at the 5% level. In fact, because $z > 2.58$ we reject the null hypothesis at the 1% level; p value $< .01$ (It should be noted that the sample sizes of 7 and 8 in this example may be not large enough.)

Note: An SAS program would include these instructions:

```
DATA;
INPUT GROUP $ COTININE;
DATALINES;
U 8
```

```
...
U 111
E 35
...
E 208;
PROC NPAR1WAY WILCOXON; CLASS GROUP;
VAR COTININE;
```

7.4.2. The Wilcoxon Signed-Rank Test

The idea of using the *ranks*, instead of measured values, to form statistical tests to compare population means applies to the analysis of pair-matched data as well. As with the one-sample t test for pair-matched data, we begin by forming differences. Then the absolute values of the differences are assigned ranks; if there are ties in the differences, the average of the appropriate ranks is assigned. Next, we attach a $+$ or a $-$ sign back to each rank, depending on whether the corresponding difference is positive or negative. This is achieved by multiplying each of the ranks by $+1$, -1, or 0 because the corresponding difference is positive, negative, or zero. The results are *n signed ranks*, one for each pair of observations; for example, if the difference is zero, its signed rank is zero. The basic idea is that if the *mean difference* is positive, there would be more and larger *positive signed ranks*. If this were the case, most differences would be positive and larger in magnitude than the few negative differences. Most of the ranks—especially the larger ones—would then be positively signed. In other words, we can base the test on the *sum R* of the *positive signed ranks*. We test the null hypothesis of no difference by calculating the *standardized test statistic*:

$$z = \frac{R - \mu_R}{\sigma_R}$$

where

$$\mu_R = \frac{(n)(n+1)}{4}$$

is the mean and

$$\sigma_R = \sqrt{\frac{(n)(n+1)(2n+1)}{24}}$$

is the standard deviation of R under the null hypothesis. This normal approximation applies for relatively large samples, $n \geq 20$; the null hypothesis is rejected at the 5% level, against a two-sided alternative, if

$$z < -1.96 \quad \text{or} \quad z > 1.96$$

This test is referred to as the *Wilcoxon's signed-rank test*.

Example 7.10

Ultrasounds were taken at the time of liver transplant and again 5–10 years later to determine the systolic pressure of the hepatic artery. Results for 21 transplants for 21 children are shown in following table:

Child	Later	At Transplant	Difference	Absence of Difference	Rank	Signed Rk
1	46	35	11	11	13	13
2	40	40	0	0	2	0
3	50	58	-8	8	9	-9
4	50	71	-19	19	17.5	-17.5
5	41	33	8	8	9	9
6	70	79	-9	9	11	-11
7	35	20	15	15	15.5	15.5
8	40	19	21	21	20	20
9	56	56	0	0	2	0
10	30	26	4	4	5.5	5.5
11	30	44	-14	14	14	-14
12	60	90	-30	30	21	-21
13	43	43	0	0	2	0
14	45	42	3	3	4	4
15	40	55	-15	15	15.5	-15.5
16	50	60	-10	10	12	-12
17	66	62	4	4	5.5	5.5
18	45	26	19	19	17.5	17.5
19	40	60	-20	20	19	-19
20	35	27	-8	8	9	-9
21	25	31	-6	6	7	-7

The sum of the positive signed ranks is

$$13 + 9 + 15.5 + 20 + 5.5 + 4 + 5.5 + 17.5 = 90$$

Its mean and standard deviation under the null hypothesis are

$$\mu_R = \frac{(21)(22)}{4}$$
$$= 115.5$$
$$\sigma_R = \sqrt{\frac{(21)(22)(43)}{24}}$$
$$= 28.77$$

leading to a standardized z score of

$$z = \frac{90 - 115.5}{28.77}$$
$$= -.89$$

The result indicates that the systolic pressure of the hepatic artery measured 5 years after the liver transplant, as compared to the measurement at transplant, is lower on the average; however, the difference is not statistically significant at the 5% level $(-.89 > -1.96)$.

Note: An SAS program would include these instructions:

```
DATA;
INPUT POST PRE;
DIFF = POST - PRE;
DATALINES;
46 35
...
35 27
25 31;
PROC UNIVARIATE;
```

for which we'll get, among many other things, the test statistic (SGN RANK) and the p-value $(\text{Prob} > |S|)$.

7.5. ONE-WAY ANALYSIS OF VARIANCE (ANOVA)

Suppose that the goal of a research project is to discover whether there are differences in the means of several independent groups. The problem is how we will measure the extent of differences among the means. If we had two groups then we would measure the difference by the distance between sample means $(\overline{x} - \overline{y})$ and use the two-sample t test. Here we have more than two groups; we could take all possible pairs of means and do many two-sample t tests. What is the matter with this approach of doing many two-sample t tests, one for each pair of samples? As the number of groups increases, so does the number of tests to perform; for example, we would have to do 45 tests if we have 10 groups to compare. Obviously, the amount of work is greater, but that should not be the critical problem—especially with technological aids such as the use of calculators and computers. So, what is the problem? The answer is that performing many tests increases the probability that one or more of the comparisons will result in a Type I error (i.e., a significant test result when the null hypothesis is true). This statement should make sense intuitively. For example, suppose the null hypothesis is true and we perform 100 tests—each with a 0.05 probability of resulting in a Type I error; then 5 of these 100 tests would be statistically significant as the results of Type I errors. Of course, we usually do not need to do that many tests; however, every time we do more than one, then the probability that at least one will result in a Type I error exceeds 0.05, indicating a falsely significant difference! What is needed is a different way to summarize the differences between several means and a method of *simultaneously* comparing these means in one step. This method is called ANOVA or one-way ANOVA, which is an abbreviation of "ANalysis Of VAriance." The method, as well as the name ANOVA, can be described as follows.

We have continuous measurements Xs from k independent samples; the sample sizes may or may not be equal. We assume that these are samples from k normal distributions with a common variance σ^2, but the means μ_i may or may not be the same. The case where we apply the two-sample t test is a special case of this one-way ANOVA model with $k = 2$. Data from the ith sample can be summarized into sample size n_i, sample mean $\bar{x}_i$, and sample variance s_i^2. And if we pool data together, the (grand) mean of this combined sample can be calculated from

$$\bar{x} = \frac{\sum (n_i)(\bar{x}_i)}{\sum (n_i)}$$

In that combined sample of size $n = \sum n_i$, the variation in X is conventionally measured in terms of the deviations $x_{ij} - \bar{x}$ (where x_{ij} is the jth measurement from the ith sample); the total variation, denoted by *SST*, is the sum of squared deviations:

$$SST = \sum_{i,j} (x_{ij} - \bar{x})^2$$

For example, $SST = 0$ when all observations x'_{ij}s are the same. *SST* is the numerator of the sample variance of the combined sample, the greater the *SST*, the greater the variation among all X values. The total variation in the combined sample can be decomposed into two components:

$$x_{ij} - \bar{x} = (x_{ij} - \bar{x}_i) + (\bar{x}_i - \bar{x})$$

(i) The first term reflects the variation *within* the ith sample; the sum

$$SSW = \sum_{i,j} (x_{ij} - \bar{x}_i)^2$$
$$= \sum_i (n_i - 1)s_i^2$$

is called the *within sum of squares*.

(ii) The difference between the above two sums of squares,

$$SSB = SST - SSW$$
$$= \sum_{i,j} (\bar{x}_i - \bar{x})^2$$
$$= \sum_i n_i (\bar{x}_i - \bar{x})^2$$

is called the *between sum of squares*. *SSB* represents the variation or differences between the sample means, a measure very much similar to the numerator of a sample variance; the n_i's serve as *weights*.

Corresponding to the partitioning of the total sum of squares *SST*, there is partitioning of the associated degrees of freedom (*df*). We have $(n-1)$ degrees of freedom associated with *SST*, the denominator of the variance of the combined sample; *SSB* has $(k-1)$ degrees of freedom representing the differences between k groups, the remaining $(n-k = \sum(n_i-1))$ degrees of freedom are associated with *SSW*. These results lead to the usual presentation of the ANOVA process:

(a) The *within mean square*

$$MSW = \frac{SSW}{n-k}$$

$$= \frac{\sum_i (n_i - 1)s_i^2}{\sum(n_i - 1)}$$

serves as an estimate of the common variance σ^2 as stipulated by the one-way ANOVA *model*. In fact, it can be seen that *MSW* is a natural extension of the pooled estimate s_p^2 as used in the two-sample t test; It is a measure of the average variation within the k samples.

(b) The *between mean square*

$$MSB = \frac{SSB}{k-1}$$

represents the *average* variation (or differences) between the k sample means.

(c) The breakdowns of the total sum of squares and its associated degree of freedom are *displayed* in the form of an *analysis of variance table* (ANOVA table) as follows.

Source of Variation	SS	df	MS	F-stat	p-value
Between samples	SSB	$k-1$	MSB	$\frac{MSB}{MSW}$	p
Within samples	SSW	$n-k$	MSW		
Total	SST	$n-1$			

The test statistic F for the above one-way analysis of variance compares *MSB* (the *average* variation—or differences—between the k sample means) and *MSE* (the average variation within the k samples); a value near 1 supports the null hypothesis of *no differences between the k population means*. Decisions are made by referring the observed value of the test statistic F to the F table in Appendix E with $(k-1, n-k)$ degress of freedom. In fact, when $k=2$, we have

$$F = t^2$$

where t is the test statistic for comparing the two population means. In other words, when $k = 2$, the F test is equivalent to the two-sided two-sample t test.

Example 7.11

Vision, or more specifically visual acuity, depends on a number of factors. A study was undertaken in Australia to determine the effect of one of these factors: racial variation. Visual acuity of recognition as assessed in clinical practice has a defined normal value of 20/20 (or zero in log scale). The following summarized the data on monocular visual acuity (expressed in log scale); part of this data set were given in Example 7.6:

1. Australian males of European origin

$$n_1 = 89$$
$$\bar{x}_1 = -.20$$
$$s_1 = .18$$

2. Australian males of Aboriginal origin

$$n_2 = 107$$
$$\bar{x}_2 = -.26$$
$$s_2 = .13$$

3. Australian females of European origin

$$n_3 = 63$$
$$\bar{x}_3 = -.13$$
$$s_3 = .17$$

4. Australian females of Aboriginal origin

$$n_4 = 54$$
$$\bar{x}_4 = -.24$$
$$s_4 = .18$$

To proceed with a one-way ANOVA, we calculate the mean of the combined sample:

$$\bar{x} = \frac{(89)(-.20) + (107)(-.26) + (63)(-.13) + (54)(-.24)}{89 + 107 + 63 + 54}$$
$$= -.213$$

and

$$SSB = (89)(-.20 + .213)^2 + (107)(-.26 + .213)^2 + (63)(-.13 + .213)^2$$
$$+ (54)(-.24 + .213)^2$$
$$= .7248$$
$$MSB = \frac{.7248}{3}$$
$$= .2416$$
$$SSW = (88)(.18)^2 + (106)(.13)^2 + (62)(.17)^2 + (53)(.18)^2$$
$$= 8.1516$$
$$MSW = \frac{8.1516}{309}$$
$$= .0264$$
$$F = \frac{.2416}{.0264}$$
$$= 9.152$$

The results are summarized in the following ANOVA table:

Source of Variation	SS	df	MS	F Statistic	p-Value
Between samples	.7248	3	.2416	9.152	< .0001
Within samples	8.1516	309	.0264		
Total	8.8764	312			

The resulting F test indicates that the overall differences between the four population means is highly significant ($p < .00001$).

Example 7.12

A study was conducted to test the question as to whether cigarette smoking is associated with reduced serum-testosterone levels in men aged 35 to 45. The study involved the following four groups:

1. Nonsmokers who had never smoked.
2. Former smokers who had quit for at least 6 months prior to the study.
3. Light smokers, defined as those who smoked 10 or fewer cigarettes per day.
4. Heavy smokers, defined as those who smoked 30 or more cigarettes per day.

Each group consisted of 10 men and the following table shows raw data, where serum-testosterone levels were measured in μg/dl.

Nonsmokers	Former Smokers	Light Smokers	Heavy Smokers
.44	.46	.37	.44
.44	.50	.42	.25
.43	.51	.43	.40
.56	.58	.48	.27
.85	.85	.76	.34
.68	.72	.60	.62
.96	.93	.82	.47
.72	.86	.72	.70
.92	.76	.60	.60
.87	.65	.51	.54

An application of the one-way ANOVA yields

Source of Variation	SS	df	MS	F Statistic	p-Value
Between samples	0.3406	3	0.1135	3.82	0.0179
Within samples	1.0703	36	0.0297		
Total	1.4109	39			

The resulting F test indicates that the overall differences between the four population means is statistically significant at the 5% level but not at the 1% level ($p = 0.0179$).

Note: An SAS program would include these instructions:
```
DATA;
INPUT GROUP $ SERUMT;
DATALINES;
N .44
...
N .87
F .46
...
F .65
L .37
...
L .51
H .44
...
H .54;
PROC ANOVA;
CLASS GROUP;
MODEL SERUMT = GROUP;
MEANS GROUP;
```
The row is an option to provide the sample mean of each group.

7.6. NOTES ON COMPUTATIONS

Samples of SAS program instructions were provided for all procedures, at the end of Examples 7.2, 7.7, 7.9, 7.10 and 7.12. All p-values provided by SAS for t tests are for two-sided alternatives; if you choose to perform your test as one-sided, divide the obtained p-value by 2. The one-sample t test and the two-sample t test can also be implemented easily using Microsoft's Excel. The first two steps are the same as those used to obtain descriptive statistics: (1) Click the *paste function icon*, f*, and (2) click *Statistical*. Among functions available, choose TTEST. A box appears with four rows to be filled. The first two are for data in the two groups to be compared; in each you identify the range of cells, say B2:B23. The third box asks for "tails," enter "1" ("2") for a one-sided (two-sided) alternative. Enter the "type" of test on the last row, "1" ("2") for one-sample (two-sample) t test.

EXERCISES

7.1. The criterion for issuing a smog alert is established at greater than 7 ppm of a particular pollutant. Samples collected from 16 stations in a certain city give an $\bar{x}$ of 7.84 ppm with a standard deviation of $s = 2.01$ ppm. Do these findings indicate that the smog alert criterion has been exceeded? State clearly your null and alternative hypotheses, and state your choice of the test size.

7.2. The purpose of an experiment is to investigate the effect of vagal nerve stimulation on insulin secretion. The subjects are mongrel dogs with varying body weights. The following table gives the amount of immunoreactive insulin in pancreatic venous plasma just before stimulation of the left vagus and gives the amount measured 5 minutes after stimulation for 7 dogs.

	Blood Levels of Immunoreactive Insulin (μU/ml)	
Dog	Before	After
1	350	480
2	200	130
3	240	250
4	290	310
5	90	280
6	370	1450
7	240	280

Test the null hypothesis that the stimulation of the vagus nerve has no effect on the blood level of immunoreactive insulin, that is,

$$H_0 : \mu_{\text{before}} = \mu_{\text{after}}$$

State your alternative hypothesis and your choice of the test size, and draw appropriate conclusion.

7.3. In a study of saliva cotinine, seven subjects—all of whom had abstained from smoking for a week—were asked to smoke a single cigareete. The cotinine levels at 12 hours and 24 hours after smoking are provided below:

	Cotinine Levels (mmol/liter)	
Subject	After 12 hours	After 24 hours
1	73	24
2	58	27
3	67	49
4	93	59
5	33	0
6	18	11
7	147	43

Test to compare the mean cotinine levels at 12 hours and 24 hours after smoking; state clearly your null and alternative hypotheses, and state your choice of the test size.

7.4. Dentists often make many people nervous. To see if such nervousness elevates blood pressure, systolic blood pressure of 60 subjects were measured in a dental setting and then again in a medical setting. Data for 60 matched pairs (dental–medical) are summarized as follows:

$$\text{Mean} = 4.47$$

$$\text{Standard deviation} = 8.77$$

Test to compare the mean blood pressure under two different settings; name the test and state clearly your null and alternative hypotheses, and state your choice of the test size.

7.5. In Example 7.10 a study with 21 transplants for 21 children was reported where ultrasounds were taken at the time of liver transplant and again 5–10 years later to determine systolic pressure of the hepatic artery. In that example, the Wilcoxon's signed rank test was applied to compare the hepatic systolic pressures measured at two different times. The following table gives the diastolic presures obtained from the same study. Test to compare the mean diastolic hepatic pressure; name the test and state clearly your null and alternative hypotheses, and state your choice of the test size.

	Diastolic Hepatic Pressure	
Subject	After 5–10 years	At Transplant
1	14	25
2	10	10
3	20	23
4	10	14
5	4	19

	Diastolic Hepatic Pressure	
Subject	After 5–10 years	At Transplant
6	20	12
7	10	5
8	18	4
9	12	23
10	18	8
11	10	10
12	10	20
13	15	12
14	10	10
15	10	19
16	15	20
17	26	26
18	20	8
19	10	10
20	10	11
21	10	16

7.6. A study was conducted to investigate whether oat bran cereal helps to lower serum cholesterol in men with high cholesterol levels. Fourteen men were randomly placed on a diet that included either oat bran or corn flakes; after 2 weeks, their low-density lipoprotein cholesterol levels were recorded. Each man was then switched to the alternative diet. After a second 2-week period, the LDL cholesterol level of each individual was again recorded. The data were as follows:

	LDL (mmol/liter)	
Subject	Corn Flakes	Oat Bran
1	4.61	3.84
2	6.42	5.57
3	5.40	5.85
4	4.54	4.80
5	3.98	3.68
6	3.82	2.96
7	5.01	4.41
8	4.34	3.72
9	3.80	3.49
10	4.56	3.84
11	5.35	5.26
12	3.89	3.73
13	2.25	1.84
14	4.24	4.14

Test to compare the means LDL cholesterol level; name the test and state clearly your null and alternative hypotheses, and state your choice of the test size.

7.7. Data in epidemiologic studies are sometimes self-reported. Screening data from the hypertension detection and follow-up program in Minneapolis, Minnesota (1973–1974) provided an opportunity to evaluate the accuracy of self-reported height and weight. The following table gives the percent discrepancy between self-reported and measured height:

$$x = \frac{\text{Self-reported height} - \text{Measured height}}{\text{Measured height}} \times 100\%.$$

	Men			Women		
Education	n	Mean	SD	n	Mean	SD
≤ High school	476	1.38	1.53	323	.66	1.53
≥ College	192	1.04	1.31	62	.41	1.46

Example 7.4 was focused on the sample of men with high school education; using the same procedure, investigate the difference between self-reported height and measured height among

(a) Men with college education

(b) Women with high-school education

(c) Women with college education

In each case, name the test and state clearly your null and alternative hypotheses, and state your choice of the test size. Also, compare the mean difference in percent discrepancy between

(a) Men with different education levels

(b) Women with different education levels

(c) Men versus women at each educational level

In each case, name the test and state clearly your null and alternative hypotheses, and state your choice of the test size.

7.8. A case–control study was undertaken to study the relationship between hypertension and obesity. Persons aged 30–49 years who were clearly nonhypertensive at their first multiphasic health checkup and became hypertensive by age 55 were sought and identified as cases. Controls were selected from among participants in a health plan, those who had the first checkup and no sign of hypertension in subsequent checkups. One control was matched to each case based on sex, race, year of birth, and year of entrance into the health plan. Data for 609 matched pairs are summarized as follows.

	Paired Difference	
Variable	Mean	Standard Deviation
Systolic blood pressure (mmHg)	6.8	13.86
Diastolic blood pressure (mmHg)	5.4	12.17
Body mass index (kg/m^2)	1.3	4.78

Compare the cases versus the controls using each measured characteristic; in each case, name the test and state clearly your null and alternative hypotheses, and state your choice of the test size.

7.9. The Australian study of Example 6.13 also provided these data on monocular acuity (expressed in log scale) for two female groups of subjects:

- Australian females of European origin

$$n_1 = 63$$
$$\bar{x}_1 = -.13$$
$$s_1 = .17$$

- Australian females of Aboriginal origin

$$n_2 = 54$$
$$\bar{x}_2 = -.24$$
$$s_2 = .18$$

Do these indicate a racial variation among women? Name your test and state clearly your null and alternative hypotheses, and state your choice of the test size.

7.10. The ages (in days) at time of death for samples of 11 girls and 16 boys who died of sudden infant death syndrome are shown below:

Females	Males	
53	46	115
56	52	133
60	58	134
60	59	175
78	77	175
87	78	
102	80	
117	81	
134	84	
160	103	
277	114	

Do these indicate a gender difference? Name your test and state clearly your null and alternative hypotheses, and state your choice of the test size.

7.11. An experimental study was conducted with 136 5-year-old children in four Quebec schools to investigate the impact of simulation games designed to teach children to obey certain traffic safety rules. The transfer of learning was measured by observing children's reactions to a quasi-real-life model of traffic risks. The scores on the transfer of learning for the control and attitude/behavior simulation game groups are summarized below:

Summarized Data	Control	Simulation Game
n	30	33
$\bar{x}$	7.9	10.1
s	3.7	2.3

Test to investigate the impact of simulation games; name your test and state clearly your null and alternative hypotheses, and state your choice of the test size.

7.12. In a trial to compare a stannous fluoride dentifrice (A) with a commercially available fluoride-free dentifrice (D), 270 children received A and 250 received D for a period of 3 years. The number x of DMFS increments (that is, the number of new decayed, missing, and filled tooth surfaces) was obtained for each child. Results were as follows:

$$\text{Dentifrice A:} \quad \bar{x}_A = 9.78$$
$$s_A = 7.51$$
$$\text{Dentifrice D:} \quad \bar{x}_D = 12.83$$
$$s_D = 8.31$$

Do the results provide strong enough evidence to suggest a real effect of fluoride in *reducing* the mean DMFS?

7.13. An experiment was conducted at the University of California at Berkeley to study the psychological environment effect on the anatomy of the brain. A group of 19 rats was randomly divided into two groups. Twelve animals in the treatment group lived together in a large cage, furnished with playthings that were changed daily, while animals in the control group lived in isolation with no toys. After a month, the experimental animals were killed and dissected. The following table gives the cortex weights (the thinking part of the brain) in milligrams:

Treatment	Control
707	669
740	650
745	651
652	627
649	656
676	642
699	698
696	
712	
708	
749	
690	

Use the two-sample t test to compare the means of the two groups and draw appropriate conclusion.

7.14. Depression is one of the most commonly diagnosed conditions among hospitalized patients in mental institutions. The occurrence of depression was determined during the summer of 1979 in a multiethnic probability sample of 1000 adults in Los Angeles County, as part of a community survey of the epidemiology of depression and help-seeking behavior. The primary measure of depression was the CES-D scale developed by the Center for Epidemiologic Studies. On a scale of 0 to 60, a score of 16 or higher was classified as depression. The following table gives the average CES-D score for the two sexes.

	CES-D Score		
	Cases	$\bar{x}$	s
Male	412	7.6	7.5
Female	588	10.4	10.3

Use a t test to compare the males versus the females and draw appropriate conclusion.

7.15. A study was undertaken to study the relationship between exposure to polychlorinated biphenyls (PCBs) and reproduction among women occupationally exposed to PCBs during the manufacture of capacitors in upstate New York. Interviews were conducted in 1982 with women who had held jobs with direct exposure and women who had never held a direct-exposure job, in order to ascertain information on reproductive outcomes. Data are summarized in the following table.

Variable	Exposure			
	Direct ($n = 172$)		Indirect ($n = 184$)	
	Mean	SD	Mean	SD
Weight gain during pregnancy (lbs)	25.5	14.0	29.0	14.7
Birth weight (g)	3313	456	3417	486
Gestational age (days)	279.0	17.0	279.3	13.5

Test to evaluate the effect of direct exposure (as compared to indirect exposure) using each measured characteristic; in each case, name the test and state clearly your null and alternative hypotheses, and state your choice of the test size.

7.16. The following data are taken from a study that compares adolescents who have bulimia to healthy adolescents with similar body compositions and levels of physical activity. The following table provides measures of daily caloric intake for random samples of 23 bulimic adolescents and 15 healthy ones.

Daily Caloric Intake (kcal/kg)				
Bulimic Adolescents			Healthy Adolescents	
15.9	17.0	18.9	30.6	40.8
16.0	17.6	19.6	25.7	37.4
16.5	28.7	21.5	25.3	37.1
18.9	28.0	24.1	24.5	30.6
18.4	25.6	23.6	20.7	33.2
18.1	25.2	22.9	22.4	33.7
30.9	25.1	21.6	23.1	36.6
29.2	24.5		23.8	

Use the Wilcoxon test to compare the two populations.

7.17. A group of 19 rats was randomly divided into two groups. The 12 animals in the experimental group lived together in a large cage, furnished with playthings that were changed daily, while the seven animals in the control group lived in isolation without toys. The following table provides the cortex weights (the thinking part of the brain) in milligrams:

Experimental Group	Control Group
707, 740, 745, 652, 649, 676, 699, 696, 712, 708, 749, 690	669, 650, 651, 627, 656, 642, 698

Use the Wilcoxon test to compare the two populations.

7.18. College students were assigned to three study methods in an experiment to determine the effect of study technique on learning. The three methods are Read only, Read and underline, and Read and take notes, and the test scores are as follows:

Technique	Test Score					
Read only	15	14	16	13	11	14
Read and underline	15	14	25	10	12	14
Read and take notes	18	18	18	16	18	20

Test to compare the three groups simultaneously; name your test and state clearly your null and alternative hypotheses, and state your choice of the test size.

7.19. Four different brands of margarine were analyzed to determine the level of some unsaturated fatty acids (as percentage of fats). Results are as follows:

Brand	Fatty Acids (Percent)				
A	13.5	13.4	14.1	14.2	
B	13.2	12.7	12.6	13.9	
C	16.8	17.2	16.4	17.3	18.0
D	18.1	17.2	18.7	18.4	

Test to compare the four groups simultaneously; name your test and state clearly your null and alternative hypotheses, and state your choice of the test size.

7.20. A study was done to determine if simplification of smoking literature improved patient comprehension. All subjects were administered a pretest. Subjects were then randomized into three groups. One group received no booklet, one group received one written at the fifth grade reading level, and the third received one written at the tenth grade reading level. After booklets were received, all subjects were administered a second test. The mean score differences (postscore − prescore) are given below along with their standard deviations and sample sizes.

	No Booklet	Fifth Grade Level	Tenth Grade Level
$\bar{x}$:	0.25	1.57	0.63
s:	2.28	2.54	2.38
n:	44	44	41

Test to compare the three groups simultaneously; name your test and state clearly your null and alternative hypotheses, and state your choice of the test size.

7.21. A study was conducted to investigate the risk factors for peripheral arterial disease among persons 55–74 years of age. The following table provides data on LDL cholesterol levels (mmol/liter) from four different subgroups of subjects:

Group	n	$\bar{x}$	s
1. Patients with intermittent claudication	73	6.22	1.62
2. Major asymptotic disease cases	105	5.81	1.43
3. Minor asymptotic disease cases	240	5.77	1.24
4. Those with no disease	1080	5.47	1.31

Test to compare the three groups simultaneously; name your test and state clearly your null and alternative hypotheses, and state your choice of the test size.

7.22. A study was undertaken in order to clarify the relationship between heart disease and occupational carbon disulfide exposure along with another important factor, elevated diastolic blood pressure (DBP), in a data set obtained from a 10-year prospective follow-up of two cohorts of over 340 male industrial workers in Finland. Carbon disulfide is an industrial solvent that is used all over the world in the production of viscose rayon fibers. The following table gives the mean and standard deviation (SD) of serum cholesterol (mg/100 ml) among exposed and nonexposed cohorts, by diastolic blood pressure (DBP).

DBP (mmHg)	Exposed			Nonexposed		
	n	Mean	SD	n	Mean	SD
< 95	205	220	50	271	221	42
95–100	92	227	57	53	236	46
≥ 100	20	233	41	10	216	48

Test to compare simultaneously, separately for the exposed and nonexposed groups, the means serum cholesterol level at the three DBP levels using one-way ANOVA. Also, compare serum cholesterol levels between exposed and nonexposed cohorts at each level of DBP by using the two-sample t tests. Draw your conclusions.

7.23. When a patient is diagnosed as having cancer of the prostate, an important question in deciding on treatment strategy for the patient is whether or not the cancer has spread to the neighboring lymph nodes. The question is so critical in prognosis and treatment that it is customary to operate on the patient (i.e., perform a laparotomy) for the sole purpose of examining the nodes and removing tissue samples to examine under the microscope for evidence of cancer. However, certain variables that can be measured without surgery are predictive of the nodal involvement; and the purpose of the study presented here was to examine the data for 53 prostate cancer patients receiving surgery, to determine which of five preoperative variables are predictive of nodal involvement. Table 7.3 presents the comple data set. For each of the 53 patients, there are two continuous independent variables, age at diagnosis and level of serum acid phosphatase (× 100; called "acid"), and three binary variables, X-ray reading, pathology reading (grade) of a biopsy of the tumor obtained by needle before

Table 7.3. Prostate Cancer Data

X-ray	Grade	Stage	Age	Acid	Nodes
0	1	1	64	40	0
0	0	1	63	40	0
1	0	0	65	46	0
0	1	0	67	47	0
0	0	0	66	48	0
0	1	1	65	48	0
0	0	0	60	49	0
0	0	0	51	49	0
0	0	0	66	50	0
0	0	0	58	50	0
0	1	0	56	50	0
0	0	1	61	50	0
0	1	1	64	50	0
0	0	0	56	52	0
0	0	0	67	52	0
1	0	0	49	55	0
0	1	1	52	55	0
0	0	0	68	56	0
0	1	1	66	59	0
1	0	0	60	62	0
0	0	0	61	62	0
1	1	1	59	63	0
0	0	0	51	65	0
0	1	1	53	66	0
0	0	0	58	71	0
0	0	0	63	75	0
0	0	1	53	76	0
0	0	0	60	78	0
0	0	0	52	83	0
0	0	1	67	95	0
0	0	0	56	98	0
0	0	1	61	102	0
0	0	0	64	187	0
1	0	1	58	48	1
0	0	1	65	49	1
1	1	1	57	51	1
0	1	0	50	56	1
1	1	0	67	67	1
0	0	1	67	67	1
0	1	1	57	67	1
0	1	1	45	70	1
0	0	1	46	70	1
1	0	1	51	72	1
1	1	1	60	76	1
1	1	1	56	78	1
1	1	1	50	81	1

(cont.)

X-ray	Grade	Stage	Age	Acid	Nodes
0	0	0	56	82	1
0	0	1	63	82	1
1	1	1	65	84	1
1	0	1	64	89	1
0	1	0	59	99	1
1	1	1	68	126	1
1	0	0	61	136	1

surgery, and a rough measure of the size and location of the tumor (stage) obtained by palpation with the fingers via the rectum. In addition, the sixth column presents the finding at surgery—the primary outcome of interest which is binary: a value of 1 denotes nodal involvement, and a value of 0 denoting no nodal involvement found at surgery. The three binary factors have been previously investigated; this exercise is focussed on the effects of the two continuous factors (age and acid phosphatase). Test to compare the group with nodal involvement and the group without using

(a) The two-sample t test

(b) The Wilcoxon rank-sum test

8

Regression Analysis

Methods discussed in Chapters 6 and 7 are tests of significance; they provide analyses of data where a single measurement was made on each element of a sample, and the study may involve one, two, or several samples. If the measurement made is binary or categorical, we are often concerned with a comparison of proportions—the topics of Chapter 6. If the measurement made is continuous, we are often concerned with a comparison of means—the topics of Chapter 7. The main focus of both chapters was the *difference* between populations or subpopulations. In many other studies, however, the purpose of the research is to assess relationships among a set of variables. For example, the sample consists of pairs of values, say a mother's weight and her newborn's weight measured from each of 50 sets of mother-and-baby, and the research objective is concerned with the association between these weights. Regression analysis is the technique for investigating relationships between variables; it can be used for assessment of association as well as for prediction. Consider, for example, an analysis of whether or not a woman's age is predictive of her systolic blood pressure. As another example, the research question could be whether or not a leukemia patient's white blood count is predictive of his survival time. Research designs may be classified as experimental or observational. Regression analyses are applicable to both types; yet the confidence one has in the results of a study can vary with the research type. In most cases, one variable is usually taken to be the response or dependent variable—that is, a variable to be predicted from or explained by other variables. The other variables are called predictors, or explanatory variables or independent variables. The above examples, as well as others, show a wide range of applications in which the dependent variable is a continuous measurement. Such a variable is often assumed to be normally distributed and a *model* is formulated to express the *mean* of this normal distribution as a function of potential independent variables under investigation. The dependent variable is denoted by Y, and the study often involves a number of *risk factors* or *predictor variables*: $X_1, X_2, \ldots, X_k$.

8.1. SIMPLE REGRESSION ANALYSIS

In this section we will discuss the basic ideas of simple regression analysis when only one predictor or independent variable is available for predicting the response of interest. In the interpretation of the primary parameter of the model, we will discuss both scales of measurement, discrete and continuous, even though in practical applications the independent variable under investigation is often on a continuous scale.

8.1.1. The Simple Linear Regression Model

Choosing an appropriate model and analytical technique depends on the type of variable under investigation. In a variety of applications, the dependent variable of interest is a continuous variable that we can assume, maybe after an appropropriate transformation, to be normally distributed. The *regression model* describes the *mean* of that normally distributed dependent variable Y as a function of the predictor or independent variable X,

$$Y_i = \beta_0 + \beta_1 x_i + \epsilon_i$$

where

- Y_i is the value of the response or dependent variable from the ith pair.
- β_0 and β_1 are the two unknown parameters.
- x_i is the value of the independent variable from the ith pair.
- ϵ_i is a random error term that is distributed as normal with mean zero and variance σ^2, so that $(\beta_0 + \beta_1 x_i)$ is the mean μ_i of Y_i.

The above model is referred to as the *simple linear regression model*. It is *simple* because it contains only one independent variable. It is *linear* because the independent variable appears only in the first power; if we graph the mean of Y versus X, the graph is a *straight line* with *intercept* β_0 and *slope* β_1.

8.1.2. The Scatter Diagram

As mentioned above, and stipulated by the *simple linear regression model*, if we graph the mean of Y versus X, the graph is a *straight line*. But that is the line for the means of Y; at each level of X, the *observed value* of Y may exceed or fall short of its mean. Therefore, when we graph the *observed* value of Y versus X, the points do not fall perfectly on any line. This is an important characteristic for *statistical* relationships as pointed out in Chapter 2. If we let each pair of numbers (x, y) be represented by a dot in a diagram with the x's on the horizontal axis, we have the figure called a *scatter diagram* as seen in parts of Chapter 2 and again in the next few examples. The scatter diagram is a useful diagnostic tool for checking out the validity of features of the simple linear regression model. For example, if dots fall around a curve, not a straight line, then the *linearity* assumption may be violated. In addition, the model stipulates that for each level of X, the normal distribution for Y has constant variance not depending on the value of X. That would lead to a scatter diagram with dots spreading out—around the line—evenly across levels of X. Most of the times, an appropriate transformation, such as taking logarithm, of Y or X would improve and bring the data closer to fitting the model.

8.1.3. Meaning of Regression Parameters

The parameters β_0 and β_1 are called regression coefficients. The parameter β_0 is the intercept of the regression line. If the scope of the model includes $X = 0$, β_0 gives the mean of Y when $X = 0$; when the scope of the model does not cover $X = 0$, β_0 does not have any particular meaning as a separate term in the regression model. As for the meaning of β_1, our more important parameter, it can be seen as follows. We first consider the case of a binary dependent variable with the conventional coding

$$X_i = \begin{cases} 0 & \text{if the patient is not exposed} \\ 1 & \text{if the patient is exposed} \end{cases}$$

Here, the term "exposed" may refer to a risk factor such as smoking, or a patient's characteristic such as race (white/nonwhite) or sex (male/female). It can be seen that

(i) For a nonexposed subject, that is, $X = 0$, we have

$$\mu_y = \beta_0$$

(ii) For an exposed subject, that is, $X = 1$, we obtain

$$\mu_y = \beta_0 + \beta_1$$

Hence, β_1 represents the *increase* (or *decrease*, if β_1 is negative) in the mean of Y associated with the exposure. Similarly, for a continuous covariate X and any value x of X, we have the following:

(i) When $X = x$,

$$\mu_y = \beta_0 + \beta_1 x$$

(ii) Whereas if $X = x + 1$,

$$\mu_y = \beta_0 + \beta_1(x + 1)$$

It can be seen that, by taking the difference, β_1 represents the *increase* (or *decrease*, if β_1 is negative) in the mean of Y associated with *one unit increase* in the value of X, $X = x + 1$ versus $X = x$. For m units increase in the value of X, say $X = x + m$ versus $X = x$, the corresponding increase (or decrease) in the mean of Y is $m\beta_1$.

8.1.4. Estimation of Parameters

To find *good* estimates of the unknown parametrs β_0 and β_1, statisticians use a method called *least squares*, which is described as follows. For each subject or pair of values (X_i, Y_i), we consider the deviation from the observed value Y_i to its *expected value*, the mean $\beta_0 + \beta_1 X_i$:

$$Y_i - (\beta_0 + \beta_1 X_i) = \epsilon_i$$

In particular, the method of least squares requires that we consider the *sum of squared deviations*:

$$S = \sum_{i=1}^{n} (Y_i - \beta_0 - \beta_1 X_i)^2$$

According to the method of least squares, the good estimates of β_0 and β_1 are values b_0 and b_1, respectively, which *minimize* the sum S. The results are

$$b_1 = \frac{\sum xy - \frac{(\sum x)(\sum y)}{n}}{\sum x^2 - \frac{(\sum x)^2}{n}}$$

$$b_0 = \bar{y} - b\bar{x}$$

Given the estimates b_0 and b_1 obtained from the sample, we estimate the mean response by

$$\hat{Y} = b_0 + b_1 X$$

This is our *predicted value* for (the mean of) Y at a given level/value of X.

Example 8.1

In the following table, the first two columns give the values for the birth weight (x, in ounces) and the increase in weight between the 70th and 100th days of life, expressed as a percentage of the birth weight (y) for 12 infants. We first let each pair of numbers (x, y) be represented by a dot in a diagram with the x's on the horizontal axis, we have the scatter diagram shown below. The dots do not fall perfectly on a straight line, but rather scatter around one, very typical for statistical relationships. However, a straight line seems to fit very well. Generally, the 12 dots go from upper left to lower right, and we have a negative association. We obtained, as shown in Example 2.11, a Pearson's correlation coefficient of $r = -.946$, indicating a very strong negative association.

	x	y	x^2	y^2	xy
	112	63	12,544	3,969	7,056
	111	66	12,321	4,356	7,326
	107	72	11,449	5,184	7,704
	119	52	14,161	2,704	6,188
	92	75	8,464	5,625	6,900
	80	118	6,400	13,924	9,440
	81	120	6,561	14,400	9,720
	84	114	7,056	12,996	9,576
	118	42	13,924	1,764	4,956
	106	72	11,236	5,184	7,632
	103	90	10,609	8,100	9,270
	94	91	8,836	8,281	8,554
Totals:	1,207	975	123,561	86,487	94,322

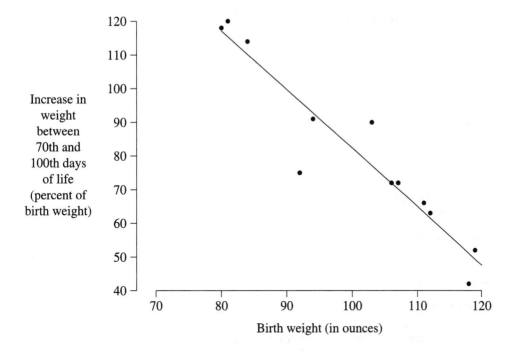

Increase in weight between 70th and 100th days of life (percent of birth weight)

Birth weight (in ounces)

Applying the formulas we obtain the estimates for the slope and intercept as follows:

$$b_1 = \frac{94,322 - \frac{(1,207)(975)}{12}}{123,561 - \frac{(1,207)^2}{12}}$$

$$= -1.74$$

$$\bar{x} = 1,207/12$$

$$= 100.6$$

$$\bar{y} = 975/12$$

$$= 81.3$$

$$b_0 = 81.3 - (-1.74)(100.6)$$

$$= 256.3$$

For example, if the birth weight is 95 ounces, it is predicted that the increase between the 70th and 100th days of life would be

$$\hat{y} = 256.3 + (-1.74)(95)$$

$$= 90.1\% \text{ of birth weight}$$

Note: An SAS program would include these instructions:

```
DATA;
INPUT WEIGHT GAIN;
DATALINES;
112 63
111 66
...
103 90
94 91
;
PROC REG;
MODEL = WEIGHT;
PLOT GAIN*WEIGHT;
```

for which we will get the analysis as well as the scatter diagram.

Example 8.2

In the table below, the first two columns give the values for age (x, in years) and systolic blood pressure (y, in mmHg) for 15 women. We first let each pair of numbers (x, y) be represented by a dot in a diagram with the x's on the horizontal axis, we have the scatter diagram shown below. Again the dots do not fall perfectly on a straight line, but rather scatter around one, very typical for statistical relationships. In this example, a straight line still seems to fit too; however, the dots spread more and cluster less around the line, indicating a weaker association. Generally, the 15 dots go from lower left to upper right, and we have a positive association. We obtained, as shown in Example 2.12, a Pearson's correlation coefficient of $r = .566$, indicating a moderate positive association, thereby confirming the above observation from the graph.

	x	y	x^2	y^2	xy
	42	130	1,764	16,900	5,460
	46	115	2,116	13,225	5,290
	42	148	1,764	21,904	6,216
	71	100	5,041	10,000	7,100
	80	156	6,400	24,336	12,480
	74	162	5,476	26,224	11,988
	70	151	4,900	22,801	10,570
	80	156	6,400	24,336	12,480
	85	162	7,225	26,224	13,770
	72	158	5,184	24,964	11,376
	64	155	4,096	24,025	9,920
	81	160	6,561	25,600	12,960
	41	125	1,681	15,625	5,125
	61	150	3,721	22,500	9,150
	75	165	5,625	27,225	12,375
Totals	984	2,193	67,954	325,889	146,260

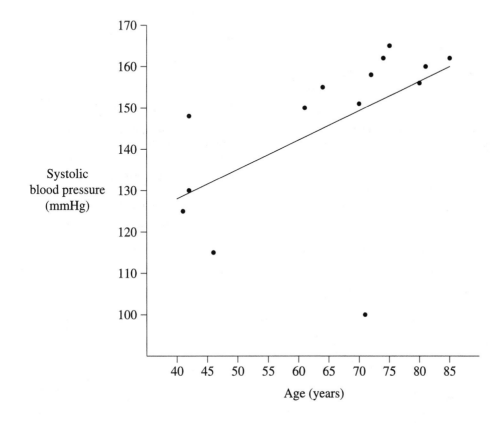

Applying the formulas we obtain the estimates for the slope and intercept as follows:

$$b_1 = \frac{146,260 - \frac{(984)(2,193)}{15}}{67,954 - \frac{(984)^2}{15}}$$

$$= .71$$

$$\bar{x} = 984/15$$

$$= 65.6$$

$$\bar{y} = 2,193/15$$

$$= 146.2$$

$$b_0 = 146.2 - (.71)(65.6)$$

$$= 99.6$$

For example, for a 50-year-old woman, it is predicted that her systolic blood pressure would be about

$$\hat{y} = 99.6 + (.71)(50)$$

$$= 135 \text{ mmHg}$$

8.1.5. Testing for Independence

In addition to being able to *predict* the (mean) response at various levels of the independent variable, regression data can also be used to test for the independence between the two variables under investigation. Such a statistical test can be viewed or approached in two different ways: through the coefficient of correlation or through the slope.

1. The correlation coefficient r measures the strength of the relationship between two variables. It is an estimate of an unknown population correlation coefficient ρ (rho), the same way the sample mean $\bar{x}$ is used as an estimate of some unknown population mean μ. We are usually interested in knowing if we may conclude that $\rho \neq 0$, that is, that the two variables under investigation are really correlated. The test statistic is

$$t = r\sqrt{\frac{n-2}{1-r^2}}$$

The procedure is often performed as two-sided, that is,

$$H_A : \rho \neq 0$$

and it is a t test with $(n-2)$ degrees of freedom; the same t test as used in the comparisons of population means in Chapter 7.

2. The role of the slope β_1 can be seen as follows. Because the regression model describes the mean of the dependent variable Y as a function of the predictor or independent variable X,

$$\mu_y = \beta_0 + \beta_1 x$$

Y and X would be independent if $\beta_1 = 0$. The test for

$$H_0 : \beta_1 = 0$$

can be performed similar to the method for one-sample problems in Chapters 6 and 7 (Sections 6.1 and 7.1). In that process, the observed/estimated value b_1 is converted to standard unit: the number of standard errors away from the hypothesized value of zero. The formula for standard error of b_1 is rather complicated; fortunately, the resulting test is *identical* to the above t test. Whenever needed—for example, in the computation of confidence intervals for the slope—we can always obtain the numerical value of its standard error from computer output.

When the above t test for independence is significant, the value of X has a real effect on the distribution of Y. To be more precise, the square of the correlation coefficient, r^2, represents the proportion of the variability of Y accountable for by X. For example, a $r^2 = .25$ indicates that the total variation in Y is reduced by 25 percent by the use of information about X. In other words, if we have a sample- of the same size, with all the n subjects having the same X value, the variation in Y (say, measured by its variance) is 25% less than the variation of Y in the current sample. It is interesting to note that an $r = .5$ would give an impression of greater association between X and Y, but a 25% reduction in variation is not. The parameter r^2 is called the coefficient of determination, an index with a clear operational interpretation than the coefficient of correlation r.

Example 8.3

For the birth weight problem of Example 2.11 and Example 8.1, we have

$$n = 12$$

$$r = -.946$$

leading to

$$t = (-.946)\sqrt{\frac{10}{1 - (-.946)^2}}$$

$$= -9.23$$

At $\alpha = .05$ and $df = 10$ degrees of freedom, the tabulated t coefficient is 2.228, indicating that the null hypothesis of independence should be rejected ($t = -9.23 < -2.228$). In this case, the birth weight (X) would account for

$$r^2 = .895$$

or 89.5% of the variation in growth rates between the 70th and 100th days of life.

Example 8.4

For the blood pressure problem of Example 2.12 and Example 8.2, we have

$$n = 15$$
$$r = .566$$

leading to

$$t = (.566)\sqrt{\frac{13}{1 - (.566)^2}}$$
$$= 2.475$$

At $\alpha = .05$ and $df = 13$ degrees of freedom, the t tabulated value is 2.16. Because

$$t > 2.16$$

we have to conclude that the null hypothesis of independence should be rejected; that is, the relationship between age and systolic blood pressure is real. However, a woman's age (X) would account for only

$$r^2 = .32$$

or 32% of the variation among systolic blood pressures.

8.1.6. Analysis of Variance Approach

The variation in Y is conventionally measured in terms of the deviations $(Y_i - \bar{Y})$'s; the total variation, denoted by SST, is the sum of squared deviations:

$$SST = \sum (Y_i - \bar{Y})^2$$

For example, $SST = 0$ when all observations are the same; SST is the numerator of the sample variance of Y, the greater SST the greater the variation among Y values.

When we use the regression approach, the variation in Y is decomposed into two components:

$$Y_i - \bar{Y} = (Y_i - \hat{Y}_i) + (\hat{Y}_i - \bar{Y})$$

1. The first term reflects the *variation around the regression line*; the part then cannot be explained by the regression itself with the sum of squared deviations:

$$SSE = \sum(Y_i - \hat{Y}_i)^2$$

called the *error sum of squares*,.

2. The difference between the above two sums of squares,

$$SSR = SST - SSE$$
$$= \sum(\hat{Y}_i - \bar{Y})^2$$

is called the *regression sum of squares*. *SSR* may be considered a measure of the variation in Y associated with the regression line. In fact, we can express the coefficient of determination as

$$r^2 = \frac{SSR}{SST}$$

Corresponding to the partitioning of the total sum of squares *SST*, there is partitioning of the associated degrees of freedom (df). We have $(n - 1)$ degrees of freedom associated with *SST*, the denominator of the sample variance of Y; *SSR* has one degree of freedom representing the slope, and the remaining $(n - 2)$ are associated with *SSE*. These results lead to the usual presentation of regression analysis by most computer programs:

1. The *error mean square*

$$MSE = \frac{SSE}{n - 2}$$

serves as an estimate of the constant variance σ^2 as stipulated by the regression *model*.

2. The breakdowns of the total sum of squares and its associated degree of freedom are *displayed* in the form of an *analysis of variance table* (ANOVA table) as follows.

Source of Variation	SS	df	MS	F Statistic	p-Value
Regression	SSR	1	$MSR = \frac{SSR}{1}$	$F = \frac{MSR}{MSE}$	p
Error	SSE	$n - 2$	$MSE = \frac{SSE}{n-2}$		
Total	SST	$n - 1$			

The test statistic F for the above analysis of variance approach compares MSR and MSE; a value near 1 supports the null hypothesis of independence. In fact, we have

$$F = t^2$$

where t is the test statistic for testing whether or not $\beta_1 = 0$; the F test is equivalent to the two-sided t test when referred to the F table in Appendix E with $(1, n - 2)$ degrees of freedom.

Example 8.5

For the birth weight problem of Examples 8.1 and 8.3, we have the following:

Source of Variation	SS	df	MS	F Statistic	p-Value
Regression	6508.43	1	6508.43	85.657	0.0001
Error	759.82	10	75.98		
Total	7268.25	11			

Example 8.6

For the blood pressure problem of Examples 8.2 and 8.4, we have the following:

Source of Variation	SS	df	MS	F Statistic	p-Value
Regression	1691.20	1	1691.20	6.071	0.0285
Error	3621.20	13	278.55		
Total	5312.40	14			

8.2. MULTIPLE REGRESSION ANALYSIS

The effect of some factor on a dependent or response variable may be influenced by the presence of other factors because of redundancies or effect modifications—that is, interactions. Therefore, in order to provide a more comprehensive analysis, it may be desirable to consider a large number of factors and sort out which ones are most closely related to the dependent variable. In this section we will discuss a multivariate method for this type of risk determination. This method, which is multiple regression analysis, involves a linear combination of the explanatory or independent variables, also called *covariates*; the variables must be quantitative with particular numerical values for each subject in the sample. A covariate or independent variable—such as a patient characteristic—may be dichotomous, polytomous, or continuous (categorical factors will be represented by dummy variables). Examples of dichotomous covariates are (a) sex and (b) presence or absence of certain co-morbidity. Polytomous covariates include race and different grades of symptoms; these can be covered by the use of *dummy* variables. Continuous covariates include patient age, blood pressure, and so on; in many cases, data transformations (e.g., taking the logarithm) may be needed to satisfy the linearity assumption.

8.2.1. Regression Model with Several Independent Variables

Suppose we want to consider k independent variables simultaneously, the simple linear model of previous section can be easily generalized and expressed as

$$Y_i = \beta_0 + \sum_{j=1}^{k} \beta_j x_{ji} + \epsilon_i$$

where

- Y_i is the value of the response or dependent variable from the ith subject.
- $\beta_0, \beta_1, \ldots, \beta_k$ are the $(k+1)$ unknown parameters; β_0 is the intercept and $\beta_i's$ are the slopes, one for each independent variable.
- x_{ij} is the value of the jth independent variable ($j = 1$ to k) from the ith subject ($i = 1$ to n).
- ϵ_i is a random error term which is distributed as normal with mean zero and variance σ^2, so that the mean of Y_i is

$$\mu_i = \beta_0 + \sum_{j=1}^{k} \beta_j x_{ji}$$

The above model is referred to as the *multiple linear regression model*. It is *multiple* because it contains several independent variables. It is still *linear* because the independent variables appear only in the first power; this feature is rather difficult to check because we do not have a scatter diagram to rely on as in the case of simple linear regression. In addition, the model can modified to include higher powers of independent variables as well as their various products as seen in subsequent subsections.

8.2.2. Meaning of Regression Parameters

Similar to the univariate case, β_i represents

1. the *increase* (or *decrease*, if β_i is negative) in the mean of Y associated with the exposure if X_i is binary (exposed $X_i = 1$ versus unexposed $X_i = 0$), *assuming* that other independent variables are fixed, or

2. the *increase* (or *decrease*, if β_i is negative) in the mean of Y associated with *one unit increase* in the value of X_i, $X_i = x + 1$ versus $X_i = x$. For m units increase in the value of X_i, say $X_i = x + m$ versus $X_i = x$, the corresponding increase (or decrease) in the mean of Y is $m\beta_i$, *assuming* that other independent variables are fixed. In other words, β_i represents the *additional contribution* of X_i in the explanation of variation among y values. Of course, before such analyses are done, the problem and the data have to be examined carefully. If some of the variables are highly correlated, then one or a few of the correlated factors are likely to be as good a predictor as all of them; information from other, similar studies also has to be incorporated so as to drop some of these correlated explanatory variables.

8.2.3. Effect Modifications

Consider the multiple regression model involving *two* independent variables:

$$Y_i = \beta_0 + \beta_1 x_{1i} + \beta_2 x_{2i} + \beta_3 x_{1i} x_{2i} + \epsilon_i$$

It can be seen that the meaning of β_1 and β_2 here is not the same as that given earlier because of the cross-product term $\beta_3 x_1 x_2$. Suppose, for simplicity, that both X_1 and X_2 are binary, then:

1. For $X_2 = 1$ or exposed, we have

$$\mu_y = \beta_0 + \beta_1 + \beta_3 \qquad \text{if exposed to } X_1$$
$$\mu_y = \beta_0 \qquad \text{if not exposed to } X_1$$

so that the increase (or decrease) in the mean of Y due to an exposure to X_1 is $\beta_1 + \beta_3$, whereas

2. For $X_2 = 0$ or not exposed, we have

$$\mu_y = \beta_0 + \beta_1 \qquad \text{if exposed to } X_1$$
$$\mu_y = \beta_0 \qquad \text{if not exposed to } X_1$$

so that the increase (or decrease) in the mean of Y due to an exposure to X_1 is β_1.

In other words, the effect of X_1 depends on the level (presence or absence) of X_2 and vice versa. This phenomenon is called *effect modification*; that is, one factor modifies the effect of the other. The cross-product term $x_1 x_2$ is called an interaction term; the use of these products will help in the investigation of possible effect modifications. If $\beta_3 = 0$, the effect of two factors acting together (represented by $\beta_1 + \beta_2$) is equal to the combined effects of two factors acting separately. If $\beta_3 > 0$, we have a synergistic interaction; if $\beta_3 < 0$, we have an antagonistic interaction.

8.2.4. Polynomial Regression

Consider the multiple regression model involving *one* independent variable:

$$Y_i = \beta_0 + \beta_1 x_i + \beta_2 x_i^2 + \epsilon_i$$

or it can be written as a multiple model:

$$Y_i = \beta_0 + \beta_1 x_{1i} + \beta_2 x_{2i}^2 + \epsilon_i$$

with $X_1 = X$ and $X_2 = X^2$ where X is a continuous independent variable. The meaning of β_1 here is not the same as that given earlier because of the quadratic term $\beta_2 x_i^2$. We have, for example,

$$\mu_y = \beta_0 + \beta_1 x + \beta_2 x^2 \qquad \text{when } X = x$$

$$\mu_y = \beta_0 + \beta_1(x+1) + \beta_2(x+1)^2 \qquad \text{when } X = x+1.$$

so that the difference is

$$\beta_1 + \beta_2(2x + 1)$$

a function of x.

Polynomial models with an independent variable present in higher powers than the second are not often used. The second-order or quadratic model has two basic types of uses: (i) when the true relationship is a second-degree polynomial or when the true relationship is unknown but the second-degree polynomial provides a better fit than a linear one, but (ii) more often, a quadratic model is fitted for the purpose of establishing the linearity. The key item to look for is whether $\beta_2 = 0$. The use of polynomial models, however, is not without drawbacks. The most potential drawback is that X and X^2 are strongly related, especially if X is restricted to a narrow range; in this case the standard errors are often very large.

8.2.5. Estimation of Parameters

To find *good* estimates of the $(k + 1)$ unknown parameters β_0 and β_i, statisticians use the same method of *least squares* which was described in the previous section. For each subject with data values (Y_i, X_i), we consider the deviation from the observed value Y_i to its *expected value*,

$$\mu_y = \beta_0 + \sum_{j=1}^{k} \beta_j x_{ji}$$

In particular, the method of least squares requires that we consider the *sum of squared deviations*:

$$S = \sum_{i=1}^{n} \left(Y_i - \beta_0 - \sum_{j=1}^{k} \beta_j x_{ji} \right)^2$$

According to the method of least squares, the good estimates of β_0 and β_i are values b_0 and b_i, respectively, which *minimize* the sum S. The method is the same, but the results are much more difficult to obtain; fortunately, these results are provided by most standard computer programs such as Excel and SAS. In addition, computer output also provides standard errors for all estimates of regression coefficients.

8.2.6. Analysis of Variance Approach

The total sum of squares

$$SST = \sum (Y_i - \bar{Y})^2$$

and its associated degree of freedom $(n - 1)$ are defined and partitioned the same as in the case of simple linear regression The results are *displayed* in the form of an *analysis of variance table* (ANOVA table) of the same form:

Source of Variation	SS	df	MS	F Statistic	p-Value
Regression	SSR	k	$MSR = \frac{SSR}{k}$	$F = \frac{MSR}{MSE}$	p
Error	SSE	$n - k - 1$	$MSE = \frac{SSE}{n-k-1}$		
Total	SST	$n - 1$			

where k is the number of independent variables. In addition:

1. The coefficient of multiple determination is defined as

$$R^2 = \frac{SSR}{SST}$$

It measures the proportionate reduction of total variation in Y associated with the use of the set of independent varables. As for r^2 of the simple linear regression, we have

$$0 \le R^2 \le 1$$

and R^2 only assumes the value 0 when all $\beta_i = 0$.

2. The *error mean square*

$$MSE = \frac{SSE}{n - 2}$$

serves as an estimate of the constant variance σ^2 as stipulated by the regression *model*.

8.2.7. Testing Hypotheses in Multiple Linear Regression

Once we have fit a multiple regression model and obtained estimates for the various parameters of interest, we want to answer questions about the contributions of various factors to the prediction of the binary response variable. There are three types of such questions:

1. *An Overall Test:* Taken collectively, does the entire set of explatory or independent variables contribute significantly to the prediction of the response? (or the explanation of variation among responses).
2. *Test for the Value of a Single Factor:* Does the addition of one particular variable of interest add significantly to the prediction of response over and above that achieved by other independent variables?
3. *Test for Contribution of a Group of Variables:* Does the addition of a group of variables add significantly to the prediction of response over and above that achieved by other independent variables?

Overall Regression Tests

We now consider the first question stated above concerning an overall test for a model containing k factors.

The null hypothesis for this test may stated as follows: "All k independent variables *considered together* do not explain the variation in the responses." In other words,

$$H_0 : \beta_1 = \beta_2 = \cdots = \beta_k = 0$$

This *global* null hypothesis can tested using the F statistic in the above ANOVA table:

$$F = \frac{MSR}{MSE}$$

an F test at $(k, n - k - 1)$ degrees of freedom.

Tests for a Single Variable

Let us assume that we now wish to test whether the addition of one particular independent variable of interest adds significantly to the prediction of the response over and above that achieved by other factors already present in the model. The null hypothesis for this test may stated as: "Factor X_i does not have any value added to the prediction of the response *given that other factors are already included in the model*." In other words,

$$H_0 : \beta_i = 0$$

To test such a null hypothesis, one can use

$$t_i = \frac{\hat{\beta}_i}{SE(\hat{\beta}_i)}$$

in a t test with $n - k - 1$ degrees of freedom, where $\hat{\beta}_i$ is the corresponding estimated regression coefficient and $SE(\hat{\beta}_i)$ is the estimate of the standard error of $\hat{\beta}_i$, both of which are printed by standard computer packaged programs.

Example 8.7

Ultrasounds were taken at the time of liver transplant and again 5–10 years later to determine the systolic pressure of the hepatic artery. Results for 21 transplants for 21 children are shown in following table; also available are sex (M = male, F = female) and age at the second measurement.

Child	After 5–10 years	At Transplant	Sex	Age
1	46	35	F	16
2	40	40	F	19
3	50	58	F	19
4	50	71	M	23
5	41	33	M	16
6	70	79	M	23
7	35	20	M	13
8	40	19	M	19
9	56	56	M	11
10	30	26	F	14
11	30	44	M	15
12	60	90	F	12
13	43	43	F	15
14	45	42	M	14
15	40	55	M	14
16	50	60	F	17
17	66	62	F	21
18	45	26	F	21
19	40	60	M	11
20	35	27	M	9
21	25	31	M	9

Using the second measurement of the systolic pressure of the hepatic artery as our dependent variable, the resulting ANOVA table is as follows:

Source of Variation	SS	df	MS	F Statistic	p-Value
Regression	1810.93	3	603.64	12.158	0.0002
Error	844.02	17	49.65		
Total	2654.95	20			

The result of the overall F test ($p = 0.0002$) indicates that, taken collectively, the three independent variables (systolic pressure at transplant, sex, and age) contribute significantly to the prediction of the dependent variable. In addition, we have the following:

Variable	Coefficient	Standard Error	t Statistic	p-Value
Pressure at transplant	0.381	0.082	4.631	0.0002
Sex	1.740	3.241	0.537	0.5982
Age	0.935	0.395	2.366	0.0301

The effects of pressure at transplant and age are significant at the 5% level, whereas the effect of sex is not ($p = 0.5982$).

Note: An SAS program would include these instructions:
```
DATA;
INPUT POST PRE SEX AGE;
DATALINES;
46 35 2 16
40 40 2 19
...
35 27 1 9
25 31 1 9
;
PROC REG;
MODEL POST = PRE SEX AGE;
```
which gives us all of the above results.

Example 8.8

There have been times that the city of London experienced periods of dense fog. The following table shows such data for a 15-day very severe period which include the number of deaths in each day (y), the mean atmospheric smoke (x_1, in mg/m^3), and the mean atmospheric sulfur dioxide content (x_2, in parts/million):

Number of Deaths	Smoke	Sulfur Dioxide
112	0.30	0.09
140	0.49	0.16
143	0.61	0.22
120	0.49	0.14
196	2.64	0.75
294	3.45	0.86
513	4.46	1.34

Number of Deaths	Smoke	Sulfur Dioxide
518	4.46	1.34
430	1.22	0.47
274	1.22	0.47
255	0.32	0.22
236	0.29	0.23
256	0.50	0.26
222	0.32	0.16
213	0.32	0.16

Using the number of deaths in each day as our dependent variable, the resulting ANOVA table is as follows:

Source of Variation	SS	df	MS	F Statistic	p-Value
Regression	205097.52	2	102548.76	36.566	0.0001
Error	33654.20	12	2804.52		
Total	238751.73	14			

The result of the overall F test ($p = 0.0001$) indicates that, taken collectively, the two independent variables contribute significantly to the prediction of the dependent variable. In addition, we have the following:

Variable	Coefficient	Standard Error	t Statistic	p-Value
Smoke	−220.324	58.143	−3.789	0.0026
Sulfur	1051.816	212.596	4.947	0.0003

The effects of both factors, the mean atmospheric smoke and the mean atmospheric sulfur dioxide content, are significant even at the 1% level (both $p < 0.001$).

Contribution of a Group of Variables

This testing procedure addresses the more general problem of assessing the additional contribution of two or more factors to the prediction of the response over and above that made by other variables already in the regression model. In other words, the null hypothesis is of the form

$$H_0 : \beta_1 = \beta_2 = \cdots = \beta_m = 0$$

To test such a null hypothesis, one can fit two regression models: one with all X's included to obtain the regression sum of squares ($SSR1$) and one with all other X's with X's under investigation deleted to obtain the regression sum of squares ($SSR2$). Define the mean square due to H_0 as

$$MSR = \frac{SSR1 - SSR2}{m}$$

Then H_0 can be tested using

$$F = \frac{MSR}{MSE}$$

an F test at $(m, n-k-1)$ degrees of freedom. This *multiple contribution* procedure is very useful for assessing the importance of potential explanatory variables. In particular, it is often used to test whether a similar group of variables, such as *demographic characteristics*, is important for the prediction of the response; these variables have some trait in common. Another application would be a collection of powers and/or product terms (referred to as interaction variables). It is often of interest to assess the interaction effects collectively before trying to consider individual interaction terms in a model as previously suggested. In fact, such use reduces the total number of tests to be performed, and this, in turn, helps to provide better control of overall Type I error rates that may be inflated due to multiple testing.

Example 8.9

Refer to the data on liver transplants of Example 8.7 consisting of three independent variables: hepatic systolic pressure at transplant time (called pressure1), age (at the second measurement time, and sex of the child. Let consider all five quadratic terms and products of these three original factors ($x1 = $ pressure1^2, $x2 = $ age^2, $x3 = $ pressure$1 *$ age, $x4 = $ pressure$1 *$ sex, and $x5 = $ age $*$ sex). Using the second measurement of the systolic pressure of the hepatic artery as our dependent variable and fitting the multiple regression model with all eight (8) independent variables (three original plus five newly defined terms), we have

$$SSR = 1944.70 \text{ with 8 degrees of freedom}$$
$$SSE = 710.25 \text{ with 12 degrees of freedom}$$

or

$$MSE = 19.19$$

as compared to the results from Example 8.7:

$$SSR = 1810.93 \text{ with 3 degrees of freedom}$$

The significance of the additional contribution of the five new factors, considered together, is judged using the F statistic:

$$F = \frac{\frac{1944.70 - 1810.93}{5}}{19.19}$$

$$= .80 \text{ at } (5, 12) \text{ degrees of freedom}$$

In other words, all five quadratic and product terms considered together do not contribute significantly to the prediction/explanation of the second measurement of the systolic pressure of the hepatic artery; the model with three original factors is adequate.

Stepwise Regression

In many applications, our major interest is to identify important risk factors. In other words, we wish to identify from many available factors a small subset of factors that relate significantly to the outcome—for example, the disease under investigation. In that identification process, of course, we wish to avoid a large Type I (false positive) error. In a regression analysis, a Type I error corresponds to including a predictor that has no real relationship to the outcome; such an inclusion can greatly confuse the interpretation of the regression results. In a standard multiple regression analysis, this goal can be achieved by using a strategy that adds into or removes from a regression model one factor at a time according to a certain order of relative importance. Therefore the two important steps are as follows:

1. Specify a criterion or criteria for selecting a model.
2. Specify a strategy for applying the chose criterion or criteria.

Strategies This is concerned with specifying the strategy for selecting variables. Traditionally, such a strategy is concerned with whether a particular variable should be added to a model or whether any variable should be deleted from a model at a particular stage of the process. As computers became more accessible and more powerful, these practices became more popular.

Forward Selection Procedure In the forward selection procedure, we proceed as follows:

Step 1 Fit a simple linear regression model to each factor, one at a time.

Step 2 Select the most important factor according to certain predetermined criteria.

Step 3 Test for the significance of the factor selected in step 2 and determine, according to certain predetermined criteria, whether or not to add this factor to the model.

Step 4 Repeat steps 2 and 3 for those variables not yet in the model. At any subsequent step, if none meets the criteria in step 3, no more variables are included in the model and the process is terminated.

Backward Elimination Procedure   In the backward elimination procedure, we proceed as follows:

Step 1   Fit the multiple regression model containing all available independent variables.

Step 2   Select the least important factor according to certain predetermined criteria; this is done by considering one factor at a time and treating it as though it were the last variable to enter.

Step 3   Test for the significance of the factor selected in step 2 and determine, according to certain predetermined criteria, whether or not to delete this factor from the model.

Step 4   Repeat steps 2 and 3 for those variables still in the model. At any subsequent step, if none meets the criteria in step 3, no more variables are removed in the model and the process is terminated.

Stepwise Regression Procedure   Stepwise regression is a modified version of forward regression that permits reexamination, at every step, of the variables incorporated in the model in previous steps. A variable entered at an early stage may become superfluous at a later stage because of its relationship with other variables now in the model; the information it provides becomes redundant. That variable may be removed, if meeting the elimination criteria, and the model is refitted with the remaining variables, and the forward process goes on. The whole process, one step forward followed by one step backward, continues until no more variables can be added or removed.

Criteria   For the first step of the forward selection procedure, decisions are based on individual score test results (t test, $(n - 2)df$). In subsequent steps, both forward and backward, the decision is made as follows. Suppose there are r independent variables already on the model and a decision is needed in the forward selection process. Two regression models are now fitted, one with all r current X's included to obtain the regression sum of squares ($SSR1$) and one with all $r X$'s plus the X under investigation to obtain the regression sum of squares ($SSR2$). Define the mean square due to addition or elimination as

$$MSR = \frac{SSR2 - SSR1}{1}$$

Then the decision concerning the candidate variable is based on

$$F = \frac{MSR}{MSE}$$

an F test at $(1, n - r - 1)$ degrees of freedom.

The following example is used to illustrate the process; however, the process is most useful when we have a large number of independent variables.

Example 8.10

Refer to the data on liver transplants of Example 8.7 consisting of three independent variable: hepatic systolic pressure at transplant time (called pressure1), age (at the second measurement time), and sex of the child. The results for individual terms were shown in Example 8.7; these indicate that the pressure at transplant time (pressure1) is the most significant variable. Thus we do the following:

Step 1 Variable PRESSURE1 is entered. The model with only pressure at transplant time yields

$$SSR = 1460.47 \quad \text{with 1 } df$$

Analysis of Variables Not in the Model: With the addition of age, we have

$$SSR = 1796.61 \text{ with } 2df$$

$$MSE = 47.69(df = 18)$$

leading to an F statistic of 7.05 ($p = 0.0161$). Variable AGE is entered next; the remaining variage (sex) does not meet the criterion of .1 (or 10%) level to enter the model.

Step 2 Variable AGE is entered. The final model consists of two independent variables with the following results:

Factor	Coefficient	Standard Error	F Statistic	p-Value
Pressure1	0.3833	0.0806	22.60	0.0002
Age	0.9918	0.3735	7.05	0.0161

Note: The SAS program of Example 8.7 should be changed to
```
PROC REG;
PMODEL POST = PRE SEX AGE/SELECTION = STEPWISE;
```
to specify the stepwise process.

8.3. NOTES ON COMPUTATIONS

Samples of SAS program instructions were provided for all procedures, at the end of Examples 8.1, 8.7, and 8.10. Regression analyses can also be implemented easily using Microsoft's Excel; however, you need *Data Analysis*. "Data analysis" is an Excel add-in option that is available from the Excel installation CD; after installation, it is listed in your "*Tools*" menu. The process is rather simple: (1) Click the *Tools* and then (2) use *Data Analysis*. Among functions available, choose REGRESSION. A box appears, use the cursor to fill in the ranges of Y and X's. The results include all items mentioned in this chapter, plus confidence intervals for regression coefficients.

EXERCISES

8.1. Trace metals in drinking water affect the flavor of the water, and unusually high concentration can pose a health hazard. The following table shows trace-metal concentrations (zinc, in mg/liter) for both surface water and bottom water at six different river locations. Our aim is to see if surface water concentration (x) is predictive of bottom water concentration (y).

Location	Zinc concentration (mg/liter)	
	Bottom	Surface
1	.430	.415
2	.266	.238
3	.567	.390
4	.531	.410
5	.707	.605
6	.716	.609

(a) Draw a scatter diagram to show a possible association between the concentrations, and check to see if a linear model is justified.

(b) Estimate the regression parameters, estimate the bottom water concentration for location with a surface water concentration of .5 mg/L, and draw the regression line on the same graph with the scatter diagram.

(c) Test to see if the two concentrations are independent; state your hypotheses and your choice of the test size.

(d) Calculate the coefficient of determination and provide your interpretation.

8.2. In a study of saliva cotinine, seven subjects—all of whom had abstained from smoking for a week—were asked to smoke a single cigarette. The cotinine levels at 12 hours and 24 hours after smoking are provided below:

Subject	Cotinine Levels (mmol/liter)	
	After 12 Hours	After 24 Hours
1	73	24
2	58	27
3	67	49
4	93	59
5	33	0
6	18	11
7	147	43

(a) Draw a scatter diagram to show a possible association between the cotinine levels (24-hour measurement as the dependent variable), and check to see if a linear model is justified.

(b) Estimate the regression parameters, estimate the 24-hour measurement for a subject with a 12-hour cotinine level of 60 mmol/liter, and draw the regression line on the same graph with the scatter diagram.

(c) Test to see if the two cotinine levels are independent; state your hypotheses and your choice of the test size.

(d) Calculate the coefficient of determination and provide your interpretation.

8.3. The following data give the net food supply (x, number of calories per person per day) and the infant mortality rate (y, number of infant deaths per 1000 live births) for certain selected countries before World War II:

Country	x	y	Country	x	y
Argentina	2730	98.8	Iceland	3160	42.4
Australia	3300	39.1	India	1970	161.6
Austria	2990	87.4	Ireland	3390	69.6
Belgium	3000	83.1	Italy	2510	102.7
Burma	1080	202.1	Japan	2180	60.6
Canada	3070	67.4	New Zealand	3260	32.2
Chile	2240	240.8	Netherlands	3010	37.4
Cuba	2610	116.8	Sweden	3210	43.3
Egypt	2450	162.9	England	3100	55.3
France	2880	66.1	USA	3150	53.2
Germany	2960	63.3	Uruguay	2380	94.1

(a) Draw a scatter diagram to show a possible association between the infant mortality rate (used as the dependent variable) and the net food supply, and check to see if a linear model is justified.

(b) Estimate the regression parameters, estimate the infant mortality rate for a country with a net food supply of 2900 calories per person per day, and draw the regression line on the same graph with the scatter diagram.

(c) Test to see if the two factors are independent; state your hypotheses and your choice of the test size.

(d) Calculate the coefficient of determination and provide your interpretation.

8.4. Refer to the data in Exercise 8.3, but in the context of a multiple regression problem with two independent variables: the net food supply ($x_1 = x$) and its square ($x_2 = x^2$).

(a) Taken collectively, do the two independent variables contribute significantly to the variation in the number of infant deaths?

(b) Calculate the coefficient of multiple determination and provide your interpretation.

(c) Fit the multiple regression model to obtain estimates of individual regression coefficients and their standard errors, and draw your conclusion—especially the conditional contribution of the quadratic term.

8.5. The following are the heights (measured to the nearest 2 cm) and the weights (measured to the nearest kg) of 10 men and 10 women.

Men:

Height:	162	168	174	176	180	180	182	184	186	186
Weight:	65	65	84	63	75	76	82	65	80	81

Women:

Height:	152	156	158	160	162	162	164	164	166	166
Weight:	52	50	47	48	52	55	55	56	60	60

Separately for each group, men and women, do the following:

(a) Draw a scatter diagram to show a possible association between the weight (used as the dependent variable) and the height and check to see if a linear model is justified.

(b) Estimate the regression parameters, estimate the weight for a subject who is 160 cm (does the gender have an effect on this estimate?), and draw the regression line on the same graph with the scatter diagram.

(c) Test to see if the two factors are independent; state your hypotheses and your choice of the test size.

(d) Calculate the coefficient of determination and provide your interpretation.

(e) Is there evidence of an effect modification? (Compare the two coefficients of determination/correlation, informally.)

8.6. Refer to the data in Exercise 8.5, but in the context of a multiple regression problem with three independent variables: height, gender, and product height-by-gender.

(a) Fit the multiple regression model to obtain estimates of individual regression coefficients and their standard errors. Draw your conclusion concerning the conditional contribution of each factor.

(b) Within the context of the multiple regression model in (a), does gender alter the effect of height on weight?

(c) Taken collectively, do the three independent variables contribute significantly to the variation in weights?

(d) Calculate the coefficient of multiple determination and provide your interpretation.

8.7. In an assay of heparin, a standard preparation is compared with a test preparation by observing the log clotting times (y, in seconds) of blood containing different doses of heparin (x is log dose, replicate readings are made at each dose level):

Log Clotting Times				Log Dose
Standard		Test		
1.806	1.756	1.799	1.763	0.72
1.851	1.785	1.826	1.832	0.87
1.954	1.929	1.898	1.875	1.02
2.124	1.996	1.973	1.982	1.17
2.262	2.161	2.140	2.100	1.32

Separately for each preparation, standard and test, do the following:

(a) Draw a scatter diagram to show a possible association between the log clotting time (used as the dependent variable) and the log dose and check to see if a linear model is justified.

(b) Estimate the regression parameters, estimate the log clotting time for a log dose of 1.0 (Are estimates for different preparations different?), and draw the regression line on the same graph with the scatter diagram.

(c) Test to see if the two factors are independent; state your hypotheses and your choice of the test size.

(d) Calculate the coefficient of determination and provide your interpretation.

(e) Is there evidence of an effect modification? (Compare the two coefficients of determination/correlation, informally.)

8.8. Refer to the data in Exercise 8.7, but in the context of a multiple regression problem with three independent variables: log dose, preparation, and product log dose-by-preparation.

(a) Fit the multiple regression model to obtain estimates of individual regression coefficients and their standard errors. Draw your conclusion concerning the conditional contribution of each factor.

(b) Within the context of the multiple regression model in (a), does preparation alter the effect of log dose on the log clotting time?

(c) Taken collectively, do the three independent variables contribute significantly to the variation in log clotting times?

(d) Calculate the coefficient of multiple determination and provide your interpretation.

8.9. Data are shown below for two groups of patients who died of acute myelogenous leukemia. Patients were classified into the two groups according to the presence or absence of a morphologic characteristic of white cells. Patients termed "AG positive" were identified by the presence of Auer rods and/or significant granulature of the leukemic cells in the bone marrow at diagnosis. For the AG-negative patients these factors were absent. Leukemia is a cancer characterized by an overproliferation of white blood cells; the higher the white blood count (WBC), the more severe the disease. Separately for each morphologic group, AG positive and AG negative, do the following:

(a) Draw a scatter diagram to show a possible association between the log survival time (take log yourself and use as the dependent variable) and the log WBC (take log yourself), and check to see if a linear model is justified.

(b) Estimate the regression parameters, estimate the survival time for a patient with a WBC of 20,000 (Are estimates for different groups different?), and draw the regression line on the same graph with the scatter diagram.

(c) Test to see if the two factors are independent; state your hypotheses and your choice of the test size.

(d) Calculate the coefficient of determination and provide your interpretation.

(e) Is there evidence of an effect modification? (Compare the two coefficients of determination/correlation, informally.)

AG Positive ($N = 17$)		AG Negative ($N = 16$)	
White Blood Count (WBC)	Survival Time (weeks)	White Blood Count (WBC)	Survival Time (weeks)
2,300	65	4,400	56
750	156	3,000	65
4,300	100	4,000	17
2,600	134	1,500	7
6,000	16	9,000	16
10,500	108	5,300	22
10,000	121	10,000	3
17,000	4	19,000	4
5,400	39	27,000	2
7,000	143	28,000	3
9,400	56	31,000	8
32,000	26	26,000	4
35,000	22	21,000	3
100,000	1	79,000	30
100,000	1	100,000	4
52,000	5	100,000	43
100,000	65		

8.10. Refer to the data in Exercise 8.9, but in the context of a multiple regression problem with three independent variables: log WBC, the morphologic characteristic (AG, represented by a binary indicator: 0 of AG negative and 1 if AG positive), and product log WBC-by-morphologic characteristic (AG).

(a) Fit the multiple regression model to obtain estimates of individual regression coefficients and their standard errors. Draw your conclusion concerning the conditional contribution of each factor.

(b) Within the context of the multiple regression model in (a), does the morphologic characteristic (AG) alter the effect of log WBC on log survival time?

(c) Taken collectively, do the three independent variables contribute significantly to the variation in log survival times?

(d) Calculate the coefficient of multiple determination and provide your interpretation.

8.11. The purpose of this study was to examine the data for 44 physicians working for an emergency service at a major hospital so as to determine which of a number of factors are related to the number of complaints received during the previous year. In addition to the number of complaints, data available consist of the number of visits—which serves as the *size* for the observation unit, the physician—and four other factors under investigation. Table 8.1 presents the comple data set. For each of the 44 physicians there are two continuous explanatory factors, the revenue (dollars per hour) and work load at the emergency service (hours) and two binary variables, gender (Female/Male) and residency training in emergency services (No/Yes).

Table 8.1. Emergency Service Data

N Visits	Complaint	Residency	Gender	Revenue	Hours
2014	2	Y	F	263.03	1287.25
3091	3	N	M	334.94	1588.00
879	1	Y	M	206.42	705.25
1780	1	N	M	226.32	1005.50
3646	11	N	M	288.91	1667.25
2690	1	N	M	275.94	1517.75
1864	2	Y	M	295.71	967.00
2782	6	N	M	224.91	1609.25
3071	9	N	F	249.32	1747.75
1502	3	Y	M	269.00	906.25
2438	2	N	F	225.61	1787.75
2278	2	N	M	212.43	1480.50
2458	5	N	M	211.05	1733.50
2269	2	N	F	213.23	1847.25
2431	7	N	M	257.30	1433.00
3010	2	Y	M	326.49	1520.00
2234	5	Y	M	290.53	1404.75
2906	4	N	M	268.73	1608.50
2043	2	Y	M	231.61	1220.00
3022	7	N	M	241.04	1917.25
2123	5	N	F	238.65	1506.25
1029	1	Y	F	287.76	589.00
3003	3	Y	F	280.52	1552.75
2178	2	N	M	237.31	1518.00
2504	1	Y	F	218.70	1793.75
2211	1	N	F	250.01	1548.00
2338	6	Y	M	251.54	1446.00

Table 8.1. (Continued)

N Visits	Complaint	Residency	Gender	Revenue	Hours
3060	2	Y	M	270.52	1858.25
2302	1	N	M	247.31	1486.25
1486	1	Y	F	277.78	933.75
1863	1	Y	M	259.68	1168.25
1661	0	N	M	260.92	877.25
2008	2	N	M	240.22	1387.25
2138	2	N	M	217.49	1312.00
2556	5	N	M	250.31	1551.50
1451	3	Y	F	229.43	973.75
3328	3	Y	M	313.48	1638.25
2927	8	N	M	293.47	1668.25
2701	8	N	M	275.40	1652.75
2046	1	Y	M	289.56	1029.75
2548	2	Y	M	305.67	1127.00
2592	1	N	M	252.35	1547.25
2741	1	Y	F	276.86	1499.25
3763	10	Y	M	308.84	1747.50

Divide the number of complaints by the number of visits and use this ratio (number of complaints per visit) as the primary *outcome* or dependent variable Y. Individually for each of the two continuous explanatory factors, the revenue (dollars per hour) and work load at the emergency service (hours), do the following

(a) Draw a scatter diagram to show a possible association with the number of complaints per visit, and check to see if a linear model is justified.

(b) Estimate the regression parameters, estimate the number of complaints per visit for a physician having the (sample) *mean* level of the explanatory factor, and draw the regression line on the same graph with the scatter diagram.

(c) Test to see if the factor and the number of complaints per visit are independent; state your hypotheses and your choice of the test size.

(d) Calculate the coefficient of determination and provide your interpretation.

8.12. Refer to the data in Exercise 8.11, but consider all four explanatory factors and the product residency training-by-workload simultaneously.

(a) Fit the multiple regression model to obtain estimates of individual regression coefficients and their standard errors. Draw your conclusion concerning the conditional contribution of each factor.

(b) Within the context of the multiple regression model in (a), does the residency training alter the effect of workload on the number of complaints per visit?

(c) Taken collectively, do the five independent variables contribute significantly to the variation in log survival times?

(d) Calculate the coefficient of multiple determination and provide your interpretation.

Bibliography

Ahlquist, D. A., McGill, D. B., Schwartz, S., and Taylor, W. F. (1985). Fecal blood levels in health and disease: A study using HemoQuant. *New England Journal of Medicine* 314:1422.

Anderson, J. W., et al. (1990). Oat bran cereal lowers serum cholesterol total and LDL cholesterol in hypercholesterolemic men. *American Journal of Clinical Nutrition* 52:495–499.

Arsenault, P. S. (1980). Maternal and antenatal factors in the risk of sudden infant death syndrome. *American Journal of Epidemiology* 111:279–284.

Begg, C. B. and McNeil, B. (1988). Assessment of radiologic tests: Control of bias and other design considerations. *Radiology* 167:565–569.

Berkowitz, G. S. (1981). An epidemiologic study of pre-term delivery. *American Journal of Epidemiology* 113:81–92.

Blot, W. J., et al. (1978). Lung cancer after employment in shipyards during World War II. *New England Journal of Medicine* 299:620–624.

Brown, B. W. (1980). Prediction analyses for binary data. In: *Biostatistics Casebook*, edited by R. G. Miller, B. Efron, B. W. Brown, and L. E. Moses. New York: John Wiley & Sons, pp. 3–18.

Centers for Disease Control (1990). *Summary of Notifiable Diseases: United States 1989 Morbidity and Mortality Weekly Report* 38.

Cohen, J. (1960). A coefficient of agreement for nominal scale. *Educational and Psychological Measuments* 20:37–46.

Coren, S. (1989). Left-handedness and accident-related injury risk. *American Journal of Public Health* 79:1040–1041.

D'Angelo, L. J., Hierholzer, J. C., Holman, R. C., and Smith, J. D. (1981). Epidemic keratoconjunctivitis caused by adenovirus Type 8: Epidemiologic and laboratory aspects of a large outbreak. *American Journal of Epidemiology* 113:44–49.

Daniel, W. W. (1987). *Biostatistics: A Foundation for Analysis in The Health Sciences*. New York: John Wiley and Sons.

Dienstag, J. L., and Ryan, D. M. (1982). Occupational exposure to hepatitis B virus in hospital personnel: Infection or immunization. *American Journal of Epidemiology* 15:26–39.

Douglas, G. (1990). Drug therapy. *New England Journal of Medicine* 322:443–449.

Einarsson, K., et al. (1985). Influence of age on secretion of cholesterol and synthesis of bile acids by the liver. *New England Journal of Medicine* 313:277–282.

Engs, R. C., and Hanson, D. J. (1988). University students' drinking patterns and problems: Examining the effects of raising the purchase age. *Public Health Reports* 103:667–673.

Fiskens, E. J. M. and Kronshout, D. (1989). Cardiovascular risk factors and the 25 year incidence of diabetes mellitus in middle-aged men. *American Journal of Epidemiology* 130:1101–1108.

Fowkes, F. G. R., et al. (1992). Smoking, lipids, glucose intolerance, and blood pressure as risk factors for peripheral atherosclerosis compared with ischemic heart disease in the Edinburgh Artery Study. *American Journal of Epidemiology* 135:331–340.

Fox, A. J., and Collier, P. F. (1976). Low mortality rates in industrial cohort studies due to selection for work and survival in the industry. *British Journal of Preventive and Social Medicine* 30:225–230.

Freeman, D. H. (1980). *Applied Categorical Data Analysis*. New York: Marcel Deekker.

Freireich, E. J., et al. (1963). The effect of 6–mercaptopurine on the duration of steroid-induced remissions in acute leukemia: A model for evaluation of other potentially useful therapy. *Blood* 21:699–716.

Frerichs, R. R., et al. (1981). Prevalence of depression in Los Angeles County. *American Journal of Epidemiology* 113:691–699.

Fulwood, R., et al. (1986). Total serum cholesterol levels of adults 20–74 years of age: United States, 1976–1980. *Vital and Health Statistics, Series M: #236.*

Grady, W. R., et al. (1986). Contraceptives failure in the United States: Estimates from the 1982 National Survey of Family Growth. *Family Planning Perspectives* 18:200–209.

Graham, S., et al. (1988). Dietary epidemiology of cancer of the colon in western New York. *American Journal of Epidemiology* 128:490–503.

Gwirtsman, H. E., et al. (1989). Decreased caloric intake in normal weight patients with bulimia: Comparison with female volunteers. *American Journal of Clinical Nutrition* 49:86–92.

Helsing, K. J., and Szklo, M. (1981). Mortality after bereavement. *American Journal of Epidemiology* 114:41–52.

Herbst, A. L., Ulfelder, H., and Poskanzer, D. C. (1971). Adenocarcinoma of the vagina. *New England Journal of Medicine* 284:878–881.

Hiller, R., and Kahn, A. H. (1976). Blindness from glaucoma. *British Journal of Ophthalmology* 80:62–69.

Hollows, F. C., and Graham, P. A. (1966). Intraocular pressure, glaucoma, and glaucoma suspects in a defined population. *British Journal of Ophthalmology* 50:570–586.

Hosmer, D. W., Jr., and Lemeshow, S. (1989). *Applied Logistic Regression*. New York: John Wiley and Sons.

Jackson, R., et al. (1992). Does recent alcohol consumption reduce the risk of acute myocardial infarction and coronary death in regular drinkers? *American Journal of Epidemiology* 136:819–824.

Kaplan, E. L. and Meier, P. (1958). Nonparametric estimation from incomplete observations. *Journal of the American StatisticalAssociation* 53:457–481.

Kelsey, J. L., Livolsi, V. A., Holford, T. R., Fischer, D. B., Mostow, E. D., Schartz, P. E., O'Connor, T., and White, C. (1982). A case–control study of cancer of the endometrium. *American Journal of Epidemiology* 116:333–342.

Khabbaz, R., et al. (1990). Epidemiologic assessment of screening tests for antibody to human T lymphotropic virus type I. *American Journal of Public Health* 80:190–192.

Kleinbaum, D. G., Kupper, L. L., and Muller, K. E. (1988). *Applied Regression Analysis and Other Multivariate Methods*. Boston: PWS-Kent Publishing Company.

Kleinman, J. C., and Kopstein, A. (1981). Who is being screened for cervical cancer? *American Journal of Public Health* 71:73–76.

Klinhamer, P. J. J. M., et al. (1989). Intraobserver and interobserver variability in the quality assessment of cervical smears. *Acta Cytologica* 33:215–218.

Knowler, W. C., et al. (1981). Diabetes incidence in Pima Indians: Contributions of obesity and parental diabetes. *American Journal of Epidemiology* 113:144–156.

Koenig, J. Q., et al. (1990). Prior exposure to ozone potentiates subsequent response to sulfur dioxide in adolescent asthmatic subjects. *American Review of Respiratory Disease* 141:377–380.

Kono, S., et al. (1992). Prevalnce of gallstone disease in relation to smoking, alcohol use, obesity, and glucose tolerance: A study of self-defense officials in Japan. *American Journal of Epidemiology* 136:787–805.

Kushi, L. H., et al. (1988). The association of dietary fat with serum cholesterol in vegetarians: The effects of dietary assessment on the correlation coefficient. *American Journal of Epidemiology* 128:1054–1064.

Le, C. T. (1997). *Applied Survival Analysis*. New York: John Wiley and Sons.

Lee, M. (1989). Improving patient comprehension of literature on smoking. *American Journal of Public Health* 79:1411–1412.

Li, D. K., et al. (1990). Prior condom use and the risk of tubal pregnancy. *American Journal of Public Health* 80:964–966.

Mack, T. M., et al. (1976). Estrogens and endometrial cancer in a retirement community. *New England Journal of Medicine* 294:1262–1267.

Makuc, D., et al. (1989). National trends in the use of preventive health care by women. *American Journal of Public Health* 79:21–26.

Mantel, N., and Haenszel, W. (1959). Statistical aspects of the analysis of data from retrospective studies of disease. *Journal of the National Cancer Institute* 22:719-748.

Matinez, F. D., et al. (1992). Maternal age as a risk factor for wheezing lower respiratory illness in the first year of life. *American Journal of Epidemiology* 136:1258–1268.

May, D. (1974). Error rates in cervical cytological screening tests. *British Journal of Cancer* 29:106–113.

McCusker, J., et al. (1988). Association of electronic fetal monitoring during labor with caesarean section rate with neonatal morbidity and mortality. *American Journal of Public Health* 78:1170–1174.

Negri, E., et al. (1988). Risk factors for breast cancer: Pooled results from three Italian case–control studies. *American Journal of Epidemiology* 128:1207–1215.

Nischan, P., et al. (1988). Smoking and invasive cervical cancer risk: Results from a case–control study. *American Journal of Epidemiology* 128:74–77.

Nurminen, M., et al. (1982). Quantitated effects of carbon disulfide exposure, elevated blood pressure and aging on coronary mortality. *American Journal of Epidemiology* 115:107–118.

Ockene, J. (1990). The relationship of smoking cessation to coronary heart disease and lung cancer in the Multiple Risk Factor Intervention Trial. *American Journal of Public Health* 80:954–958.

Padian, N. S. (1990). Sexual histories of heterosexual couples with one HIV-infected partner. *American Journal of Public Health* 80:990–991.

Palta, M., et al. (1982). Comparison of self-reported and measured height and weight. *American Journal of Epidemiology* 115:223–230.

Pappas, G., et al. (1990). Hypertension prevalence and the status of awareness, treatment, and control in the Hispanic health and nutrition examination survey (HHANES). *American Journal of Public Health* 80:1431–1436.

Renaud, L., and Suissa, S. (1989). Evaluation of the efficacy of simulation games in traffic safety education of kindergarten children. *American Journal of Public Health* 79:307–309.

Renes, R., et al. (1981). Transmission of multiple drug-resistant tuberculosis: Report of a school and community outbreaks. *American Journal of Epidemiology* 113:423–435.

Rosenberg L., et al. (1981). Case–control studies on the acute effects of coffee upon the risk of myocardial infarction: Problems in the selection of a hospital control series. *American Journal of Epidemiology* 113:646–652.

Rossignol, A. M. (1989). Tea and premenstrual syndrome in the People's Republic of China. *American Journal of Public Health* 79:67–68.

Rousch, G. C., et al. (1982). Scrotal carcinoma in Connecticut metal workers: Sequel to a study of sinonasal cancer. *American Journal of Epidemiology* 116:76–85.

Salem-Schatz, S., et al. (1990). Influence of clinical knowledge, organization context and practice style on transfusion decision making. *Journal of the American Medical Association* 25:476–483.

Sandek, C. D., et al. (1989). A preliminary trial of the programmable implantable medication system for insulin delivery. *The New England Journal of Medicine* 321:574–579.

Schwarts, B., et al. (1989). Olfactory function in chemical workers exposed to acrylate and methacrylate vapors. *American Journal of Public Health* 79:613–618.

Selby, J. V., et al. (1989). Precursors of essential hypertension: The role of body fat distribution. *American Journal of Epidemiology* 129:43–53.

Shapiro, S., et al. (1979). Oral contraceptive use in relation to myocardial infarction. *Lancet* 1:743–746.

Strader, C. H., et al. (1988). Vasectomy and the incidence of testicular cancer. *American Journal of Epidemiology* 128:56–63.

Strogatz, D. (1990). Use of medical care for chest pain differences between blacks and whites. *American Journal of Public Health* 80:290–293.

Taylor, H. (1981). Racial variations in vision. *American Journal of Epidemiology* 113:62–80.

Taylor, P. R., et al. (1989). The relationship of polychlorinated biphenyls to birth weight and gestational age in the offspring of occupationally exposed mothers. *American Journal of Epidemiology* 129:395–406.

Thompson, R. S., et al. (1989). A case–control study of the effectiveness of bicycle safety helmets. *TNew England Journal of Medicine* 320:1361–1367.

True, W. R., et al. (1988). Stress symptomology among Vietnam veterans. *American Journal of Epidemiology* 128:85–92.

Tuyns, A. J., et al. (1977). Esophageal cancer in Ille-et-Vilaine in relation to alcohol and tobacco consumption: Multiplicative risks. *Bulletin of Cancer* 64:45–60.

Umen, A. J., and Le, C. T. (1986). Prognostic factors, models, and related statistical problems in the survival of end-stage renal disease patients on hemodialysis. *Statistics in Medicine* 5:637–652.

Weinberg, G. B., et al. (1982). The relationship between the geographic distribution of lung cancer incidence and cigarette smoking in Allegheny County, Pennsylvania. *American Journal of Epidemiology* 115:40–58.

Whittemore, A. S., et al. (1988). Personal and environmental characteristics related to epithelial ovarian cancer. *American Journal of Epidemiology* 128:1228–1240.

Whittemore, A. S. et al. (1992). Characteristics relating to ovarian cancer risk: Collaborative analysis of 12 U.S. case–control studies. *American Journal of Epidemiology* 136:1184–1203.

Yassi, A., et al. (1991). An analysis of occupational blood level trends in Manitoba: 1979 through 1987. *American Journal of Public Health* 81:736–740.

Yen, S., Hsieh, C., and MacMahon, B. (1982). Consumption of alcohol and tobacco and other risk factors for pancreatitis. *American Journal of Epidemiology* 116:407–414.

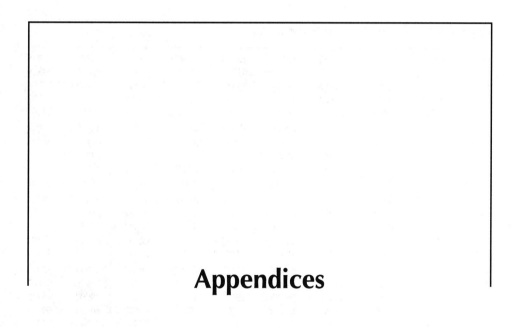

Appendices

Appendix A: Table of Random Numbers

63271	59986	71744	51102	15141	80714	58683	93108	13554	79945
88547	09896	95436	79115	08303	01041	20030	63754	08459	28364
55957	57243	83865	09911	19761	66535	40102	26646	60147	15704
46276	87453	44790	67122	45573	84358	21625	16999	13385	22782
55363	07449	34835	15290	76616	67191	12777	21861	68689	03263
69393	92785	49902	58447	42048	30378	87618	26933	40640	16281
13186	29431	88190	04588	38733	81290	89541	70290	40113	08243
17726	28652	56836	78351	47327	18518	92222	55201	27340	10493
36520	64465	05550	30157	82242	29520	69753	72602	23756	54935
81628	36100	39254	56835	37636	02421	98063	89641	64953	99337
84649	48968	75215	75498	49539	74240	03466	49292	36401	45525
63291	11618	12613	75055	43915	26488	41116	64531	56827	30825
70502	53225	03655	05915	37140	57051	48393	91322	25653	06543
06426	24771	59935	49801	11082	66762	94477	02494	88215	27191
20711	55609	29430	70165	45406	78484	31639	52009	18873	96927
41990	70538	77191	25860	55204	73417	83920	69468	74972	38712
72452	36618	76298	26678	89334	33938	95567	29380	75906	91807
37042	40318	57099	10528	09925	89773	41335	96244	29002	46453
53766	52875	15987	46962	67342	77592	57651	95508	80033	69828
90585	58955	53122	16025	84299	53310	67380	84249	25348	04332
32001	96293	37203	64516	51530	37069	40261	61374	05815	06714
62606	64324	46354	72157	67248	20135	49804	09226	64419	29457
10078	28073	85389	50324	14500	15562	64165	06125	71353	77669
91561	46145	24177	15294	10061	98124	75732	00815	83452	97355
13091	98112	53959	79607	52244	63303	10413	63839	74762	50289
73864	83014	72457	22682	03033	61714	88173	90835	00634	85169
66668	25467	48894	51043	02365	91726	09365	63167	95264	45643
84745	41042	29493	01836	09044	51926	43630	63470	76508	14194
48068	26805	94595	47907	13357	38412	33318	26098	82782	42851
54310	96175	97594	88616	42035	38093	36745	56702	40644	83514
14877	33095	10924	58013	61439	21882	42059	24177	58739	60170
78295	23179	02771	43464	59061	71411	05697	67194	30495	21157
67524	02865	39593	54278	04237	92441	26602	63835	38032	94770
58268	57219	68124	73455	83236	08710	04284	55005	84171	42596
97158	28672	50685	01181	24262	19427	52106	34308	73685	74246
04230	16831	69085	30802	65559	09205	71829	06489	85650	38707
94879	56606	30401	02602	57658	70091	54986	41394	60437	03195
71446	15232	66715	26385	91518	70566	02888	79941	39684	54315
32886	05644	79316	09819	00813	88407	17461	73925	53037	91904
62048	33711	25290	21526	02223	75947	66466	06232	10913	75336
84534	42351	21628	53669	81352	95152	08107	98814	72743	12849
84707	15885	84710	35866	06446	86311	32648	88141	73902	69981
19409	40868	64220	80861	13860	68493	52908	26374	63297	45052
57978	48015	25973	66777	45924	56144	24742	96702	88200	66162
57295	98298	11199	96510	75228	41600	47192	43267	35973	23152
94044	83785	93388	07833	38216	31413	70555	03023	54147	06647
30014	25879	71763	96679	90603	99396	74557	74224	18211	91637
07265	69563	64268	88802	72264	66540	01782	08396	19251	83613
84404	88642	30263	80310	11522	57810	27627	78376	36240	48952
21778	02085	27762	46097	43324	34354	09369	14966	10158	76089

Appendix B: Area Under the Standard Normal Curve

Entries in the table give the area under the curve between the mean and z standard deviations above the mean. For example, for $z = 1.25$ the area under the curve between the mean and z is .3944.

z	.00	.01	.02	.03	.04	.05	.06	.07	.08	.09
.0	.0000	.0040	.0080	.0120	.0160	.0199	.0239	.0279	.0319	.0359
.1	.0398	.0438	.0478	.0517	.0557	.0596	.0636	.0675	.0714	.0753
.2	.0793	.0832	.0871	.0910	.0948	.0987	.1026	.1064	.1103	.1141
.3	.1179	.1217	.1255	.1293	.1331	.1368	.1406	.1443	.1480	.1517
.4	.1554	.1591	.1628	.1664	.1700	.1736	.1772	.1808	.1844	.1879
.5	.1915	.1950	.1985	.2019	.2054	.2088	.2123	.2157	.2190	.2224
.6	.2257	.2291	.2324	.2357	.2389	.2422	.2454	.2486	.2518	.2549
.7	.2580	.2612	.2642	.2673	.2704	.2734	.2764	.2794	.2823	.2852
.8	.2881	.2910	.2939	.2967	.2995	.3023	.3051	.3078	.3106	.3133
.9	.3159	.3186	.3212	.3238	.3264	.3289	.3315	.3340	.3365	.3389
1.0	.3413	.3438	.3461	.3485	.3508	.3531	.3665	.3577	.3599	.3621
1.1	.3643	.3554	.3686	.3708	.3729	.3749	.3770	.3790	.3810	.3830
1.2	.3849	.3869	.3888	.3907	.3925	.3944	.3962	.3980	.3997	.4015
1.3	.4032	.4049	.4066	.4082	.4099	.4115	.4131	.4147	.4162	.4177
1.4	.4192	.4207	.4222	.4236	.4251	.4265	.4279	.4292	.4306	.4319
1.5	.4332	.4345	.4357	.4370	.4382	.4394	.4406	.4418	.4429	.4441
1.6	.4452	.4463	.4474	.4484	.4495	.4505	.4515	.4525	.4535	.4545
1.7	.4554	.4564	.4573	.4582	.4591	.4599	.4608	.4616	.4625	.4633
1.8	.4641	.4649	.4656	.4664	.4671	.4678	.4686	.4693	.4699	.4706
1.9	.4713	.4719	.4726	.4732	.4738	.4744	.4750	.4756	.4761	.4767
2.0	.4772	.4778	.4783	.4788	.4793	.4798	.4803	.4808	.4812	.4817
2.1	.4821	.4826	.4830	.4834	.4838	.4842	.4846	.4850	.4854	.4857
2.2	.4861	.4864	.4868	.4871	.4875	.4878	.4881	.4884	.4887	.4890
2.3	.4893	.4896	.4898	.4901	.4904	.4906	.4909	.4911	.4913	.4916
2.4	.4918	.4920	.4922	.4925	.4927	.4929	.4931	.4932	.4934	.4936
2.5	.4938	.4940	.4941	.4943	.4945	.4946	.4948	.4949	.4951	.4942
2.6	.4953	.4955	.4956	.4957	.4959	.4960	.4961	.4962	.4963	.4964
2.7	.4965	.4966	.4967	.4968	.4969	.4970	.4971	.4972	.4973	.4974
2.8	.4974	.4975	.4976	.4977	.4977	.4978	.4979	.4979	.4980	.4981
2.9	.4981	.4982	.4982	.4983	.4984	.4984	.4985	.4985	.4986	.4986
3.0	.4986	.4987	.4987	.4988	.4988	.4989	.4989	.4989	.4990	.4990

Appendix C: Percentiles of the *t* Distribution

Entries in the table give t_α values, where α is the area or probability in the upper tail of the *t* distribution. For example, with 10 degrees of freedom and a .05 area in the upper tail, $t_{.05} = 1.812$.

Degrees of Freedom	Area in Upper Tail				
	.10	.05	.025	.01	.005
1	3.078	6.314	12.706	31.821	63.657
2	1.886	2.920	4.303	6.965	9.925
3	1.638	2.353	3.182	4.541	5.841
4	1.533	2.132	2.776	3.747	4.604
5	1.476	2.015	2.571	3.365	4.032
6	1.440	1.943	2.447	3.143	3.707
7	1.415	1.895	2.365	2.998	3.499
8	1.397	1.860	2.306	2.896	3.355
9	1.383	1.833	2.262	2.821	3.250
10	1.372	1.812	2.228	2.764	3.169
11	1.363	1.796	2.201	2.718	3.106
12	1.356	1.782	2.179	2.681	3.055
13	1.350	1.771	2.160	2.650	3.012
14	1.345	1.761	2.145	2.624	2.977
15	1.341	1.753	2.131	2.602	2.947
16	1.337	1.746	2.120	2.583	2.921
17	1.333	1.740	2.110	2.567	2.898
18	1.330	1.734	2.101	2.552	2.878
19	1.328	1.729	2.093	2.539	2.861
20	1.325	1.725	2.086	2.528	2.845
21	1.323	1.721	2.080	2.518	2.831
22	1.321	1.717	2.074	2.508	2.819
23	1.319	1.714	2.069	2.500	2.807
24	1.318	1.711	2.064	2.492	2.797
25	1.316	1.708	2.060	2.485	2.787
26	1.315	1.706	2.056	2.479	2.779
27	1.314	1.703	2.052	2.473	2.771
28	1.313	1.701	2.048	2.467	2.763
29	1.311	1.699	2.045	2.462	2.756
30	1.310	1.697	2.042	2.457	2.750
40	1.303	1.684	2.021	2.423	2.704
60	1.296	1.671	2.000	2.390	2.660
120	1.289	1.658	1.980	2.358	2.617
∞	1.282	1.645	1.960	2.326	2.576

Appendix D: Percentiles of Chi-Square Distribution

Entries in the table give χ_α^2 values, where α is the area or probability in the upper tail of the chi-square distribution. For example, with 10 degrees of freedom and a .01 area in the upper tail, $\chi_{.01}^2 = 23.2093$.

Degrees of Freedom	Area in Upper Tail	
	.05	.01
1	3.841	6.35
2	5.991	9.210
3	7.815	11.350
4	9.488	13.277
5	11.071	15.086
6	12.592	16.812
7	14.067	18.475
8	15.507	20.090
9	16.919	21.666
10	18.307	23.209
11	19.675	24.725
12	21.026	26.217
13	22.362	27.688
14	23.685	29.141
15	24.996	30.578
16	26.296	32.000
17	27.587	33.408
18	28.869	34.805
19	30.144	36.191
20	31.410	37.566
21	32.671	38.932
22	33.924	40.289
23	35.173	41.638
24	36.415	42.980
25	37.653	44.314
26	38.885	45.642
27	40.113	46.963
28	41.337	48.278
29	42.557	49.588
30	43.773	50.892
40	55.759	63.691
50	67.505	76.154
60	79.082	88.380
70	90.531	100.425
80	101.879	112.329
90	113.145	124.116
100	124.342	135.807

Appendix E: Percentiles of the *F* Distribution

Entries in the table give F_α values, where α is the area or probability in the upper tail of the *F* distribution. For example, with 3 numerator degrees of freedom, 20 denominator degrees of freedom, and a .01 area in the upper tail, $F_{.01} = 4.94$ at $df = (3, 20)$.

Denominator Degrees of Freedom	(Numerator Degrees of Freedom, Area in Upper Tail)							
	(2,.05)	(2,.01)	(3,.05)	(3,.01)	(4,.05)	(4,.01)	(5,.05)	(5,.01)
5	5.79	13.27	5.41	12.06	5.19	11.39	4.82	10.97
6	5.14	10.92	4.76	9.78	4.53	9.15	4.39	8.75
7	4.74	9.55	4.35	8.45	4.12	7.85	3.97	7.46
8	4.46	8.65	4.07	7.59	3.84	7.01	3.69	6.63
9	4.26	8.02	3.86	6.99	3.63	6.42	3.48	6.06
10	4.10	7.56	3.71	6.55	3.48	5.99	3.33	5.64
11	3.98	7.21	3.59	6.22	3.36	5.67	3.20	5.32
12	3.89	6.93	3.49	5.95	3.26	5.41	3.11	5.06
13	3.81	6.70	3.41	5.74	3.18	5.21	3.03	4.86
14	3.74	6.51	3.34	5.56	3.11	5.24	2.96	4.69
15	3.68	6.36	3.29	5.42	3.06	4.89	2.90	4.56
16	3.63	6.23	3.24	5.29	3.01	4.77	2.85	4.44
17	3.59	6.11	3.20	5.18	2.96	4.67	2.81	4.34
18	3.55	6.01	3.16	5.09	2.93	4.58	2.77	4.25
19	3.52	5.93	3.13	5.01	2.90	4.50	2.74	4.17
20	3.49	5.85	3.10	4.94	2.87	4.43	2.71	4.10
21	3.47	5.78	3.07	4.87	2.84	4.37	2.68	4.04
22	3.44	5.72	3.05	4.82	2.82	4.31	2.66	3.99
23	3.42	5.66	3.03	4.76	2.80	4.26	2.64	3.94
24	3.40	5.61	3.01	4.72	2.78	4.22	2.62	3.90
25	3.39	5.57	2.99	4.68	2.76	4.18	2.60	3.85
26	3.37	5.53	2.98	4.64	2.74	4.14	2.59	3.82
27	3.35	5.49	2.96	4.60	2.73	4.11	2.57	3.78
28	3.34	5.45	2.95	4.57	2.71	4.07	2.56	3.75
29	3.33	5.42	2.93	4.54	2.70	4.04	2.55	3.73
30	3.32	5.39	2.92	4.51	2.69	4.02	2.53	3.70
35	3.27	5.27	2.87	4.40	2.64	3.91	2.49	3.59
40	3.23	5.18	2.84	4.31	2.61	3.83	2.45	3.51
50	3.18	5.06	2.79	4.20	2.56	3.72	2.40	3.41
60	3.15	4.98	2.76	4.13	2.53	3.65	2.37	3.34
80	3.11	4.88	2.72	4.04	2.49	3.56	2.33	3.26
100	3.09	4.82	2.70	3.98	2.46	3.51	2.31	3.21
120	3.07	4.79	2.68	3.95	2.45	3.48	2.29	3.17
∞	3.00	4.61	2.60	3.78	2.37	3.32	2.21	3.02

Answers to Exercises

CHAPTER 1

1.1. For left-handed: $p = .517$. For right-handed: $p = .361$.

1.2. For factory workers: $x = 49$. For nursing students: $x = 73$.

1.3. For cases: $p = .775$. For controls: $p = .724$.

1.4. For Nursing Home A: $p = .250$. For Nursing Home B: $p = .025$.
   The proportion in Nursing Home A where the "index" nurse worked is 10 times higher than the proportion in Nursing Home B.

1.5. (a) For high exposure level: $p = .488$. For low exposure level: $p = .111$.
      Students in the high exposure group has a much higher proportion of cases, more than four times higher.
   (b) $OR = 7.66$; it supports the conclusion in (a) showing that high exposure is associated with higher odds, and thus higher proportion, of positive cases.

1.6. (a) With EFM: $p = .126$. Without EFM: $p = .077$.
      The EFM-exposed group has a higher proportion of caesarean deliveries.
   (b) $OR = 1.72$; it supports the conclusion in (a), showing that EFM exposure is associated with higher odds, and thus higher proportion, of caesarean deliveries.

1.7. (a) With helmet: $p = .116$. Without helmet: $p = .338$.
      The group without helmet protection has a higher proportion of head injuries.
   (b) $OR = .26$; it supports the conclusion in (a), showing that helmet protection is associated with reduced odds, and thus lower proportion, of head injuries.

1.8. (a) Men: $OR = .94$, indicating a slightly lower risk of myocardial infarction.
      Women: $OR = .55$, indicating a lower risk of myocardial infarction.

(b) The effect of drinking is stronger in women, reducing the risk more: 45% versus 6%.

(c) Men: $OR = .57$, indicating a lower risk of coronary death.
Women: $OR = .39$, indicating a lower risk of coronary death.

(d) The effect of drinking is stronger in women, reducing the risk more: 61% versus 43%.

1.9. (a) Zero or one partners: $OR = 2.70$.

(b) Two or more partners: $OR = 1.10$.

(c) Both odds ratios indicate an elevated risk associated with smoking, but the effect on those with zero or one partners is clearer.

(d) Combined estimate of odds ratio: $OR_{MH} = 1.26$.

1.10. Chart is not available.

1.11. Chart is not available.

1.12. Chart is not available.

1.13. Chart is not available.

1.14. Chart is not available.

1.15. Sensitivity $= .733$; Specificity $= .972$.

1.16. For Dupont's EIA: Sensitivity $= .938$; specificity $= .988$. For cellular product's EIA: Sensitivity $= 1.0$; specificity $= .952$.

1.17. (a) Heart disease: 30.2%; cancer: 24.1%; Cerebrovascular disease: 8.2%; Accidents: 4.0% Others: 33.4%

(b) Population size: 3,525,297.

(c) Rates per 100,000: Cancer $= 235.4$; cerebrovasculardisease $= 80.3$; accidents $= 39.2$; others $= 325.5$.

1.18. Chart is not available.

1.19. Odds ratio $OR = 1.43$.

1.20. (a) For nonsmokers: $OR = 1.28$.

(b) For smokers: $OR = 1.61$.

(c) The risk seems to be higher for smokers.

(d) Combined estimate: $OR_{MH} = 1.53$.

1.21. (a) Odds ratios associated with race (black vs. white, nonpoor): 25–44, 1.07; 45–64, 2.00; 65+, 1.54. Different ratios indicate possible effect modifications by age.

(b) Odds ratios associated with income (poor vs. nonpoor, black): 25–44: 2.46, 45–64, 1.65; 65+, 1.18. Different ratios indicate a possible effect modification by age.

(c) Odds ratios associated with race (black vs. white) for 65 + years + poor, 1.18; for 65 + years + nonpoor, 1.54. The difference ($1.18 \neq 1.52$) indicates a possible effect modification by income.

1.22. (a)

Age Group	Odds Ratio
25–44	7.71
45–64	6.03
65+	3.91

(b) The odds ratios decrease with increasing age;

(c) $OR_{MH} = 5.40$.

1.23. (a)

Weight Group	Odds Ratio
< 57	5.00
57–75	2.75
> 75	1.30

(b) The odds ratios decrease with increasing weight;

(c) $OR_{MH} = 2.78$.

1.24. • For age at first live birth,

Age	Odds Ratio
22–24	1.26
25-27	1.49
28 +	1.95

General odds is 1.43.

• For Age at menopause,

Age	Odds Ratio
45–49	1.10
50+	1.40

General odds is 1.27.

1.25. Results for (b) and (c) parts:

• For smoking,

Status	Odds Ratio
Past	1.24
Current	1.40

General odds is 1.23.

• For alcohol,

Status	Odds Ratio
Past	1.08
Current	.87

General odds is .88.

- For body mass index,

BMI level	Odds Ratio
22.5–24.9	1.41
25+	1.39

General odds is 1.22.

1.26. • For duration of unprotected intercourse,

Years	Odds Ratio
2–9	.94
10–14	1.04
15+	1.54

General odds is 1.21 showing an upward trend of risks.

- For history of infertility,

History	Odds Ratio
Yes, no drug use	1.13
Yes, with drug use	3.34

General odds is 1.33 showing an upward trend of risks.

1.27. • For boys,

Maternal Age	Odds Ratio
21–25	.97
26–30	.67
30+	.43

General odds is .62, showing a downward trend of risks, decreasing with increasing maternal age.

- For girls,

Maternal Age	Odds Ratio
21–25	.80
26–30	.81
30+	.62

General odds is .84, showing a downward trend of risks, decreasing with increasing maternal age, but the trend is weaker than that for boys.

1.28. Sensitivity = .650; specificity = .917.

1.29. (a) For 1987, 24,027; for 1986, 15,017.

(b) Number of cases of AIDS transmitted from mothers to newborns in 1988: 468.

1.30. Follow-up death rates:

Age (years)	Deaths/1000 Months
21–30	3.95
31–40	5.05
41–50	11.72
51–60	9.80
61–70	10.19
70+	20.09

RR (70+ years vs. 51–60 years) = 2.05.

1.31. Death rates for Georgia (per 100,000)

(a) Crude rate for Georgia: 908.3
(b) Adjusted rate (U.S. as standard), Georgia: 1060.9
    vs. Adjusted rate for Alaska: 788.6
    vs. Adjusted rate for Floria: 770.6
(c) Adjusted rate (Alaska as standard): 560.5
    vs. Crude rate for Alaska: 396.8

1.32. With Georgia as standard:

Alaska = 668.4; Florida = 658.5 vs. crude rate for Georgia of 908.3.

1.33. Standardized mortality ratios

Years since entering the industry:	1–4	5–9	10–14	15+
SMR:	.215	.702	.846	.907
RR(15+ years vs. 1–4 years):	422			

1.34. Chart is not available.

1.35. Charts are not available; (c) General odds is 1.31, showing an upward trend with coffee consumption: given two persons who were admitted for different conditions, the odds that the one with an acute condition consumes more coffee is 1.31.

1.36. (a)

Group	Proportion of HBV-Positive Workers
Physicians	
Frequent	.210
Infrequent	.079
Nurses	
Frequent	.212
Infrequent	.087

(b) Odds ratios associated with frequent contacts

For physicians: 3.11
For nurses: 2.80

(c) Odds ratios are similar but larger for physicians.

(d) $OR_{MH} = 2.93$.

1.37. Graphs are not available.

1.38. (a) For age

Group	Odds Ratio
14–17	2.09
18–19	1.96
20–24	1.69
25–29	1.02

Yes, the younger the mother, the higher the risk.

(b) For socioeconomic level:

Group	Odds Ratio
Upper	.30
Upper middle	.34
Middle	.56
Lower middle	.71

Yes, the poorer the mother, the higher the risk.

(c) General odds is .57: Given two mothers with different economic levels, the odds that the richer one having premature delivery is .57. Yes, it supports the results in (b).

1.39. (a)

Group	SMR
Male	1.22
Female	.78
Black	2.09
White	.85

(b) Relative risks: Associated with gender, 1.57; associated with race, 2.47.

1.40.

Group	Odds Ratios
For Protestants:	.50
For Catholics:	4.69
For others:	.79

Yes, there is clear evidence of an effect modification (4.69 $\neq$ .50, .79).

1.41. • For age at first live birth, with "28 or older" group as baseline:

Age	Odds Ratio
< 22	.51
22–24	.65
25–27	.76

• For age at menopause, with "50 or older" group as baseline:

Age	Odds Ratio
< 45	.72
45–49	.79

1.42.

Symptom	Odds Ratio
Nightmares	3.72
Sleep problems	1.54
Troubled memories	3.46
Depression	1.46
Temper control problems	1.78
Life goal association	1.50
Omit feelings	1.39
Confusion	1.57

1.43.

Group	Odds Ratio
Males	
Low fat, low fiber	1.15
High fat, high fiber	1.80
High fat, low fiber	1.81
Females	
Low fat, low fiber	1.72
High fat, high fiber	1.85
High fat, low fiber	2.20

Yes, there are evidences of effect modifications: For example:

(i) For males: high vs. low fat, the odds ratio is 1.8 with high fiber and 1.57 (= 1.81/1.15) with low fiber.

(ii) For females: high vs. low fat, the odds ratio is 1.85 with high fiber and 1.28 (= 2.20/1.72) with low fiber.

1.44. Graph is not available.

1.45. (a) Choosing "never" as baseline, here are the odds ratios associated with being a resident (vs. attending physician):

Action Level	Odds Ratio
Rarely	1.93
Occasionally	24.3
Frequent	33.8
Very frequent	5.2

(b) The general odds is 6.15: given two physician of different types, the odds that the resident committing more unnecessary transfusion is 6.15. Yes, this agrees with the results in (a).

1.46. Results are:

Factor	Odds Ratio
X ray	8.86
Stage	5.25
Grade	3.26

CHAPTER 2

2.1. Graphs are not available; median = 193.

2.2. Graphs are not available; median for 1979 is 47.6, median for 1987 is 27.8.

2.3. Graphs are not available.

2.4. Graphs are not available.

2.5. Graphs are not available.

2.6. Graphs are not available.

2.7. Graphs are not available.

2.8. Graphs are not available; median from graph is 83, exact is 86.

2.9. Graphs are not available.

	$\bar{x}$	s^2	s	$s/\bar{x}$
Men:	84.71	573.68	23.95	28.3%
Women:	88.51	760.90	27.58	31.2%

2.10. Graphs are not available.

2.11. $\bar{x} = 168.75$; $s^2 = 1372.75$; $s = 37.05$.

2.12. $\bar{x} = 3.05$; $s^2 = .37$; $s = .61$.

2.13. $\bar{x} = 112.78$; $s^2 = 208.07$; $s = 14.42$.

2.14. $\bar{x} = 100.58$; $s^2 = 196.08$; $s = 14.00$.

2.15. $\bar{x} = .718$; $s^2 = .261$; $s = .511$.

2.16.

	$\bar{x}$	s^2	s
Age:	65.6	243.11	15.19
SBP:	146.2	379.46	19.48

2.17.

	$\bar{x}$	s^2	s
Females:	107.6	4373.5	66.1
Males:	97.8	1635.9	40.4

2.18. $\bar{x} = .22$; $s^2 = .44$; $s = .66$.

2.19.

	$\bar{x}$	s^2	s
Treatment:	651.9	31394.3	177.2
Control:	656.1	505.1	22.5

2.20. $\bar{x} = 169.0$, mean is lower than LA's; $s^2 = 81.5$; $s = 9.0$; $CV = 5\%$.

2.21. $\bar{x} = 2.5$; $s^2 = 9.5$; $s = 3.1$.

2.22. Mean $= 14.1$; geometric mean $= 10.3$; median $= 12.5$.

2.23. Graph is not available.

2.24. Mean $= 21.3$; geometric mean $= 10.6$; median $= 10.0$.

2.25. Mean $= 98.5$; geometric mean $= 93.4$; median $= 92.5$.

2.26. Graph is not available.

2.27.

	$\bar{x}$	s^2
Bulimic:	22.1	21.0
Healthy:	29.7	42.1

Bulimic group has smaller mean and smaller variance.

2.28.

	$\bar{x}$	s^2	s	Median
Drug A:	133.9	503.8	22.4	130.0
Drug R:	267.4	4449.0	66.7	253.0

2.29. (a) For survival time:

	$\bar{x}$	s^2	s
AG positive:	62.5	2954.3	54.4
AG negative:	17.9	412.2	20.3

(b) For WBC:

	$\bar{x}$	Geometric Mean	Median
AG positive:	29073.5	12471.9	10000
AG negative:	29262.5	15096.3	20000

2.30. Graphs are not available.

2.31. Graph is not available.

2.32. Graph is not available.

2.33. Graphs are not available.

2.34. Graph is not available.

2.35. Results:

Measure	Value
Pearson's	.931
Kendall's	.875
Spearman's	.963

2.36. Graph is not available.

Measure	Men	Women
Pearson's	.514	.718
Kendall's	.282	.714
Spearman's	.377	.849

2.37. Graph is not available.

Measure	Value
Pearson's	−.786
Kendall's	−.619
Spearman's	−.767

2.38. Graph is not available.

Measure	Standard	Test
Pearson's	.940	.956
Kendall's	.896	.955
Spearman's	.960	.988

2.39. 20 patients with nodes, 33 patients without nodes.

Factor	$\bar{x}$	s^2	s
Age			
Without node	60.1	31.4	5.6
With node	58.3	49.1	7.0
Acid			
Without node	64.5	744.2	27.3
With node	77.5	515.3	22.7

2.40. All patients, .054; with nodes, .273; without nodes, −.016. Nodal involvement seems to change the strength of the relationship.

2.41. (a) 12 females, 32 males; 20 with residency, 24 without.

Factor	$\bar{x}$	s
Gender		
Females	.00116	.00083
Males	.00139	.00091
Residency		
Without	.00147	.00099
With	.00116	.00073

(b) Between complaints and revenue: .031. Between complaints and work load: .279.

(c) Graph is not available.

2.42. Between y and x_1 is .756. Between y and x_2 is .831.

CHAPTER 3

3.1. Odds ratio $= .62$; Pr(Pap $=$ yes) $= .82$, Pr(Pap $=$ yes | black) $= .75 \neq .82$.

3.2. Odds ratio $= 5.99$; Pr(second $=$ present) $= .65$,
Pr(second $=$ present | first $=$ present) $= .78 \neq .65$.

3.3. (a) .202

(b) .217

(c) .376

(d) .268

3.4. Positive predictive value for Population A, .991; for Population B, .900.

3.5. (a) Sensitivity $= .733$, specificity $= .972$.

(b) .016

(c) .301

3.6. Results:

Prevalence	Positive Predictive Value
.2	.867
.4	.946
.6	.975
.7	.984
.8	.991
.9	.996

Yes:

$$\text{Prevalence} = \frac{(\text{PPV})(1 - \text{specificity})}{(\text{PPV})(1 - \text{specificity}) + (1 - \text{PPV})(\text{sensitivity})}$$

$$= .133 \qquad \text{if PPV} = .8$$

3.7. (a) .1056
   (b) .7995

3.8. (a) .9500
   (b) .0790
   (c) .6992

3.9. (a) .9573
   (b) .1056

3.10. (a) 1.645
   (b) 1.96
   (c) .84

3.11. $102.8 = 118.4 - (1.28)(12.17)$

3.12. 20–24 years: 101.23   106.31   141.49   146.57
   25–29 years: 104.34   109.00   141.20   145.86

   For example, $123.9 - (1.645)(13.74) = 101.3$.

3.13. (a) 200+ days: .1587; 365 + days: $\cong 0$
   (b) .0228

3.14. (a) .0808
   (b) 82.4

3.15. (a) 17.2
   (b) 19.2%
   (c) .0409

3.16. (a) .5934
   (b) .0475
   (c) .0475

3.17. (a) $\cong 0(z = 3.79)$
   (b) $\cong 0(z = -3.10)$

3.18. (a) .2266
   (b) .0045
   (c) .0014

3.19. (a) .0985
   (b) .0019

3.20. Rate $= 13.89$ per 1000 live births; $z = 13.52$.

3.21. For t distribution, 20 df:
    (a) Left of 2.086: .975; left of 2.845: .995.
    (b) Right of 1.725: .05; right of 2.528: .01.
    (c) Beyond ± 2.086: .05; beyond ± 2.845: .01.

3.22. For Chi-square distribution, 2 df:
    (a) Right of 5.991: .05; right of 9.210: .01.
    (b) Right of 6.348: between .01 and .05.
    (c) Between 5.991 and 9.210: .04.

3.23. For F distribution, (2, 30) df:
    (a) Right of 3.32: .05; right of 5.39: .01.
    (b) Right of 2.61: $< .01$.
    (c) Between 3.32 and 5.39: .04.

3.24. Kappa $= .399$, marginally good agreement.

3.25. Kappa $= .734$, good agreement—almost excellent.

CHAPTER 4

4.1. $\mu = .5$; 6 possible samples with $\mu_{\bar{x}} = .5 (= \mu)$.

4.2.

$$\Pr(\mu - 1 \le \bar{x} \le \mu + 1) = \Pr(-2.33 \le z \le 2.33)$$
$$= .9802$$

4.3. Confidence intervals:

Group	95% Confidence Interval
Left-handed	(.444, .590)
Right-handed	(.338, .384)

4.4. Confidence intervals:

Group	95% Confidence Interval
Students	(.320, .460)
Workers	(.667, .873)

4.5. Confidence intervals:

Year	95% Confidence Interval
1983	(.455, .493)
1987	(.355, .391)

4.6. Confidence intervals:

Level	95% Confidence Interval
High	(.402, .574)
Low	(.077, .145)

4.7. Confidence intervals:

For whites:	$25.3 \pm (1.96)(.9) = (23.54\%, 27.06\%)$	
For blacks:	$38.6 \pm (1.96)(1.8) = (35.07\%, 42.13\%)$	

No, sample sizes were already incorporated into standard errors.

4.8. Confidence intervals:

Parameter	95% Confidence Interval
Sensitivity	(.575, .891)
Specificity	(.964, .980)

4.9. Confidence intervals:

Assay	Parameter	95% Confidence Interval
Dupont's	Sensitivity	(.820, 1.0)
	Specificity	(.971, 1.0)
Cellular Product's	Sensitivity	Not available
	Specificity	(.935, .990)

Note: sample sizes are very small here.

4.10. Confidence intervals:

Personnel	Exposure	95% Confidence Interval
Physicians	Frequent	(.121, .299)
	Infrequent	(.023, .135)
Nurses	Frequent	(.133, .291)
	Infrequent	(.038, .136)

4.11. (a) Proportion: (.067, .087); odds ratio: (1.44, 2.05).

4.12. (a) Proportion: (.302, .374); odds ratio: (.15, .44).

4.13. Confidence intervals:

Event	Gender	95% Confidence Interval for *OR*
Myocardial infarction	Men	(.69, 1.28)
	Women	(.30, .99)
Coronary death	Men	(.39, .83)
	Women	(.12, 1.25)

No clear evidence of effect modification, intervals are overlapsed.

4.14. Confidence intervals:

Religion Group	95% Confidence Interval for *OR*
Protestant	(.31, .84)
Catholic	(1.50, 13.94)
Others	(.41, 1.51)

The odds ratio for the Catholics is much higher.

4.15. (a) Proportion: (.141, .209); odds ratio: (1.06, 1.93).

4.16. (a) Cases vs. hospital controls

$$\text{Odds ratio} = \frac{(177)(31)}{(11)(249)}$$

$$= 2.0$$

$$\text{Exp}\left[\ln 2.0 \pm 1.96\sqrt{\frac{1}{177} + \frac{1}{31} + \frac{1}{11} + \frac{1}{249}}\right] = (.98, 4.09)$$

(b) Cases vs. population controls

$$\text{Odds ratio} = \frac{(177)(26)}{(11)(233)}$$

$$= 1.78$$

$$\text{Exp}\left[\ln 1.78 \pm 1.96\sqrt{\frac{1}{177} + \frac{1}{26} + \frac{1}{11} + \frac{1}{233}}\right] = (.86, 3.73)$$

4.17. Confidence intervals:

Maternal Age (years)	OR (95% Confidence Interval) Boys	Girls
< 21	2.32 (.90, 5.99)	1.62 (.62, 4.25)
21–25	2.24 (1.23, 4.09)	1.31 (.74, 2.30)
26–30	1.55 (.87, 2.77)	1.31 (.76, 2.29)

4.18. (a)

Duration (years)	OR (95% Confidence Interval)	
2–9	.94	(.74, 1.20)
10–14	1.04	(.71, 1.53)
≥ 15	1.54	(1.17, 2.02)

(b)

Group	OR (95% Confidence Interval
No drug use	1.13 (.83, 1.53)
Drug use	3.34 (1.59, 7.02)

4.19.

$$\overline{x} = 3.05$$

$$s = .61$$

$$SE(\overline{x}) = .19$$

$$3.05 \pm (2.262)(.19) = (2.61, 3.49)$$

4.20.

$$\overline{x} = 112.78$$

$$s = 14.42$$

$$SE(\overline{x}) = 3.40$$

$$112.78 \pm (2.110)(3.40) = (105.61, 119.95)$$

4.21.

$$\overline{x} = 100.58$$

$$s = 14.00$$

$$SE(\overline{x}) = 4.04$$

$$100.58 \pm (2.201)(4.04) = (91.68, 120.48)$$

4.22.

Group	95% Confidence Interval
Females	(63.2, 152.0)
Males	(76.3, 119.3)

4.23.

$$\overline{x} = .22$$

$$s = .66$$

$$SE(\overline{x}) = .18$$

$$.22 \pm (2.160)(.18) = (-.16, .60)$$

4.24. Confidence intervals:

Group	95% Confidence Interval
Treatment	(653.3, 676.9)
Control	(681.1, 722.7)

4.25. (a) Mean: (.63, 4.57); correlation coefficient: (.764, .981).

4.26. (a) On log scale: (1.88, 2.84); in weeks: (6.53, 17.19).

4.27. Control: $\qquad$ $7.9 \pm (1.96)(3.7)/\sqrt{30} = (6.58, , 9.22)$
Simulation game: $\quad 10.1 \pm (1.96)(2.3)/\sqrt{33} = (9.32, 10.88)$

4.28. (a) $25.0 \pm (1.96)(2.7)/\sqrt{58} = (24.31, 25.69)$
(b) On the average, people with large body mass index are more likely to develop diabetes mellitus.

4.29. Confidence intervals:

DBP Level	Exposure	95% Confidence Interval
< 95:	Yes	(213.2, 226.8)
	No	(216.0, 226.0)
95–100:	Yes	(215.3, 238.6)
	No	(223.6,248.4)
≥ 100:	Yes	(9215.0, 251.0)
	No	(186.2, 245.8)

4.30. 95% confidence interval: $(-.220, .320)$.

4.31. 95% confidence interval: $(.545, .907)$.

4.32. Standard: $(.760, .986)$; Test: $(.820, .990)$.

4.33. With smoke: $(.398, .914)$; with sulfur dioxide: $(.555, .942)$.

4.34. Men: $(-.171, .864)$; women: $(.161, .928)$.

4.35. AG-positive: $(.341, .886)$; AG-negative: $(-.276, .666)$.

CHAPTER 5

5.1. (a) $H_0: \mu = 30$; $H_A: \mu > 30$.
(b) $H_0: \mu = 11.5$; $H_A: \mu \neq 11.5$.
(c) Hypotheses are for population parameters.
(d) $H_0: \mu = 31.5$; $H_A: \mu < 31.5$.
(e) $H_0: \mu = 16$; $H_A: \mu \neq 16$.
(f) Same as (c).

5.2. $H_0: \mu = 74.5$.

5.3. $H_0: \mu = 7250$; $H_A: \mu < 7250$.

5.4. $H_0: \pi = 38$; $H_A: \pi > 38$.

5.5. $H_0: \pi = .007$; $H_A: \mu > .007$.
$$p\text{-value} = Pr(\geq 20 \text{ cases out of } 1000 \mid H_0)$$

$$H_0: \text{mean} = (1000)(.007) = 7$$

$$\text{variance} = (1000)(.007)(.993) = (2.64)^2$$

$$z = \frac{20 - 7}{2.64}$$

$$= 4.92; \qquad p\text{-value} \cong 0$$

5.6. The mean difference.

$$H_0: \mu_d = 0$$

$$H_A: \mu_d \neq 0 \quad \text{(two-sided)}$$

5.7.

$$H_0: \pi = \frac{20.5}{5000}$$

$$H_A: \pi > \frac{20.5}{5000} \quad \text{(one-sided)}$$

5.8. $H_0: \sigma = 20$; $H_A: \sigma \neq 20$.

5.9. One-sided.

5.10. Under $H_0: \pi = .25$; variance $= \pi(1 - \pi)/100 = (.043)^2$

$$z = \frac{.18 - .25}{.043}$$

$$= -1.63; \qquad \alpha = .052$$

Under $H_A: \pi = .15$; variance $= \pi(1 - \pi)/100 = (.036)^2$

$$z = \frac{.18 - .15}{.036}$$

$$= .83; \qquad \beta = .2033$$

The change makes α smaller and β larger.

5.11. Under H_0:

$$z = \frac{.22 - .25}{.043}$$

$$= -.70; \qquad \alpha = .242$$

Under H_A:

$$z = \frac{.22 - .15}{.036}$$

$$= 1.94; \qquad \beta = .026$$

The new change makes α larger and β smaller.

5.12.

$$p\text{-value} = \Pr(p < .18 \text{ or } p > .32)$$

$$= 2\Pr\left(z \geq \frac{.32 - .25}{.043} = 1.63\right)$$

$$= .1032$$

5.13.

$$p = .18$$

$$SE(p) = .036$$

$$.18 \pm (1.96)(.036) = (.109, .251), \text{ which includes } .25$$

5.14. $SE(\overline{x}) = .054$

Cutpoint for $\alpha = .05$: $4.86 \pm (1.96)(.054) = 4.75$ and 4.96

$$\mu = 4.86 + .1$$

$$= 4.96$$

$$z = \frac{4.96 - 4.96}{.054}$$

$$= 0; \quad \text{power} = .5$$

5.15. $SE(\overline{x}) = 1.11$

Cutpoints for $\alpha = .05$: $128.6 \pm (1.96)(1.11) = 126.4$ and 130.8 $\mu = 135$

$$\text{Power} = 1 - \Pr(126.4 \leq \overline{x} \leq 130.8 | \mu = 135)$$

$$\cong 1.0$$

CHAPTER 6

6.1. Proportion is $p = .227$.

$z = -1.67$; p-value $= (2)(.0475) = .095$.

6.2. $\chi^2 = 75.03$; p-value $\cong 0$.

6.3.

$$z = (264 - 249)/\sqrt{264 + 249}$$

$$= .66; \quad p\text{-value} = .5092$$

or $\chi^2 = .44$.

6.4. $z = 3.77$ or $\chi^2 = 14.23$; p-value $< .01$.

6.5. $z = 4.60$; p-value $\cong 0$.

6.6. H_0: consistent report for a couple (i.e., man and woman agree)

$$z = (6 - 7)/\sqrt{6 + 7}$$
$$= -.28; \qquad p\text{-value} = .7794$$

6.7. H_0: no effects of acrylate and methacrylate vapors on olfactory function

$$z = (22 - 9)/\sqrt{22 + 9}$$
$$= 2.33; \qquad p\text{-value} = .0198$$

6.8. $z = 4.11$ or $\chi^2 = 16.89$; p-value $< .01$.

6.9. $z = 5.22$ or $\chi^2 = 27.22$; p-value $< .01$.

6.10. $z = 7.44$ or $\chi^2 = 55.36$; p-value $< .01$.

6.11. $\chi^2 = 44.49$; p-value $< .01$.

6.12. $\chi^2 = 37.73$; p-value $< .01$.

6.13. $\chi^2 = 37.95$; p-value $< .01$.

6.14. $\chi^2 = 28.26$; p-value $< .01$.

6.15. $\chi^2 = 5.58$; p-value $< .05$.

6.16. p-value $= .002$.

6.17. Pearson's: $\chi^2 = 11.35$; p-value $= .001$.
   Pearson's with Yates' correction: $\chi_c^2 = 7.11$; p-value $= .008$.
   Fisher's exact: p-value $= .013$.

6.18. p-value $= .018$.

6.19. $\chi^2 = 14.196$; $df = 3$; p-value $< .05$.

6.20. For males: $\chi^2 = 6.321$; $df = 3$; p-value $= .097$.
   For females: $\chi^2 = 5.476$; $df = 3$; p-value $= .140$.

6.21. (a) Men
   For myocardial infarction: $\chi^2 = .16$; p-value $> .05$.
   For coronary death: $\chi^2 = 8.47$; p-value $< .01$.

   (b) Women
   For myocardial infarction: $\chi^2 = 4.09$; p-value $< .05$.
   For coronary death: $\chi^2 = 2.62$; p-value $> .05$.

6.22. (a) For myocardial infarction: For men,

$$a = 197$$

$$\frac{r_1 c_1}{n} = 199.59$$

$$\frac{r_1 r_2 c_1 c_2}{n^2(n-1)} = 40.98$$

For women,

$$a = 144$$

$$\frac{r_1 c_1}{n} = 150.95$$

$$\frac{r_1 r_2 c_1 c_2}{n^2(n-1)} = 12.05$$

$$z = \frac{(197 - 199.59) + (144 - 150.95)}{\sqrt{40.98 + 12.05}}$$

$$= -1.31; \qquad p\text{-value} = .0951$$

(b) For coronary death: For men,

$$a = 135$$

$$\frac{r_1 c_1}{n} = 150.15$$

$$\frac{r_1 r_2 c_1 c_2}{n^2(n-1)} = 27.17$$

For women:

$$a = 89$$

$$\frac{r_1 c_1}{n} = 92.07$$

$$\frac{r_1 r_2 c_1 c_2}{n^2(n-1)} = 3.62$$

$$z = \frac{(135 - 150.15) + (89 - 92.07)}{\sqrt{27.17 + 3.62}}$$

$$= -3.28; \qquad p\text{-value} < .001$$

6.23. For 25.44 years:

$$a = 5$$

$$\frac{r_1 c_1}{n} = 1.27$$

$$\frac{r_1 r_2 c_1 c_2}{n^2(n-1)} = 1.08$$

For 45–64 years:

$$a = 67$$

$$\frac{r_1 c_1}{n} = 32.98$$

$$\frac{r_1 r_2 c_1 c_2}{n^2(n-1)} = 17.65$$

For 65+ years:

$$a = 24$$

$$\frac{r_1 c_1}{n} = 13.28$$

$$\frac{r_1 r_2 c_1 c_2}{n^2(n-1)} = 7.34$$

$$z = \frac{(5 - 1.27) + (67 - 32.98) + (24 - 13.28)}{\sqrt{1.08 + 17.65 + 7.34}}$$

$$= 9.49; \qquad p\text{-value} \cong 0$$

6.24. < 57 kg:

$$a = 20$$

$$\frac{r_1 c_1}{n} = 9.39$$

$$\frac{r_1 r_2 c_1 c_2}{n^2(n-1)} = 5.86$$

57–75 kgs:

$$a = 37$$

$$\frac{r_1 c_1}{n} = 21.46$$

$$\frac{r_1 r_2 c_1 c_2}{n^2(n-1)} = 13.60$$

> 75 kg:

$$a = 9$$

$$\frac{r_1 c_1}{n} = 7.63$$

$$\frac{r_1 r_2 c_1 c_2}{n^2(n-1)} = 4.96$$

$$z = \frac{(20 - 9.39) + (37 - 21.46) + (9 - 7.63)}{\sqrt{5.86 + 13.60 + 4.96}}$$

$$= 5.57; \qquad p\text{-value} \cong 0$$

6.25. For smoking: $\chi^2 = .93$; p-value $> .05$.
       For alcohol: $\chi^2 = .26$; p-value $> .05$.
       For body mass index: $\chi^2 = .87$; p-value $> .05$.

6.26.

$$C = 24{,}876$$

$$D = 14{,}159$$

$$S = 10{,}717$$

$$\sigma_S = 2{,}341.13$$

$$z = 4.58; \qquad p\text{-value} \cong 0$$

(after eliminating category "unknown")

6.27. For boys:

$$C = 19{,}478$$

$$D = 11{,}565$$

$$S = 7{,}913$$

$$\sigma_S = 2{,}558.85$$

$$z = 3.09; \qquad p\text{-value} = .001$$

For girls:

$$C = 17{,}120$$

$$D = 14{,}336$$

$$S = 2{,}784$$

$$\sigma_S = 2{,}766.60$$

$$z = 1.01; \qquad p\text{-value} = .1587$$

6.28. For duration (years):

$$C = 237{,}635$$

$$D = 240{,}865$$

$$S = 16,770$$

$$\sigma_S = 17,812.60$$

$$z = .94; \qquad p\text{-value} = .1736$$

For history of infertility:

$$C = 95,216$$

$$D = 71,846$$

$$S = 23,270$$

$$\sigma_S = 11,721.57$$

$$z = 1.99; \qquad p\text{-value} = .0233$$

6.29.

$$C = 2,442,198$$

$$D = 1,496,110$$

$$S = 946,088$$

$$\sigma_S = 95,706$$

$$z = 9.89; \qquad p\text{-value} \cong 0$$

6.30.

$$C = 364$$

$$D = 2238$$

$$S = -1874$$

$$\sigma_S = 372$$

$$z = -5.03; \qquad p\text{-value} \cong 0$$

CHAPTER 7

7.1.

$$\text{SE}(\bar{x}) = .5$$

$$t = (7.84 - 7)/(.5)$$

$$= 1.68, 15df; \qquad .05 < p\text{-value} < .10$$

7.2.

$$\overline{d} = 200$$
$$s_d = 397.2$$
$$SE(\overline{d}) = 150.1$$
$$t = (200 - 0)/(150 - 1)$$
$$= 1.33, 6df; \qquad p\text{-value} > .20$$

7.3.

$$\overline{d} = 39.4$$
$$s_d = 31.39$$
$$SE(\overline{d}) = 11.86$$
$$t = 3.32, 6df; \qquad p\text{-value} = .016$$

7.4.

$$SE(\overline{d}) = 1.13$$
$$t = 3.95, 59df; \qquad p\text{-value} = .0002$$

7.5.

$$\overline{d} = -1.10$$
$$s_d = 7.9$$
$$SE(\overline{d}) = 1.72$$
$$t = -.64, 20df; \qquad p\text{-value} > .20$$

7.6.

$$\overline{d} = .36$$
$$s_d = .41$$
$$SE(\overline{d}) = .11$$
$$t = 3.29, 13df; \qquad p\text{-value} = .006$$

7.7. For men with college education: $t = 11.00$, p-value $< .001$.
For women with high school: $t = 7.75$, p-value $< .001$.
For women with college education: $t = 2.21$, p-value $= .031$.
Other results:

(a) Men with different education levels:

$$s_p = 1.47$$
$$t = 2.70; \qquad p < .01$$

(b) Women with different education levels:

$$s_p = 1.52$$
$$t = 1.19; \qquad p > .20$$

(c) Men vs. women, $\leq$ high school:

$$s_p = 1.53$$
$$t = 6.53; \qquad p \cong 0$$

Men vs. women, $\geq$ college:

$$s_p = 1.35$$
$$t = 3.20; \qquad p \cong 0$$

7.8. SBP: $t = 12.11;$ $p \cong 0$
    DBP: $t = 10.95;$ $p \cong 0$
    BMI: $t = 6.71;$ $p \cong 0$

7.9.

$$s_p = .175$$
$$t = 3.40; \quad p \cong 0$$

7.10. $t = .54, 25df$, p-value $> .2$

7.11. $t = 2.86, 61df$, p-value $= .004$

7.12.

$$s_p = 7.9$$
$$t = 4.40; \qquad p \cong 0$$

7.13.

Treatment: $\bar{x}_1 = 701.9,$ $s_1 = 32.8$
Control: $\bar{x}_2 = 656.1,$ $s_2 = 22.5$

$$s_p = 29.6$$
$$t = 3.45, 17df; \qquad p < .01$$

7.14.

$$s_p = 9.3$$
$$t = 4.71; \qquad p \cong 0$$

7.15. Weight gain:

$$s_p = 14.4$$
$$t = 2.30; \qquad p < .05$$

Birth weight:

$$s_p = 471.1$$
$$t = 2.08; \qquad p < .05$$

Gestational age:

$$s_p = 15.3$$
$$t \cong 0; \qquad p \cong .5$$

7.16. Sum of ranks:

For bulimic adolescents: 337.5
For healthy adolescents: 403.5

$$\mu_H = \frac{15(15 + 23 + 1)}{2}$$
$$= 292.5$$
$$\sigma_H = \sqrt{\frac{(15)(23)(15 + 23 + 1)}{12}}$$
$$= 33.5$$
$$z = \frac{403.5 - 292.5}{33.5}$$
$$= 3.31; \qquad p \cong 0$$

7.17. Sum of ranks:

Experimental group: 151
Control group: 39

$$\mu_E = \frac{12(12 + 7 + 1)}{2}$$
$$= 120$$

$$\sigma_E = \sqrt{\frac{(12)(7)(12+7+1)}{12}}$$

$$= 11.8$$

$$z = \frac{151 - 120}{11.8}$$

$$= 262; \qquad p = .0088$$

7.18. An application of the one-way ANOVA yields the following:

Source of Variation	SS	df	MS	F Statistic	p-Value
Between samples	55.44	2	27.72	2.62	0.1059
Within samples	158.83	15	10.59		
Total	214.28	17			

7.19. An application of the one-way ANOVA yields the following:

Source of Variation	SS	df	MS	F Statistic	p-Value
Between samples	74.803	3	24.934	76.23	0.0001
Within samples	4.252	13	.327		
Total	79.055	16			

7.20. An application of the one-way ANOVA yields the following:

Source of Variation	SS	df	MS	F Statistic	p-Value
Between samples	40.526	2	20.263	3.509	0.0329
Within samples	527.526	126	5.774		
Total	568.052	128			

7.21. An application of the one-way ANOVA yields the following:

Source of Variation	SS	df	MS	F Statistic	p-Value
Between samples	57.184	3	19.061	37.026	< 0.0001
Within samples	769.113	1494	.515		
Total	826.297	1497			

7.22. An application of the one-way ANOVA yields the following:
For exposed group:

Source of Variation	SS	df	MS	F Statistic	p-Value
Between samples	5,310.032	2	2655.016	.987	0.3738
Within samples	845,028	314	2691.172		
Total	850,338.032	316			

For nonexposed group:

Source of Variation	SS	df	MS	F Statistic	p-Value
Between samples	10,513.249	2	5256.624	2.867	0.0583
Within samples	607,048	331	1833.982		
Total	617,561.249	333			

7.23. Factor: Age

Result of the t test: $t = 1.037$, p-value $= .3337$

Result of the Wilcoxon test: $z = -.864$, p-value $= .3875$

Factor: Acid

Result of the t test: $t = -1.785$, p-value $= .080$

Result of the Wilcoxon test: $z = 2.718$, p-value $= .0066$

CHAPTER 8

8.1. (a) Graph is not available.

(b) $\hat{\beta}_0 = .0301$, $\hat{\beta}_1 = 1.1386$, and $\hat{y} = .596$.

(c) $t = 5.622$, $p = .0049$.

(d) $r^2 = .888$.

8.2. (a) Graph is not available.

(b) $\hat{\beta}_0 = 6.08$, $\hat{\beta}_1 = .35$, and $\hat{y} = 27.08$.

(c) $t = 2.173$, $p = .082$.

(d) $r^2 = .486$.

8.3. (a) Graph is not available.

(b) $\hat{\beta}_0 = 311.45$, $\hat{\beta}_1 = -.08$, and $\hat{y} = 79.45$.

(c) $t = -5.648$, $p = .0001$.

(d) $r^2 = .618$.

8.4. (a) $F = 16.2$, $df = (2, 19)$, $p = .0001$.

(b) $R^2 = .631$.

(c) Results:

Term	$\hat{\beta}$	$SE(\hat{\beta})$	t Statistic	p-Value
x (food)	−.007	.091	−.082	.936
x^2	−.00001	.00001	−.811	.427

8.5. • For men:

• (a) Graph is not available.

(b) $\hat{\beta}_0 = -22.057$; $\hat{\beta}_1 = .538$; and $\hat{y} = 64.09$.

(c) $t = 1.697$, $p = .1282$.

(d) $r^2 = .265$.

- For women:
- (a) Graph is not available.
    - (b) $\hat{\beta}_0 = -61.624$; $\hat{\beta}_1 = .715$; and $\hat{y} = 52.78$.
    - (c) $t = 2.917$, $p = .0194$.
    - (d) $r^2 = .516$.
    - (e) Relationship is stronger and statistically significant for women but not for men.

8.6. (a) Multiple regression results:

Term	$\hat{\beta}$	$SE(\hat{\beta})$	t Statistic	p-Value
Sex	−39.573	81.462	−.486	.634
Height	.361	.650	.555	.587
Sex-by-height	.177	.492	.360	.724

- (b) No ($p = .724$)
- (c) $F = 22.39$, $df = (3, 16)$, $p = .0001$.
- (d) $R^2 = .808$.

8.7. • For standard:
- (a) Graph is not available.
    - (b) $\hat{\beta}_0 = .292$; $\hat{\beta}_1 = .362$; and $\hat{y} = 1.959$.
    - (c) $t = 7.809$, $p = .0001$.
    - (d) $r^2 = .884$.
- For test:
- (a) Graph is not available.
    - (b) $\hat{\beta}_0 = .283$; $\hat{\beta}_1 = .280$; and $\hat{y} = 1.919$.
    - (c) $t = 9.152$, $p = .0001$.
    - (d) $r^2 = .913$.
    - (e) No indication of effect modification.

8.8. (a) Multiple regression results:

Term	$\hat{\beta}$	$SE(\hat{\beta})$	t Statistic	p-Value
Preparation	−.009	.005	−1.680	.112
Logdose	.443	.088	5.051	< .001
Preparation-by-logdose	−.081	.056	−1.458	.164

- (b) No, week indication ($p = .164$).
- (c) $F = 46.23$, $df = (3, 16)$, $p = .0001$.
- (d) $R^2 = .897$.

8.9. • For AG positive:
- (a) Graph is not available.
    - (b) $\hat{\beta}_0 = 4.810$; $\hat{\beta}_1 = -.818$; and $\hat{y} = 19.58$.

(c) $t = -3.821$, $p = .002$.

(d) $r^2 = .493$.

- For AGnegative:
- (a) Graph is not available.

  (b) $\hat{\beta}_0 = 1.963$; $\hat{\beta}_1 = -.234$; and $\hat{y} = 9.05$.

  (c) $t = -.987$, $p = .340$.

  (d) $r^2 = .065$.

  (e) Relationship is stronger and statistically significant for AG positives but not so for AG negatives.

8.10. (a) Multiple regression results:

Term	$\hat{\beta}$	$SE(\hat{\beta})$	t Statistic	p-Value
AG	2.847	1.343	2.119	.043
Log WBC	-.234	.243	-.961	.345
AG-by-log WBC	-.583	.321	-1.817	.080

(b) Rather strong indication ($p = .080$).

(c) $F = 7.69$, $df = (3, 29)$, $p = .0006$.

(d) $R^2 = .443$.

8.11. • For revenue:
- (a) Graph is not available.

  (b) $\hat{\beta}_0 = (1.113)(10^{-3})$; $\hat{\beta}_1 = (.829)(10^{-6})$; and $\hat{y} = (1.329)(10^{-3})$.

  (c) $t = .198$, $p = .844$.

  (d) $r^2 = .001$.

- For workload hours:
- (a) Graph is not available.

  (b) $\hat{\beta}_0 = (.260)(10^{-3})$; $\hat{\beta}_1 = (.754)(10^{-6})$; and $\hat{y} = (1.252)(10^{-3})$.

  (c) $t = 1.882$, $p = .067$.

  (d) $r^2 = .078$.

8.12. (a) Multiple regression results:

Term	$\hat{\beta}$	$SE(\hat{\beta})$	t Statistic	p-Value
Residency	$(3.176)(10^{-3})$	$(1.393)(10^{-3})$	2.279	.028
Sex	$(.348)(10^{-3})$	$(.303)(10^{-3})$	1.149	.258
Revenue	$(1.449)(10^{-6})$	$(4.340)(10^{-6})$	.334	.741
Hours	$(2.206)(10^{-6})$	$(.760)(10^{-6})$	2.889	.006
Residency-by-hours	$(-2.264)(10^{-6})$	$(.930)(10^{-6})$	-2.436	.020

(b) Yes, rather strong indication ($p = .020$).

(c) $F = 2.14$, $df = (5, 38)$, $p = .083$.

(d) $R^2 = .219$.

Index